Cell Signaling in Vascular Inflammation

Cell Signaling in Vascular Inflammation

Edited by

Jahar Bhattacharya, MBBS, DPhil

Professor of Physiology and Cellular Biophysics,
Clinical Physiological Medicine,
and Medicine, Columbia University, New York, NY

HUMANA PRESS ✳ TOTOWA, NEW JERSEY

Production Editor: Tracy Catanese

Cover design by Patricia F. Cleary

Cover Illustration: Figure 2 from Chapter 14, "Pulmonary Vascular Barrier Regulation by Thrombin and Edg Receptors," by Jeffrey R. Jacobson and Joe G. N. Garcia.

For additional copies, pricing for bulk purchases, and/or information about other Humana titles, contact Humana at the above address or at any of the following numbers: Tel: 973-256-1699; Fax: 973-256-8341; E-mail: orders@humanapr.com, or visit our Website: www.humanapress.com

Printed in the United States of America. 10 9 8 7 6 5 4 3 2 1

e-ISBN: 1-59259-909-5

Library of Congress Cataloging in Publication Data

Cell signaling in vascular inflammation / edited by Jahar Bhattacharya.
    p. ; cm.
  Includes bibliographical references and index.
  ISBN 1-58829-525-7 (alk. paper)
 1. Vasculitis 2. Cellular signal transduction. 3. Inflammation--Mediators.
  [DNLM: 1. Vasculitis--pathology. 2. Intercellular Signaling Peptides and
Proteins. 3. Paracrine Communication--physiology. WG 515 C393 2005] I. Bhattacharya, Jahar.
  RC694.5.I53C45 2005
  616.1'3--dc22

                                                                    2004017975

Preface

Inflammatory disease of the lung vascular bed is a major cause of morbidity and mortality in both adult and pediatric age groups. A particularly devastating consequence of lung inflammation is lung injury, which alone accounts for 150,000 cases annually in the United States, and carries a mortality rate of more than 30%. Yet, in the teaching about lung inflammation and in its application to clinical practice, the importance of vascular biology has been somewhat neglected.

Lung inflammation results from the defensive responses of pulmonary vascular cells to pathogenic stimuli. The responses arise through signal transduction mechanisms, which constitute sequences of intracellular events that lead up to specific cellular responses. Secondary effects of such responses precipitate all of the phenotypic features of lung inflammatory disease, including vascular hyperpermeability, white cell accumulation, and vascular remodeling. An understanding of signal transduction pathways in lung vascular cells is therefore required not only to explain the processes of lung inflammation, but also to develop new therapeutic strategies to combat inflammatory lung diseases.

Although great strides have been made in the science of cell signaling, much of this understanding is derived from nonlung cells. Consequently, the understanding is often of tangential relevance to lung vascular biology. The lung's unique position at the systemic interface with the environment arms it with a sensitive immune defense capability, a physiologically protective feature that also carries significant pathological risk. This and other special features of the pulmonary circulation compel a studied and specific consideration of signal transduction processes in the context of lung vascular disease. It is my hope that *Cell Signaling in Vascular Inflammation* will foster better awareness of these phenomena.

My intention in assembling these chapters has been to cut across disciplines to bring together a broad-based presentation of inflammatory challenge, both in the initial phases of the inflammatory response as also in the more prolonged phase of genomic involvement. The chapters comprise a comprehensive survey of signaling processes. Hence, the book will be useful to a broad spectrum of readers, including advanced students of lung biology, investigators seeking new research directions, and clinicians and scientists involved in lung inflammation and its management.

Finally, I would like to thank several people without whose help this volume would not have been possible. I received advice and encouragement throughout from Drs. Ken Weir, Jack Reeves, and Wiltz Wagner. Ms. Paige Walker of the American Heart Association and my assistant, Ms. Rashmi Patel, provided outstanding support in getting the material together and in ensuring its preparation for publication. My wife, Sunita, supported me in many ways, not least through encouragement and patience.

Jahar Bhattacharya, MBBS, DPhil

Contents

Contributors

HAKAN AKCA, PhD • *Walther Oncology Center, Indiana University School of Medicine, Indianapolis, IN*

YUN SOO BAE, PhD • *Division of Molecular Life Sciences and Center for Cell Signaling Research , Ewha Womans University, Seoul, Korea*

ALEX BANKS • *Departments of Medicine and Microbiology, College of Physicians and Surgeons of Columbia University, New York, NY*

SUNITA BHATTACHARYA, MD • *Department of Pediatrics, College of Physicians and Surgeons of Columbia University, New York, NY*

NAVDEEP S. CHANDEL, PhD • *Department of Medicine, Northwestern University Medical School, Chicago, IL*

TONG-SHIN CHANG, PhD • *Division of Molecular Life Sciences and Center for Cell Signaling Research, Ewha Womans University, Seoul, Korea*

PETER CHEN • *Departments of Medicine and Microbiology, College of Physicians and Surgeons of Columbia University, New York, NY*

AUGUSTINE M. K. CHOI, MD • *Department of Medicine, University of Pittsburgh School of Medicine, Pittsburgh, PA*

REGINA M. DAY, PhD • *Department of Medicine, Tufts University School of Medicine, Boston, MA*

SRINIVAS DHANAKOTI, PhD • *Department of Pediatrics, University of California Los Angeles, Los Angeles, CA*

DAVID B. DONNER, PhD • *Walther Oncology Center, Indiana University School of Medicine, Indianapolis, IN*

BARRY L. FANBURG, MD • *Department of Medicine, Tufts University School of Medicine, Boston, MA*

SCOTT FAY • *Departments of Medicine and Microbiology, College of Physicians and Surgeons of Columbia University, New York, NY*

ARON B. FISHER, MD • *Institute for Environmental Medicine, University of Pennsylvania Medical Center, Philadelphia, PA*

JOE G. N. GARCIA, MD • *Division of Pulmonary and Critical Care Medicine, Johns Hopkins University School of Medicine, Baltimore, MD*

YUANSHENG GAO, MD • *Department of Pediatrics, University of California Los Angeles, Los Angeles, CA*

JASON A. GUSTIN • *Walther Oncology Center, Indiana University School of Medicine, Indianapolis, IN*

GILES E. HARDINGHAM • *Department of Preclinical Veterinary Studies, Edinburgh University, Edinburgh, UK*

MARGARET M. HARNETT, PhD • *Division of Immunology, University of Glasgow, Glasgow, Scotland*

ELIZABETH O. HARRINGTON, PhD • *Department of Medicine, Brown Medical School, Providence, RI*

ZHIGANG HONG, MD, PhD • *Department of Medicine, VA Medical Center and University of Minnesota, Minneapolis, MN*

HARRY ISCHIROPOULOS, PhD • *The Children's Hospital of Philadelphia, The Stokes Research Institute, and Department of Biochemistry and Biophysics, University of Pennsylvania, Philadelphia, PA*

JEFFREY R. JACOBSON, MD • *Division of Pulmonary and Critical Care Medicine, Johns Hopkins University School of Medicine, Baltimore, MD*

SANG WON KANG, PhD • *Division of Molecular Life Sciences and Center for Cell Signaling Research, Ewha Womans University, Seoul, Korea*

CHANDRASHEKHAR K. KORGAONKAR, PhD • *Walther Oncology Center, Indiana University School of Medicine, Indianapolis, IN*

WOLFGANG M. KUEBLER, MD, PhD • *Institute of Physiology, Charité-Universitaetsmedizin Berlin, Berlin, Germany*

SEUNG-ROCK LEE, PhD • *Division of Molecular Life Sciences and Center for Cell Signaling Research, Ewha Womans University, Seoul, Korea*

SHEU-LING LEE, PhD • *Department of Medicine, Tufts University School of Medicine, Boston, MA*

JIANZE LI • *Departments of Medicine and Microbiology, College of Physicians and Surgeons of Columbia University, New York, NY*

JULIE A. LOSMAN • *Departments of Medicine and Microbiology, College of Physicians and Surgeons of Columbia University, New York, NY*

QING LU, PhD • *Department of Medicine, Brown Medical School, Providence, RI*

ASRAR B. MALIK, PhD • *Department of Pharmacology, University of Illinois at Chicago, Chicago, IL*

LINDSEY D. MAYO, PhD • *Indiana University School of Medicine, Indianapolis, IN*

LISA MCKEAG • *Departments of Medicine and Microbiology, College of Physicians and Surgeons of Columbia University, New York, NY*

DOLLY MEHTA, PhD • *Department of Pharmacology, University of Illinois at Chicago, Chicago, IL*

RICHARD D. MINSHALL, PhD • *Department of Pharmacology, University of Illinois at Chicago, Chicago, IL*

DANIEL P. NELSON, BS • *Department of Medicine, VA Medical Center and University of Minnesota, Minneapolis, MN*

ANDREA OLSCHEWSKI • *Department of Anesthesiology, Justus-Leibig University, Giessen, Germany*

OSMAN NIDAI OZES, PhD • *Walther Oncology Center, Indiana University School of Medicine, Indianapolis, IN*

KAUSHIK PARTHASARATHI, PhD • *Department of Physiology and Cellular Biophysics, College of Physicians and Surgeons of Columbia University, New York, NY*

ROXANA PINCHEIRA, PhD • *Indiana University School of Medicine, Indianapolis, IN*

USHA RAJ, MD • *Department of Pediatrics, University of California Los Angeles, Los Angeles, CA*

SUE GOO RHEE, PhD • *National Institute of Health, National Heart, Lung, and Blood Institute, Bethesda, MD*

PAUL ROTHMAN, MD • *Departments of Medicine and Microbiology, College of Physicians and Surgeons of Columbia University, New York, NY*

SHARON ROUNDS, MD • *Department of Medicine, Brown Medical School, Providence, RI*

STEFAN W. RYTER • *Department of Medicine, University of Pittsburgh School of Medicine, Pittsburgh, PA*

SAMI I. SAID, MD • *Pulmonary and Critical Care Medicine, SUNY at Stony Brook, Stony Brook, NY*

FRED SANDER, BS • *Department of Pediatrics, University of California Los Angeles, Los Angeles, CA*

AMY R. SIMON, MD • *Department of Medicine, Tufts University School of Medicine, Boston, MA*

TROY STEVENS, PhD • *Department of Molecular and Cellular Pharmacology, University of South Alabama School of Medicine, Mobile, AL*

YUICHIRO J. SUZUKI, PhD • *Department of Medicine, Tufts University School of Medicine, and the USDA Human Nutrition Research Center on Aging at Tufts University, Boston, MA*

ANTHONY VARGHESE, PhD • *Department of Medicine, VA Medical Center and University of Minnesota, Minneapolis, MN*

BAO Q. VUONG • *Departments of Medicine and Microbiology, College of Physicians and Surgeons of Columbia University, New York, NY*

E. KENNETH WEIR, MD • *Department of Medicine, VA Medical Center and University of Minnesota, Minneapolis, MN*

Heme Oxygenase-1 and Carbon Monoxide in Vascular Regulation

Stefan W. Ryter and Augustine M. K. Choi

SUMMARY

The gaseous signaling molecules nitric oxide (NO) and carbon monoxide (CO), which are generated endogenously by the heme oxygenase (HO) and nitric oxide synthase (NOS) systems, respectively, play significant roles in the regulation of vascular function. The HO enzymes exist in both constitutive (HO-2, HO-3) and inducible (HO-1) isoforms, the latter identified as a component of the cellular stress response. HO converts heme to CO, biliverdin, and iron; and these metabolites may all contribute to the apparent cytoprotective effects of HO. Like NO, CO has potent vasodilator properties, and may regulate other vascular functions such as the aggregation of platelets and the proliferation of smooth muscle. These effects of CO typically depend on the activation of soluble guanylate cyclase activity. Although toxic at elevated concentrations, exogenous CO may exert anti-inflammatory and anti-apoptotic properties at low concentration, which depend on the modulation of mitogen-activated protein kinase pathways. Manipulation of the HO-1/CO system, either by gene transfer or application of low-dose CO, could be applied in the treatment of vascular disease. Beneficial effects of HO/CO have recently been demonstrated in the limitation of ischemia/reperfusion injury during organ transplantation.

Key Words: Carbon monoxide; heme oxygenase; cell signaling; stress response; vascular regulation.

1. INTRODUCTION

The regulation of vascular function involves a complex interplay of physiological mediators, including circulating peptides, cytokines, endocrine factors, and gaseous signaling molecules. The homeostasis maintained by these factors can be perturbed by stress, injury, and changes in pO_2 (1). Perhaps the most widely studied vasoactive agent, the endothelial-derived relaxing factor known as nitric oxide (NO), exerts a potent vasodilator action (2). NO arises during the conversion of L-arginine to L-citrulline by the activity of nitric oxide synthase (NOS) enzymes, which exist in both constitutive and inducible forms (3). The vasoregulatory properties of NO have been exploited for the treatment of sexual dysfunction, and explored for the potential treatment of pulmonary hypertension, inflammatory lung disease, and myocardial ischemia/reperfusion (I/R) injury (4–6).

A similar low-molecular-weight gaseous molecule, carbon monoxide (CO), has recently attracted widespread attention as another vasoregulator (1). Unlike its cognate gas NO, a free radical that may participate in multiple redox reactions, CO is a relatively stable gas with little reactivity except for its affinity for heme-iron centers (7–9). Like NO, the signaling effects of CO in part rely on its ability to form a complex with the heme moiety of soluble guanylate cyclase (sGC), stimulating the production of guanosine 3',5'-cyclic monophosphate (cGMP), a diffusible second messenger (10). The sGC/

From: *Cell Signaling in Vascular Inflammation*
Edited by: J. Bhattacharya © Humana Press Inc., Totowa, NJ

cGMP pathway plays a critical role in mediating the effects of CO on neurotransmission, vascular relaxation, smooth-muscle relaxation, bronchodilation, and the inhibition of platelet aggregation, coagulation, and smooth-muscle proliferation *(11–19)*. In addition to these physiological effects, low-dose CO at 10–250 ppm exerts potent anti-inflammatory and anti-apoptotic effects in cultured cells *(20,21)*. The apparent protective effects of exogenously applied CO have been demonstrated in models of organ transplantation, inflammatory and oxidative lung diseases, I/R injury, and recently, in vascular stenosis caused by balloon injury *(12,20,22–24)*.

The heme oxygenase (HO) enzymes represent the principal endogenous source of CO in humans *(25)*. The HO enzymes catalyze the rate-limiting step in the conversion of heme to its metabolites, biliverdin-IXα (BV) and ferrous iron, while releasing the α-methene bridge carbon of heme as CO *(26)*. Cytoplasmic NAD(P)H biliverdin reductase (E.C. 1:3:1:24) completes the heme degradation pathway by reducing the water-soluble BV to the hydrophobic bilirubin IXα *(27)*. Heme oxygenase-1 (HO-1), the inducible form of HO, serves as a general cytoprotectant against oxidative stress in cell culture, and in animal models of inflammatory or oxidative tissue injury *(7,28,29)*. In addition to its physiological role in heme degradation, HO-1 may affect a number of cellular processes, including growth, inflammation, and apoptosis *(7)*. The anti-inflammatory effects of HO-1 can limit tissue damage in response to pro-inflammatory stimuli *(20)*, and prevent graft rejection after transplantation *(12,22,23,30)*. The administration of CO at low concentrations can mimic the effects of HO-1 with respect to apparent anti-inflammatory and anti-apoptotic effects, suggesting a role for CO as a crucial mediator of HO-1 function *(20,21)*. The potential contributions of bile pigments, which have antioxidant properties, and heme-iron release, which triggers secondary increases in ferritin synthesis, toward the cytoprotective effects of HO have been reviewed elsewhere *(28,29)*.

This monograph will summarize current research on the role of the HO/CO system in regulation of vascular function during oxidative stress and vascular injury. We will emphasize recent findings, which suggest that HO-1 or CO applied exogenously at low concentration can protect against various forms of vascular injury, including I/R injury incurred during organ transplantation.

2. HEME OXYGENASE

2.1. Heme Oxygenase Enzymes

Heme oxygenase (E.C. 1.14.99.3) (HO) was described in 1969 by Tenhunen et al. as a hepatic microsomal mixed function oxygenase *(26)*. Three distinct isozymes have been characterized-the inducible form heme oxygenase-1 (HO-1) and two constitutive forms, heme oxygenase-2 (HO-2) and heme oxygenase-3 (HO-3) *(31–33)*. Both HO-1 and HO-2 catalyze the same biochemical reaction, but differ in physical and kinetic properties *(33,34)*. HO-3 displays a high-sequence homology with HO-2, yet the enzymatic activity of this species has not been established *(35)*.

The expression of HO-1 may occur in most tissues of the body, including the vasculature, but typically increases over an undetectable background only under inducing conditions involving shock or stress, or application of xenobiotic or pharmocologic agents *(33,34)*. HO-2 appears in most tissues, with abundant distribution in the testes and the vascular and nervous systems *(31–34,36)*. Unlike its inducible counterpart, HO-2 expression is constitutive, with the possible exception of regulation in the brain by glucocortioid hormones *(37,38)*. Although detectible in the heart and other tissues, the significance of HO-3 in the vasculature remains unclear *(35)*.

2.2. Heme Oxygenase-1: A General Response to Oxidative Cellular Stress

HO-1 induction represents a general transcriptional response to oxidative cellular stress, which can be triggered by stimulation with a large array of chemical and physical agents *(39)*. The list of inducing agents includes but is not limited to oxidants such as hydrogen peroxide or ultraviolet-A radiation, nitric oxide, pro-inflammatory cytokines and growth factors, thiol-reactive substances such as sodium arsenite and heavy metals, hemodynamic or shear stress, heat shock, and altered states of oxygen tension *(7,40)*. Heme, the substrate of HO activity and also a potent inducer of the gene *(41)*, may potentially inflict oxidative injury to endothelial cells during vascular hemolysis *(42)*.

In a comprehensive analysis of the mouse HO-1 gene 5' regulatory region, Alam et al. have discovered two upstream enhancer sequences (E1, E2) that occur respectively at -4 kb and -10 kb of the transcriptional start site *(43–46)*. These enhancers mediate the transcriptional induction of the *ho-1* gene by diverse agents, including endotoxins, heavy metal salts, phorbol esters, oxidants, and heme *(44,45)*. E1 and E2 contain repeated stress-responsive elements (StRE) consisting of recognition sequences for several transcription factors, including activator protein-1 (AP-1), v-maf oncoprotein, and Cap'n'collar/basic-leucine zipper proteins, such as NF-E2-related factor 2 (Nrf2) *(46)*. A transcriptional repressor of *ho-1* (Bach-1) has recently been charcterized *(47)*. Bach-1 potentially dimerizes with maf proteins, and antagonizes the effects of Nrf-2/maf dimers at the StRE sites of E1 and E2. The DNA-binding activity of Bach-1 is negatively regulated by heme in vitro *(48)*, and this may account for the substrate-dependent activation of *ho-1*.

2.3. Expression of HO-1 During Vascular Adaptive Responses to Hypoxia

The state of hypoxia, or lowered pO_2, generates a metabolic stress with particular physiological relevance in vascular tissues *(1,49)*. Hypoxic states occur as a result of ischemia or impaired oxygen uptake, and play a role in the pathophysiology of arteriosclerosis, fibrosis, neoplasia, and pulmonary hypertension *(50)*. Hypoxia stimulates the transcriptional upregulation of several stress proteins in vascular-derived cell lines *(51–56)*. In rat aortic vascular smooth muscle cells (VSMC), hypoxia treatment (1% O_2) induced HO-1 transcription and mRNA accumulation *(54,57)*. Hypoxia also induced HO-1 in rat pulmonary endothelial cells (PAEC), but not in rat pulmonary artery vascular smooth muscle cells. Comparative analysis of these cell types demonstrated variations in the transcription factor-binding activities underlying these responses. HO-1 mRNA induction in PAEC occurred in parallel with increased AP-1 DNA-binding activity, whereas the response in VSMC primarily involved the hypoxia-inducible factor (HIF-1), a critical mediator of transcriptional responses to hypoxia *(54,58)*. The importance of HIF-1 in *ho-1* gene activation was examined using mutant Hepa cells deficient in HIF-1α. The mutant cells failed to induce HO-1 mRNA accumulation in response to hypoxia, relative to wild-type cells *(55)*. In contrast, in mutant CHO cells deficient in HIF-1α, the *ho-1* gene still responded to hypoxic activation *(59)*. These results suggest that the transcriptional induction of HO-1 by hypoxia may involve both HIF-1, and AP-1 transcription factors, with apparent tissue-specific variation between vascular cell types *(54,58)*. The induction of HO-1 by hypoxia has been associated with glutathione (GSH) depletion, and may be inhibited by metal-chelating agents, suggesting a role for redox processes and endogenous metal ions in this response *(56,60)*. Acute or chronic hypoxia triggers HO-1 transcription in vivo in various rat organs including the heart *(54,61)*. Recent evidence implicates HO-1 as an inducible mechanism for protection against hypoxic lung injury in vivo. HO-1 null mice (*ho-1$^{-/-}$*) develop right ventricular dilation and right myocardial infarction, during chronic hypoxia (10% O_2), relative to wild-type mice that withstand the treatment, but did not differ in the development of pulmonary hypertension *(62)*. Transgenic mice with a lung-specific HO-1 overexpressing phenotype resisted the inflammatory and hypertensive effects of hypoxia *(63)*.

Nakayama et al. report a lack of HO-1 response to hypoxia in several cell types of human origin *(64)*. The transcriptional repression of HO-1 by hypoxia in human cell lines has been linked to the activation of the *ho-1* transcriptional repressor Bach-1 *(65)*. Thus, the physiological significance of HO-1 in human vascular responses to hypoxia remains uncertain. The induction of stress proteins, including HO-1, by hypoxia and other forms of oxidative stress in vascular systems may represent an adaptive response to vascular oxidative injury. By altering *ho-1* and NOS gene expression, hypoxia potentially modulates the availability of gaseous second-messengers CO and NO. Fluxes in the production of small gas signaling molecules during hypoxic stress would have potential consequences in the regulation of vascular function(s) as described in the following sections, including dilation, expression of vasoconstrictors, inhibition of platelet aggregation, and smooth-muscle proliferation *(1)*.

3. PHYSIOLOGICAL EFFECTS OF HEME OXYGENASE AND CARBON MONOXIDE

3.1. Role of CO in Vasoregulation

The putative vasoactive properties of CO depend on, in part, the stimulation of sGC and subsequent elevation of cGMP levels *(10)*. CO-mediated activation of sGC leads to a several-fold increase in cGMP production, a potency approximately 30-100 times lower than that of its cognate gas NO *(10)*. CO potentially serves as a substitute for NO, during NO-deficient states, but on the other hand may antagonize the activation of sGC by NO *(66)*. CO released from heme by the action of HO activity regulates cGMP production in vascular tissues *(16,17)*. Exposure of VSMC to exogenous CO elevated intracellular cGMP concentrations in these cells *(17)*. Exposure of VSMC to hypoxia, an inducer of HO-1 in this cell type, also increased endogenous levels of cGMP, which required HO activity and HO-derived CO, but excluded the involvement of NO *(16)*. CO released from VSMC acted in a paracrine fashion to stimulate the production of cGMP in co-cultured endothelial cells *(57)*. Morita et al. have shown that endogenous VSMC-derived CO, as well as exogenously applied CO, inhibited the proliferation of cultured VSMC *(16)*. The mechanism whereby exogenous or HO-derived CO attenuates cell growth in a cGMP-dependent fashion involved the downregulation of endothelial-derived mitogens such as platelet-derived growth factor and endothelin-1 *(57)*, and also the inhibition of E2F-1, a transcription factor involved in cell-cycle regulation *(16)*.

In vivo models have also supported a role for CO in vasorelaxation. In an isolated perfused rat-liver model, Suematsu et al. detected the presence of CO in the effluent. Treatment with metalloporphyrin HO inhibitors (i.e., ZnPPIX) diminished detectible CO levels, and increased perfusion pressure under constant flow conditions. The inhibitory effects of metalloporphyrins were reversed by the application of exogenous CO or cGMP analogs (i.e., 8-bromo-cGMP) in the perfusate *(67)*.

In isolated porcine aortic rings, the HO inhibitor SnPPIX decreased endothelium-dependent acetylcholine-dependent vasorelaxation, in the presence of the NOS inhibitor N^{ω}-nitro-L-arginine-methyl-ester (L-NAME) *(36)*. Conversely, the endothelium-dependent contractile response to phenylephrine in thoracic aortic rings was augmented in the presence of both ZnPPIX and N^{ω}-nitro-L-arginine (NNA), relative to treatment with NNA alone *(68)*. In this system, exogenously applied CO relaxed the aortic rings in a cGMP-dependent fashion. Overexpression of HO-1 by AdHO-1 infection of the vessels inhibited phenylephrine-dependent vasoconstriction in isolated aortic rings. Furthermore, Ad-HO-1 infection induced cGMP production in VSMC, which presumably was due to the generation of CO. The effects of HO-1 expression on vasoconstriction and cGMP production were subject to inhibition by ZnPPIX and occurred in the presence of NOS inhibitors (i.e., L-NNA, L-NAME) *(13)*. Thus, these effects are dependent on heme degradation and independent of NOS activity or NO generation. The effects of CO are not limited to the vascular smooth muscle, but also airway smooth muscle, whereby exogenously administered CO stimulated cGMP-dependent airway bronchodilation in guinea-pig trachea given histamine injections *(14)*. On the other hand, cGMP-independent mechanisms of vasoregulation by CO have also been proposed. CO may dilate blood vessels by directly activating calcium-dependent potassium channels (K_{Ca}) *(69–72)*. In interlobar arterial smooth muscle cells, the inhibition of HO activity by metalloporphyrins decreased endogenous CO production and decreased the number of open potassium channels (105 pS K). These effects increased vascular contractility in response to phenyephrine. The introduction of exogenous CO reversed the effects of metalloporphyrins on vascular contractility *(71)*. CO dilated porcine cerebral arterioles by increasing the effective coupling of calcium sparks to K_{Ca} channels *(72)*. The mechanism by which CO mediates these effects remains unclear.

3.2. Anti-Inflammatory Effects of CO

The mitogen-activated protein kinase (MAPK) pathways, which transduce oxidative stress and inflammatory signaling, may represent an important target of CO action *(20)*. The activation of MAPKs, a family of Ser/Thr protein kinases, responds to a variety of extracellular stimuli *(73)*. Three major MAPK signaling pathways, which include extracellular signal-regulated protein kinase (ERK), p38 MAPK (p38), and c-Jun NH_2-terminal protein kinase (JNK), have been identified in mammalian cells *(73)*.

The studies of Otterbein et al. in this laboratory showed that the anti-inflammatory properties of CO are mediated by p38 MAPK and its upstream MAPK kinase (MKK3) *(20)*. CO inhibited the expression of lipopolysaccharide (LPS)-induced pro-inflammatory cytokines in RAW 264.7 macrophages, including tumor necrosis factor (TNF)-α, interleukin (IL)-1β, and macrophage inflammatory protein-1α, while simultaneously increasing expression of the anti-inflammatory cytokine IL-10. Similar observations were made in a mouse model of lung inflammation. Using mice genetically deficient for MKK3, the upstream kinase of p38 MAPK, Otterbein et al. demonstrated the critical role of the p38 MAPK pathway in the anti-inflammatory effect of CO in vivo. In this model, the inhibitory effect of CO on TNF-α production did not require cGMP or NO production, or depend on the ERK1/2 or JNK MAPK pathways *(20)*. Sethi et al. demonstrated the inhibition of TNFα-inducible ERK1/2 activation by CO treatment in PAEC, indicating that CO can also downregulate signaling cascades initiated by pro-inflammatory cytokines *(74)*.

The mechanisms by which CO modulates the MAPKs are not clear. We hypothesize that a proximal effector, most likely a heme-containing protein, initiates the signal upon binding of the CO to the heme moiety, possibly by modulation of reactive oxygen species (ROS) production and the redox state of the cell. With respect to CO and MAPK signaling in macrophages, the identity of the upstream CO target remains elusive.

3.3. CO Inhibits Cellular Apoptosis

Apoptosis, or programmed cell death, consists of a regulated cascade of events that results in the death of a cell in response to environmental cues. Distinct from necrosis, which involves membrane disruption, apoptosis requires the action of proteases and nucleases within an intact plasma membrane, and participates in tissue development and homeostasis *(75)*. The biological significance of apoptosis varies in a tissue-specific manner. Exposure to CO has been shown to exert potent anti-apoptotic effects in vitro and in vivo in the context of I/R injury and organ transplantation (see following sections). The exogenous administration of CO or the overexpression of HO-1 prevented TNFα-induced apoptosis in murine fibroblasts *(76)*. The inhibitory effect of CO on TNFα-induced apoptosis in endothelial cells depended on the modulation of the p38 MAPK pathway, since it could be abolished with the selective chemical inhibitor SB203580, or a p38 dominant-negative mutant *(21)*. HO-1 or CO cooperated with nuclear factor (NF)-κB-dependent anti-apoptotic genes (c-IAP2 and A1) to protect against TNFα-mediated endothelial cell apoptosis *(77)*.

The anti-apoptotic effect of CO on cytokine-treated rat aortic smooth-muscle cells was partially dependent on the activation of sGC and was associated with suppression of p53 and inhibition of mitochondrial cytochrome-c release *(75)*. In this model, however, the investigators excluded a role for p38 MAPK in the anti-apoptotic effect of CO *(78)*.

3.4. CO Protects Against Ischemia/Reperfusion Injury

I/R injury has long been associated with oxidative stress resulting from the reperfusion and reoxygenation of previously ischemic tissue. HO-1 may participate in the manifestation of ischemic preconditioning, a process of acquired cellular protection against I/R injury, as observed in guinea pig transplanted lungs *(79)*. HO-1 overexpression provided potent protection against cold I/R injury in rat hearts and livers through an anti-apoptotic pathway *(80,81)*.

Exogenously applied CO at low concentrations inhibited I/R-induced apoptosis in pulmonary artery endothelial cell (PAEC) cultures, associated with the CO-dependent activation specifically of the p38α isoform with parallel suppression of ERK and JNK activation *(24)*. In addition to activation of p38α MAPK and its upstream MAPK kinase (MKK3), the anti-apoptotic effect of CO involved inhibition of Fas/FasL expression, and other apoptosis-related factors including caspases (-3, -8, -9) mitochondrial cytochrome-c release, Bcl-2 proteins, and poly (ADP-ribose) polymerase (PARP) cleavage *(82)*. CO exposure also protected against I/R-induced lung injury in vivo. Chemical inhibition of p38 MAPK activity, or the use of the *mkk3–/–* null mouse abolished the anti-apoptotic effects of CO during I/R, likely by preventing the modulation of caspase-3 activity *(24,82)*.

Similar anti-inflammatory effects of CO have now been demonstrated in models of I/R injury of the heart, kidney, and small bowel *(83)*. CO protected against liver I/R injury via activation of the p38 MAPK *(84)*. Homozygous *ho-1* null mice *(hmox-1–/–)* displayed increased mortality in a model of lung I/R injury. Inhalation of CO (1000 ppm) partially compensated for the HO-1 deficiency in *hmox-1–/–* mice, and improved survival following I/R *(15)*. In this model, the authors propose that the protection provided by CO involved the enhancement of fibrinolysis via the cGMP-dependent inhibition of plasminogen activator inhibitor-1 (PAI-1) expression *(15)*. Mice treated with a guanylate cyclase inhibitor, ODQ, were not rescued by CO from I/R-induced lethality.

3.5. Role of HO-1/CO in Atherosclerosis

HO-1 can be induced in both endothelial and vascular smooth muscle cells by pro-atherogenic stimuli, including oxidized low-density lipoprotein (LDL), lipid metabolites, shear stress, and angiotension II *(85)*. HO-1 also confers protection in animal models of arteriosclerosis, where it may be found in atherosclerotic lesions *(86)*. HO-1 is highly upregulated in the endothelium, and in the foam cells of intimal lesions from humans and apolipoprotein E-deficient mice *(86)*. Induction of endogenous HO-1 by chemical treatment (hemin) reduced the formation of atherosclerotic lesions in LDL-receptor knockout mice fed high-fat diets, relative to untreated or SnPPIX-treated controls *(87)*. The adenovirally mediated transduction of HO-1 into ApoE-deficient mice inhibited the formation of arteriosclerotic plaques relative to control mice *(88)*. The mechanism by which HO-1 protects against arterioslcerosis may involve, in part, the inhibition of platelet aggregation by HO-derived CO.

3.6. CO Inhibits Cellular Proliferation and Vascular Stenosis Associated With Balloon Injury

Under homeostatic conditions, a tightly regulated balance exists between apoptosis and cellular proliferation. Loss of growth control is typically associated with neoplasia. In the case of vascular stenosis, hyperproliferation of VSMC results in occlusion of the vascular lumen.

CO has been shown to block vascular cell proliferation in a number of models. Exogenous application of HO-1, by gene transfer or exogenous CO application, inhibited VSMC proliferation in vitro by G0/G1 arrest, which required cGMP production, the G1 cyclin-dependent protein kinase inhibitor p21[cip1], and activation of p38 MAPK *(12,13,17)*. Adenoviral-mediated overexpression of HO-1 (AdHO-1) in pigs inhibited vascular cell proliferation and lesion formation in a model of arterial injury. Conversely, HO-1–/– mice subjected to arterial injury displayed increased vascular cell proliferation, and developed hyperplastic lesions in comparison to HO-1[+/+] controls *(13)*. Employing a model of intimal hyperplasia where smooth muscle cells proliferate uncontrollably following balloon angioplasty of the carotid artery or chronic rejection of a transplanted aorta, exposure to CO completely prevented stenosis of the vessel *(12)*. Pretreatment of a rat with CO (250 ppm) for just 1 h significantly reduced the neointimal proliferation seen at 14 d after balloon angioplasty relative to control animals that did not receive CO treatment. The mechanisms involved in this effect required activation of p38 MAPK and cGMP production *(12)*. The application of HO-1 by adenovirally mediated gene transfer also protected against intimal hyperplasia following vascular balloon injury *(89)*.

3.7. Protective Roles of HO-1/CO in Organ Transplantation

Expression of the stress protein HO-1 in rodent allografts and xenografts correlates with long-term graft survival in several models of transplantation *(23,30,90)*. A higher expression of several protective genes has been observed in acute renal allograft rejection episodes in a rodent model of renal transplantation, where HO-1 expression increased in the allograft in response to immune injury *(90)*. The reduced expression of HO-1 in chronic rejection as compared with acute rejection represents either an inadequate response to injury or a consequence of prior injury that jeopardizes further tissue response to immune attack *(90)*.

Adenoviral-HO-1 gene therapy resulted in remarkable protection against rejection in rat liver transplants *(91)*. The upregulation of HO-1 protected pancreatic islet cells from Fas-mediated apoptosis in a dose-dependent fashion, supporting an anti-apoptotic function of HO-1 *(92,93)*. HO-1 may confer protection in the early phase after transplantation by inducing Th2-dependent cytokines such as IL-4 and IL-10, while suppressing interferon-gamma and IL-2 production, as demonstrated in a rat-liver allograft model *(94)*. The induction of HO-1 in rats undergoing liver transplantation with adenoviral-HO-1 gene therapy resulted in protection against I/R injury and improved survival after transplantation, possibly by suppression of Th1-cytokine production and decreased apoptosis after reperfusion *(95)*.

Beneficial effects of HO-1 modulation have been described in xeno-transplantation models, where HO-1 gene expression appears functionally associated with xenograft survival *(23,30)*. In a mouse to rat heart transplant model, the effects of HO-1 upregulation could be mimicked by CO administration, suggesting that HO-derived CO suppressed the graft rejection *(23)*. The authors proposed that CO suppressed graft rejection by inhibition of platelet aggregation, a process that facilitates vascular thrombosis and myocardial infarction. The ability of CO to suppress inflammation is likely involved in xenograft transplant models in which 400 ppm CO for 2 d prevented rejection for up to 50 d *(23)*. The modulatory effects of CO on platelet aggregation, vasodilation, and pro-inflammatory cytokines all potentially contribute to the favorable outcome in xenograft transplantation *(12)*.

Lung transplantation has become an accepted treatment modality for end-stage lung disease. After lung transplantation, there remains a persistent risk of acute and chronic graft failure, as well as of complications of the toxic immunosuppressive regimen used *(96)*. Compared to other solid organ transplants, the success of lung transplantation has been severely limited by the high incidence of acute and chronic graft rejection. The frequency and severity of episodes of acute rejection are the predominant risk factors for chronic airway rejection, manifested as obliterative bronchiolitis (OB) *(97,98)*. Data from rodent allograft studies as well as from clinical lung transplantation show that the lung, in comparison to other solid organs, is highly immunogenic. Despite advances in immunosuppression, the incidence of acute rejection in lung graft patients can be as high as 60% in the first postoperative month *(99,100)*. OB, which may develop during the first months after transplantation, is the main cause of morbidity and death following the first half-year after transplantation, despite therapeutic intervention. Once OB has developed, re-transplantation remains the only therapeutic option available *(101)*. Little is known about the pathophysiological background of OB. The possible determinants of developing OB include ongoing immunological allograft response, HLADR mismatch, cytomegalovirus infection, acute rejection episodes, organ-ischemia time, and recipient age *(101)*.

Until recently, only very limited research data were available on the possible role for HO-1 in allograft rejection after lung transplantation. Increased HO-1 expression has been detected in alveolar macrophages from lung tissue in lung-transplant recipients with either acute or chronic graft failure, when compared to stable recipients *(102)*.

In recent studies from this laboratory, Song et al. demonstrate that the level of HO-1 expression correlated to the acute rejection grade level in lung fibroblasts from a lung-transplant patient *(22)*. The effects of CO were examined in a rat model of lung transplantation. Orthotopic left lung transplantation was performed in LEW rat recipients from BN rat donors. HO-1 mRNA and protein expression were markedly elevated in transplanted rat lungs compared to sham-operated lungs. Animals were exposed to continuous inhalation CO (500 ppm) or air. Transplanted lungs developed severe intra-alveolar hemorrhage and intravascular coagulation. In the presence of continuous CO exposure (500 ppm), however, the gross anatomy and histology of transplanted lungs showed dramatic preservation relative to air-treated controls. Furthermore, transplanted lungs displayed increased apoptotic cell death compared with the transplanted lungs of CO-treated recipients, as assessed by TUNEL and caspase-3 immunostaining. CO exposure inhibited the induction of IL-6 mRNA expression in lung and serum caused by the transplantation. Gene array analysis revealed that CO also downregulated other pro-inflammatory genes, including macrophage inflammatory protein (MIP)-1α and macrophage migration inhibitory factor (MIF), and growth factors such as platelet-derived growth factor (PDGF), which were upregulated by transplantation *(22)*.

In organ transplantation, the I/R injury that occurs leads to rapid endothelial cell apoptosis. The loss of endothelial cells in the vessels serving the organ results in a rapid cascade of events including thrombosis that can ultimately result in the rejection of the organ. These data suggest CO limits lung graft injury by maintaining cell viability and suppressing inflammation.

4. CONCLUSIONS AND FUTURE PERSPECTIVES

Since the discovery that the major low-molecular-weight stress protein induced by shock or stress conditions in mammalian cells was identical to the heme metabolic enzyme HO-1 *(103)*, the potential role of this species in tissue protection has been explored in multiple models of tissue injury and disease *(7)*. Both constitutive and inducible forms of HO occur in the cardiovascular system and play significant roles in the regulation of vascular homeostasis. The studies reviewed in this chapter collectively suggest that HO can confer protection against several forms of vascular injury by inhibiting inflammation, apoptosis, platelet aggregation, and the proliferation of smooth muscle. HO-derived CO likely mediates these effects, since exogenously applied CO can exert similar protective effects as HO-1 in many model systems. Questions remain as to how best to exploit the therapeutic properties of the HO/CO system to alleviate human disease. Retroviral vector-mediated gene therapy represents one possible approach. The application of HO-1 directly, in addition to promoting increases in endogenous CO production, has additional effects related to production of bile pigments and alteration of iron metabolism. Further research is needed to completely understand all the consequences of manipulating this complex system. A more direct approach may involve the inhalation of CO in the clinic to treat human diseases. As an alternative to inhalation, pharmacological application of CO with the transition-metal carbonyl CO-releasing molecules, as described by Motterlini et al., may provide an additional therapeutic avenue *(104)*. Whether direct application of CO by either method will provide a safe modality for the treatment of human disease requires further research directed at understanding the toxicological sequelae of low-dose CO.

ACKNOWLEDGMENTS

This work was supported by an award from the American Heart Association (AHA #0335035N), to S. W. Ryter, and NIH grants R01-HL60234, R01-AI42365, and R01-HL55330 awarded to A. M. K. Choi.

REFERENCES

1. Kourembanas, S. (2002) Hypoxia and carbon monoxide in the vasculature. *Antioxid. Redox Signal* **4,** 291–299.
2. Lowenstein, C. J., Dinerman, J. L., and Snyder, S. H. (1994) Nitric oxide: a physiologic messenger. *Ann. Intern. Med.* **120,** 227–237.
3. Felley-Bosco, E., Buzard, G. S., Billiar, T. R., and Keefer, L. K. (1998) Nitric oxide, altered DNA, and mammalian disease. In Aruoma, O. I., and Halliwell, B. (eds), Molecular Biology of Free Radicals in Human Diseases. Oica International, Saint Lucia, London, pp. 287–325.
4. Andersson, K. E. (2003) Erectile physiological and pathophysiological pathways involved in erectile dysfunction. *J. Urol.* **70,** S6–13.
5. Gianetti, J., Bevilacqua, S., and De Caterina, R. (2002) Inhaled nitric oxide: more than a selective pulmonary vasodilator. *Eur. J. Clin. Invest.* **32,** 628–635.

6. Jugdutt, B. I. (2003) Nitric oxide and cardiovascular protection. *Heart Fail. Rev.* **8**, 29–34
7. Ryter, S., Otterbein, L. E., Morse, D., and Choi, A. M. K. (2002) Heme oxygenase/ carbon monoxide signaling pathways: regulation and functional significance. *Mol. Cell Biochem.* **234/235**, 249–263.
8. Wink, D. A. and Mitchell, J. B. (1998) Chemical biology of nitric oxide: insights into regulatory, cytotoxic, and cytoprotective mechanisms of nitric oxide. *Free Radic. Biol. Med.* **25**, 434–456.
9. Maines, M. D. (1997) The heme oxygenase system: a regulator of second messenger gases. *Annu. Rev. Pharmacol. Toxicol.* **37**, 517–554.
10. Furchgott, R. F. and Jothianandan, D. (1991) Endothelium-dependent and-independent vasodilation involving cyclic GMP: relaxation induced by nitric oxide, carbon monoxide and light. *Blood Vessels* **28**, 52–61.
11. Verma, A., Hirsch, D. J., Glatt, C. E., Ronnett, G. V., and Snyder, S. H. (1993) Carbon monoxide: a putative neural messenger. *Science* **259**, 381–384.
12. Otterbein, L. E., Zuckerbraun, B. S., Haga, M., et al. (2003) Carbon monoxide suppresses arteriosclerotic lesions associated with chronic graft rejection and with balloon injury. *Nat. Med.* **9**, 183–190.
13. Duckers, H. J., Boehm, M., True, A. L., et al. (2001) Heme oxygenase-1 protects against vascular constriction and proliferation. *Nat. Med.* **7**, 693–698.
14. Cardell, L. O., Ueki, I. F., Stjarne, P., et al. (1998) Bronchodilatation in vivo by carbon monoxide, a cyclic GMP related messenger. *Br. J. Pharmacol.* **124**, 1065–1068.
15. Fujita, T., Toda, K., Karimova, A., et al. (2001) Paradoxical rescue from ischemic lung injury by inhaled carbon monoxide driven by derepression of fibrinolysis. *Nat. Med.* **7**, 598–604.
16. Morita, T., Mitsialis, S. A., Koike, H., Liu, Y., and Kourembanas, S. (1997) Carbon monoxide controls the proliferation of hypoxic vascular smooth muscle cells. *J. Biol. Chem.* **272**, 32,804–32,809.
17. Morita, T., Perrella, M. A., Lee, M. E., and Kourembanas, S. (1995) Smooth muscle cell-derived carbon monoxide is a regulator of vascular cGMP. *Proc. Natl. Acad. Sci. USA* **92**, 1475–1479.
18. Brune, B. and Ullrich, V. (1987) Inhibition of platelet aggregation by carbon monoxide is mediated by activation of guanylate cyclase. *Mol. Pharmacol.* **32**, 497–504.
19. Utz, J. and Ullrich, V. (1991) Carbon monoxide relaxes ilial smooth muscle through activation of guanylate cyclase. *Biochem. Pharmacol.* **41**, 1195–2001.
20. Otterbein, L. E., Bach, F. H., Alam, J., et al. (2000) Carbon monoxide has anti-inflammatory effects involving the mitogen-activated protein kinase pathway. *Nat. Med.* **6**, 422–428.
21. Brouard, S., Otterbein, L. E., Anrather, J., et al. (2000) Carbon monoxide generated by heme oxygenase-1 suppresses endothelial cell apoptosis. *J. Exp. Med.* **192**, 1015–1026.
22. Song, R., Kubo, M., Morse, D., et al. (2003) Carbon monoxide induces cytoprotection in rat orthotopic lung transplantation via anti-inflammatory and anti-apoptotic effects. *Am. J. Pathol.* **163**, 231–242.
23. Sato, K., Balla, J., Otterbein, L., et al. (2001) Carbon monoxide generated by heme oxygenase-1 suppresses the rejection of mouse-to-rat cardiac transplants. *J. Immunol.* **166**, 4185–4194.
24. Zhang, X., Shan, P., Otterbein, L. E., et al. (2003) Carbon monoxide inhibition of apoptosis during ischemia-reperfusion lung injury is dependent on the p38 mitogen-activated protein kinase pathway and involves caspase 3. *J. Biol. Chem.* **278**, 1248–1258.
25. Vremen, H. J., Wong, R. J., and Stevenson, D. K. (2000) Carbon monoxide in breath, blood, and other tissues. In Penney, D. G. (ed), Carbon Monoxide Toxicity, CRC, Boca Raton, pp. 19–60.
26. Tenhunen, R., Marver, H., and Schmid, R. (1969) Microsomal heme oxygenase, characterization of the enzyme. *J. Biol. Chem.* **244**, 6388–6394.
27. Tenhunen, R., Ross, M. E., Marver, H. S., and Schmid, R. (1970) Reduced nicotinamide adenine dinucleotide phosphate dependent biliverdin reductase: partial purification and characterization. *Biochemistry* **9**, 298–323.
28. Ryter, S. and Tyrrell, R. M. (2000) The heme synthesis and degradation pathways, role in oxidant sensitivity. Heme oxygenase has both pro- and anti-oxidant properties. *Free Radic. Biol. Med.* **28**, 289–309.
29. Otterbein, L. E., Soares, M. P., Yamashita, K., and Bach, F. H. (2003) Heme oxygenase-1: unleashing the protective properties of heme. *Trends Immunol.* **24**, 449–455.
30. Soares, M. P., Lin, Y., Anrather, J., et al. (1998) Expression of heme oxygenase-1 can determine cardiac xenograft survival. *Nat. Med.* **4**, 1073–1077.
31. Maines, M. D., Trakshel, G. M., and Kutty, R. K. (1986) Characterization of two constitutive forms of rat liver microsomal heme oxygenase. *J. Biol. Chem.* **261**, 411–419.
32. Trakshel, G. M., Kutty, R. K., and Maines, M. D. (1986) Purification and characterization of the major constitutive form of testicular heme oxygenase. *J. Biol. Chem.* **261**, 11,131–11,137.
33. Maines, M. D. (1992) Heme Oxygenase: Clinical Applications and Functions, CRC, Boca Raton, FL.
34. Maines, M. D. (1988) Heme Oxygenase: function, multiplicity, regulatory mechanisms, and clinical applications. *FASEB J.* **2**, 2557–2568.
35. McCoubrey, W. K., Huang, T. J., and Maines, M. D. (1997) Isolation and characterization of a cDNA from the rat brain that encodes hemoprotein heme oxygenase-3. *Eur. J. Biochem.* **247**, 725–732.
36. Zakhary, R., Gaine, S. P., Dinerman, J. L., Ruat, M., Flavahan, N. A., and Snyder, S. H. (1996) Heme oxygenase 2: endothelial and neuronal localization and role in endothelium-dependent relaxation. *Proc. Natl. Acad. Sci. USA* **93**, 795–798.
37. Raju, V. S., McCoubrey, W. K., Jr., and Maines, M. D. (1997) Regulation of heme oxygenase-2 by glucocorticoids in neonatal rat brain: characterization of a functional glucocorticoid response element. *Biochim. Biophys. Acta* **1351**, 89–104.

38. Maines, M. D. (1996) Corticosterone promotes increased heme oxygenase-2 protein and transcript expression in the newborn rat brain. *Brain Res.* **722,** 83–94.

39. Keyse, S. M., Applegate, L. A., Tromvoukis, Y., and Tyrrell, R. M. (1990) Oxidant stress leads to transcriptional activation of the human heme oxygenase gene in cultured skin fibroblasts. *Mol. Cell Biol.* **10,** 4967–4969.

40. Ryter, S. W. and Tyrrell, R. M. (1997) The role of heme oxygenase-1 in the mammalian stress response: Molecular aspects of regulation and function. In Forman, H. J., and Cadenas, E. (eds), Oxidative Stress and Signal Transduction. Chapman and Hall, New York, pp. 343–386.

41. Alam, J., Shibahara, S., and Smith, A. (1989) Transcriptional activation of the heme oxygenase gene by heme and cadmium in mouse hepatoma cells. *J. Biol. Chem.* **264,** 6371–6375.

42. Balla, J., Jacob, H. S., Balla, G., Nath, K., Eaton, J. W., and Vercellotti, G. M. (1993) Endothelial-cell heme uptake from heme proteins: Induction of sensitization and desensitization to oxidant damage. *Proc. Natl. Acad. Sci. USA* **90,** 9285–9289.

43. Alam, J., Cai, J., and Smith, A. (1994) Isolation and characterization of the mouse heme oxygenase-1 gene. *J. Biol. Chem.* **269,** 1001–1009.

44. Alam, J. (1994) Multiple elements within the 5' distal enhancer of the mouse heme oxygenase-1 gene mediate induction by heavy metals. *J. Biol. Chem.* **269,** 25,049–25,056.

45. Alam, J., Camhi, S., and Choi, A. M. (1995) Identification of a second region upstream of the mouse heme oxygenase-1 gene that functions as a basal level and inducer-dependent transcription enhancer. *J. Biol. Chem.* **270,** 11,977–11,984

46. Alam, J., Wicks, C., Stewart, D., et al. (2000) Mechanism of heme oxygenase-1 gene activation by cadmium in MCF-7 mammary epithelial cells. Role of p38 kinase and Nrf2 transcription factor. *J. Biol. Chem.* **275,** 27,694–27,702.

47. Sun, J., Hoshino, H., Takaku, K., et al. (2002) Hemoprotein Bach1 regulates enhancer availability of heme oxygenase-1 gene. *EMBO J.* **21,** 5216–5224.

48. Ogawa, K., Sun, J., Taketani, S., et al. (2001) Heme mediates derepression of Maf recognition element through direct binding to transcription repressor Bach1. *EMBO J.* **20,** 2835–2843.

49. Haddad, J. J. (2002) Oxygen-sensing mechanisms and the regulation of redox-responsive transcription factors in the development and pathophysiology. *Respir. Res.* **3,** 26.

50. Semenza, G. L., Agani, F., Feldser, D., et al. (2000) Hypoxia, HIF-1, and the pathophysiology of common human diseases. *Adv. Exp. Med. Biol.* **475,** 123–130.

51. Heacock, C. S. and Sutherland, R. M. (1986) Induction characteristics of oxygen regulated proteins. *Int. J. Radiat. Oncol. Biol. Phys.* **12,** 1287–1290.

52. Graven, K. K. and Farber, H. W. (1998) Endothelial cell hypoxic stress proteins. *J. Lab. Clin. Med.* **132,** 456–463.

53. Zimmerman, L. H., Levine, R. A., and Farber, H. W. (1991) Hypoxia induces a specific set of stress proteins in cultured endothelial cells. *J. Clin. Invest.* **87,** 908–914.

54. Lee, P. J., Jiang, B. H., Chin, B. Y., et al. (1997) Hypoxia-inducible factor-1 mediates transcriptional activation of the heme oxygenase-1 gene in response to hypoxia. *J. Biol. Chem.* **272,** 5375–5381.

55. Murphy, B. J., Laderoute, K. R., Short, S. M., and Sutherland, R. M. (1991) The identification of heme oxygenase as a major hypoxic stress protein in Chinese hamster ovary cells. *Br. J. Cancer* **64,** 69–73.

56. Ryter, S., Si, M. L., Lai, C-C., and Su, C. Y. (2000) Regulation of endothelial heme oxygenase activity during hypoxia is dependent on intracellular chelatable iron. *Am. J. Physiol. Heart Circ. Physiol.* **279,** H2889–H2897.

57. Morita, T. and Kourembanas, S. (1995) Endothelial cell expression of vasoconstrictors and growth factors is regulated by smooth muscle cell-derived carbon monoxide. *J. Clin. Invest.* **96,** 2676–2682.

58. Hartsfield, C. L., Alam, J., and Choi, A. M. (1999) Differential signaling pathways of HO-1 gene expression in pulmonary and systemic vascular cells. *Am. J. Physiol.* **277,** L1133–L1141.

59. Wood, S. M., Wiesener, M. S., Yeates, K. M., et al. (1998) Selection and analysis of a mutant cell line defective in the hypoxia-inducible factor-1 alpha-subunit (HIF-1alpha). Characterization of hif-1 alpha-dependent and independent hypoxia-inducible gene expression. *J. Biol. Chem.* **273,** 8360–8368.

60. Motterlini, R., Foresti, R., Bassi, R., Calabrese, V., Clark, J. E., and Green, C. J. (2000) Endothelial heme oxygenase-1 induction by hypoxia. Modulation by inducible nitric-oxide synthase and S-nitrosothiols. *J. Biol. Chem.* **275,** 13,613–13,620.

61. Katayose, D., Isoyama, S., Fujita, H., and Shibahara, S. (1993) Separate regulation of heme oxygenase and heat shock protein 70 mRNA expression in the rat heart by hemodynamic stress. *Biochem. Biophys. Res. Commun.* **191,** 587–594

62. Yet, S. F., Perrella, M. A., Layne, M. D., et al. (1999) Hypoxia induces severe right ventricular dilatation and infarction in heme oxygenase-1 null mice. *J. Clin. Invest.* **103,** R23–R29.

63. Minamino, T., Christou, H., Hsieh, C. M., et al. (2001) Targeted expression of heme oxygenase-1 prevents the pulmonary inflammatory and vascular responses to hypoxia. *Proc. Natl. Acad. Sci. USA* **98,** 8798–8803.

64. Nakayama, M., Takahashi, K., Kitamuro, T., et al. (2000) Repression of heme oxygenase-1 by hypoxia in vascular endothelial cells. *Biochem. Biophys. Res. Commun.* **271,** 665–671.

65. Kitamuro, T., Takahashi, K., Ogawa, K., et al. (2003) Bach1 functions as a hypoxia-inducible repressor for the heme oxygenase-1 gene in human cells. *J. Biol. Chem.* **278,** 9125–9133.

66. Kajimura, M., Goda, N., and Suematsu, M. (2002) Organ design for generation and reception of CO: lessons from the liver. *Antioxid. Redox Signal* **4,** 633–637.

67. Suematsu, M., Kashiwagi, S., Sano, T., Goda, N., Shinoda, Y., and Ishimura, Y. (1994) Carbon monoxide as an endogenous modulator of hepatic vascular perfusion. *Biochem. Biophys. Res. Commun.* **205,** 1333–1337.

68. Caudill, T. K., Resta, T. C., Kanagy, N. L., and Walker, B. R. (1998) Role of endothelial carbon monoxide in attenuated vasoreactivity following chronic hypoxia. *Am. J. Physiol.* **275,** R1025–R1030.
69. Koehler, R. C. and Traystman, R. J. (2002) Cerebrovascular effects of carbon monoxide. *Antioxid. Redox Signal* **4,** 279–290.
70. Wang, R., Wu, L., and Wang, Z. (1997) The direct effect of carbon monoxide on KCa channels in vascular smooth muscle cells. *Eur. J. Physiol.* **434,** 285–291.
71. Kaide, J. I., Zhang, F., Wei, Y., et al. (2001) Carbon monoxide of vascular origin attenuates the sensitivity of renal arterial vessels to vasoconstrictors. *J. Clin. Invest.* **107,** 1163–1171.
72. Jaggar, J. H., Leffler, C. W., Cheranov, S. Y., Tcheranova, D., Shuyu, E., and Cheng, X. (2002) Carbon monoxide dilates cerebral arterioles by enhancing the coupling of Ca2+ sparks to Ca2+-activated K+ channels. *Circ. Res.* **91,** 610–617.
73. Kyriakis, J. M. and Avruch, J. (1996) Sounding the alarm: protein kinase cascades activated by stress and inflammation. *J. Biol. Chem.* **271,** 24,313–24,316.
74. Sethi, J. M., Otterbein, L. E., and Choi, A. M. (2002) Differential modulation by exogenous carbon monoxide of TNF-alpha stimulated mitogen-activated protein kinases in rat pulmonary artery endothelial cells. *Antioxid. Redox Signal* **4,** 241–248.
75. Kroemer, G., Dallaporta, B., and Resche-Rigon, M. (1998) The mitochondrial death/life regulator in apoptosis and necrosis. *Annu. Rev. Physiol.* **60,** 619–642.
76. Petrache, I., Otterbein, L. E., Alam, J., Wiegand, G. W., and Choi, A. M. (2000) Heme oxygenase-1 inhibits TNF-alpha-induced apoptosis in cultured fibroblasts. *Am. J. Physiol. Lung Cell Mol. Physiol.* **278,** L312–L319.
77. Brouard, S., Berberat, P. O., Tobiasch, E., Seldon, M. P., Bach, F. H., Soares, M. P. (2002) Heme oxygenase-1-derived carbon monoxide requires the activation of transcription factor NF-kappa B to protect endothelial cells from tumor necrosis factor-alpha-mediated apoptosis. *J. Biol. Chem.* **277,** 17,950–17,961.
78. Liu, X. M., Chapman, G. B., Peyton, K. J., Schafer, A. I., and Durante, W. (2003) Antiapoptotic action of carbon monoxide on cultured vascular smooth muscle cells. *Exp. Biol. Med.* **228,** 572–575.
79. Soncul, H., Oz, E., and Kalaycioglu, S. (1999) Role of ischemic preconditioning on ischemia-reperfusion injury of the lung. *Chest* **115,** 1672–1677.
80. Katori, M., Anselmo, D. M., Busuttil, R. W., Kupiec-Weglinski, J. W. (2002) A novel strategy against ischemia and reperfusion injury: cytoprotection with heme oxygenase system. *Transplant Immunol.* **9,** 227–233.
81. Katori, M., Buelow, R., Ke, B., et al. (2002) Heme oxygenase-1 overexpression protects rat hearts from cold ischemia/reperfusion injury via an anti-apoptotic pathway. *Transplantation* **73,** 287–292.
82. Zhang, X., Shan, P., Alam, J., Davis, R. J., Flavell, R. A., Lee, P. J. (2003) Carbon monoxide modulates Fas/Fas ligand, caspases, and Bcl-2 family proteins via the p38alpha mitogen-activated protein kinase pathway during ischemia-reperfusion lung injury. *J. Biol. Chem.* **278,** 22,061–22,070.
83. Nakao, A., Kimizuka, K., Stolz, D. B., et al. (2003) Protective effect of carbon monoxide inhalation for cold-preserved small intestinal grafts. *Surgery* **134,** 285-292.
84. Amersi, F., Shen, X. D., Anselmo, D., et al. (2002) Ex vivo exposure to carbon monoxide prevents hepatic ischemia/reperfusion injury through p38 MAP kinase pathway. *Hepatology* **35,** 815–823.
85. Siow, R. C., Sato, H., and Mann, G. E. (1999) Heme oxygenase-carbon monoxide signalling pathway in atherosclerosis: anti-atherogenic actions of bilirubin and carbon monoxide? *Cardiovasc. Res.* **41,** 385–394.
86. Wang, L. J., Lee, T. S., Lee, F. Y., Pai, R. C., and Chau, L. Y. (1998) Expression of heme oxygenase-1 in atherosclerotic lesions. *Am. J. Pathol.* **152,** 711–720.
87. Ishikawa, K., Sugawara, D., Wang, X. P., et al. (2001) Heme oxygenase-1 inhibits atherosclerotic lesion formation in ldl-receptor knockout mice. *Circ. Res.* **88,** 506–512.
88. Juan, S. H., Lee, T. S., Tseng, K. W., et al. (2001) Adenovirus-mediated heme oxygenase-1 gene transfer inhibits the development of atherosclerosis in apolipoprotein E-deficient mice. *Circulation* **104,** 1519–1525.
89. Tulis, D. A., Durante, W., Liu, X., Evans, A. J., Peyton, K. J., and Schafer, A. I. (2001) Adenovirus-mediated heme oxygenase-1 gene delivery inhibits injury-induced vascular neointima formation. *Circulation* **104,** 2710–2715.
90. Avihingsanon, Y., Ma, N., Csizmadia, E., et al. (2002) Expression of protective genes in human renal allografts: a regulatory response to injury associated with graft rejection. *Transplantation* **73,** 1079–1085.
91. Ke, B., Buelow, R., Shen, X. D., et al. (2002) Heme oxygenase-1 gene transfer prevents CD95/Fas ligand-mediated apoptosis and improves liver allograft survival via carbon monoxide signaling pathway. *Hum. Gene Ther.* **13,** 1189–1199.
92. Pileggi, A., Molano, R. D., Berney, T., et al. (2001) Heme oxygenase-1 induction in islet cells results in protection from apoptosis and improved in vivo function after transplantation. *Diabetes* **50,** 1983–1991.
93. Tobiasch, E., Gunther, L., and Bach, F. H. (2001) Heme oxygenase-1 protects pancreatic beta cells from apoptosis caused by various stimuli. *J. Invest. Med.* **49,** 566–571.
94. Ke, B., Shen, X. D., Melinek, J., et al. (2001) Heme oxygenase-1 gene therapy: a novel immunomodulatory approach in liver allograft recipients? *Transplant. Proc.* **33,** 581–582.
95. Amersi, F., Buelow, R., Kato, H., et al. (1999) Upregulation of heme oxygenase-1 protects genetically fat Zucker rat livers from ischemia/reperfusion injury. *J. Clin. Invest.* **104,** 1631–1639.
96. Hosenpud, J. D., Bennett, L. E., Keck, B. M., Boucek, M. M., and Novick, R. J. (2000) The registry of the international society for heart and lung transplantation: seventeenth official report. *J. Heart Lung Transplant.* **19,** 909–931.

97. Bando, K., Paradis, I. L., Similo, S., et al. (1995) Obliterative bronchiolitis after lung and heart-lung transplantation. An analysis of risk factors and management. *J. Thorac. Cardiovasc. Surg.* **110,** 4–13.
98. Girgis, R. E., Tu, I., Berry, G. J. et al. (1996) Risk factors for the development of obliterative bronchiolitis after lung transplantation. *J. Heart Lung Transplant.* **15,** 1200–1208.
99. Sibley, R. K., Berry, G. J., Tazelaar, H. D. et al. (1993) The role of transbronchial biopsies in the management of lung transplant recipients. *J. Heart Lung Transplant.* **12,** 308–324.
100. Trulock, E. P. (1993) Management of lung transplant rejection. *Chest* **103,** 1566–1576.
101. Estenne, M. and Hertz, M. I. (2002) Bronchiolitis obliterans after human lung transplantation. *Am. J. Respir. Crit. Care Med.* **166,** 440–444.
102. Lu, F., Zander, D. S., and Visner, G. A. (2002) Increased expression of heme oxygenase-1 in human lung transplantation. *J. Heart Lung Transplant.* **21,** 1120–1126.
103. Keyse, S. M. and Tyrrell, R. M. (1989) Heme oxygenase is the major 32-kDa stress protein induced in human skin fibroblasts by UVA radiation, hydrogen peroxide, and sodium arsenite. *Proc. Natl. Acad. Sci. USA* **86,** 99–103.
104. Motterlini, R., Clark, J. E., Foresti, R., Sarathchandra, P., Mann, B. E., and Green, C. J. (2002) Carbon monoxide-releasing molecules: characterization of biochemical and vascular activities. *Circ. Res.* **90,** E17–E24.

2

Tumor Necrosis Factor-α/Receptor Signaling Through the Akt Kinase

Osman Nidai Ozes, Hakan Akca, Jason A. Gustin, Lindsey D. Mayo,
Roxana Pincheira, Chandrashekhar K. Korgaonkar,
and David B. Donner

SUMMARY

Tumor necrosis factor (TNF) is a pleiotropic cytokine that can affect the growth, differentiation, and metabolism of virtually every nucleated cell type in the body. TNF promotes immunity, but its expression is also associated with pathologies, such as rheumatoid arthritis, type II diabetes, and cachexia. Two distinct cell-surface receptors bind TNF, the type 1 receptor (TNFR1), which contains a conserved motif called a "death domain" in its C-terminus, and the type II receptor. Binding of TNF to TNFR1 brings the death domains of TNFR1 into physical proximity, thereby promoting their interactions with cytoplasmic proteins that also contain death domains. Thus, a signal transduction cascade is initiated that coincidentally activates caspases that promote cell death and, additionally, anti-apoptotic events. The balance between these arms of the TNFR1 signaling cascade determines whether cells live or die.

We found that binding of TNF to TNFR1 activates the Akt (protein kinase B) serine threoinine kinase. In cells, Akt regulates the expression of gene products that promote cell survival or suppress apoptosis, in part through activation of a transcription factor, nuclear factor (NF)-κB. Systemically, activation of NF-κB by TNF during infections can induce a catabolic state in low-priority tissues, such as muscle and fat, thereby liberating energy reserves that permit anabolic activity in higher-priority tissues such as the liver and the immune system. Thus, TNF can coordinate the acute-phase response by acting through Akt.

Key Words: Tumor necrosis factor; Akt serine-threonine kinase; phosphatidylinositol 3-kinase; nuclear factor kappa B; immunity; apoptosis; acute-phase response.

1. INTRODUCTION

Tumor necrosis factor (TNF)-α is a multifunctional cytokine that was first identified and characterized on the basis of its ability to induce the regression of tumors in animals, and the cytotoxic response that it can elicit from some transformed cells *(1)*. Although it was originally viewed as an oncolytic agent, subsequent work showed that TNF promotes immunity, antiviral responses, the acute-phase response to infections, and the syndrome of wasting and malnutrition known as cachexia in some chronic diseases, most particularly acquired immunodeficiency syndrome (AIDS). TNF induces insulin resistance and mediates inflammation, as in rheumatoid arthritis. During overwhelming infections, overproduction of TNF induces septic shock, organ failure, and death. More positively, TNF promotes fibroblast proliferation and angiogenesis, suggesting that it plays a role in wound repair. The demonstration that the immune system produces an oncolytic agent with therapeutic potential that also induces significant, sometimes lethal, alterations in the functions of normal tissues accounts for the great interest in TNF.

From: *Cell Signaling in Vascular Inflammation*
Edited by: J. Bhattacharya © Humana Press Inc., Totowa, NJ

Many malignancies are resistant to the cytotoxic activity of TNF. Such resistance may derive from the coincident activation of signaling pathways that lead to apoptosis or cell survival *(2)*. Whether or not a cancer cell succumbs to TNF is largely determined by whether the life or death signaling events induced by the cytokine predominate in a cell. The therapeutic utility of TNF has also been limited by its ability to induce severe, dose-limiting side effects such as hypotension, liver toxicity, and metabolic derangements including insulin resistance. Thus, considerable effort has been directed towards understanding the molecular mechanisms of TNF action and how these produce cellular metabolic responses and determine whether cells live or die.

The first step in TNF action is binding to receptors expressed on essentially all nucleated cells *(2,3)*. Two distinct receptors have been identified and their cDNAs cloned—the 55-kDa type 1 receptor (TNFR1) and the 75-kDa type 2 receptor (TNFR2). The extracellular domains of the receptors share homologies with one another and with a group of cell-surface receptors that include the FAS antigen, the low-affinity nerve growth factor receptor, 4-1BB, CD40, OX40, and CD27. The intracellular domains of the TNF receptors are not similar, and TNFR1 and TNFR2 induce distinct cellular responses. TNFR1 promotes apoptosis in malignancies, fibroblast proliferation, antiviral responses, and activation of nuclear factor (NF)-κB, and plays a predominant role in the host defense against microorganisms. TNFR2 plays a poorly defined role in cytotoxicity, promotes monocyte and T-cell growth, inhibits early hematopoiesis, and activates NF-κB.

TNFR1 contains an 80-amino-acid cytoplasmic death domain, which plays an obligate role in the induction of apoptosis by promoting protein-protein interactions *(4)*. Binding of TNF to TNFR1 promotes interaction of the death domain with other proteins that also contain death domains. The TNF receptor-associated death-domain protein (TRADD) engages TNFR1 and couples the receptor to distinct pathways that promote apoptosis and survival. Apoptotic signaling is mediated by interaction of TRADD with the FAS-associated death-domain protein, FADD, and through this interaction with pro-apoptotic caspase 8. TRADD also interacts with TNF receptor-associated factor-2 (TRAF2) and another death-domain protein, RIP (receptor interacting protein). TRAF2/RIP couples the receptor to a pathway that plays a role in activation of NF-κB, which opposes apoptosis by inducing transcription of anti-apoptotic genes, as well as genes important to immunity and inflammation.

Ordinarily, NF-κB is sequestered in the cytoplasm and therefore inactive, due to its interaction with inhibitors of kappa B (IκB) proteins *(5)*. Cellular studies have indicated that once bound to TRADD, TRAF2/RIP induces a serine/threonine kinase cascade in which NF-κB-inducing kinase (NIK) phosphorylates and activates an IκB kinase (IKK) complex. The IKK complex, which can contain two related kinases, IKKα and IKKβ, phosphorylates and promotes dissociation of IκB from NF-κB. This unmasks the nuclear localization sequence of NF-κB, which moves into the nucleus, where it acts on target genes. This view of TNFR1 function and cell life-and-death decision-making has not been fully supported by developmental studies, in which genes presumed to be associated with NF-κB activation have been knocked out by homologous recombination. However, different conclusions obtained from studies with cell cultures and from animal models may suggest that TNF action remains more complex than is presently appreciated and/or that redundant pathways can complement gene defects during development. Although some details may change, it is clear that opposing signals emanate from TNFR1: one culminates in apoptosis, the other in NF-κB activation and survival (**Fig. 1**).

Mitogens, and cytokines that function as survival as well as growth factors, promote cell proliferation and viability. Binding of these factors to their receptors engages signaling cascades composed of interacting macromolecules, some of which are enzymes that produce second messengers. Phosphatidylinositol 3-kinases (PI 3-kinase) comprise a diverse family in which type 1A appears primarily responsible for conveying growth and survival signals from activated receptors *(6)*. PI 3-kinase contains an 85-kDa regulatory subunit that interacts with phosphorylated receptor tyrosine

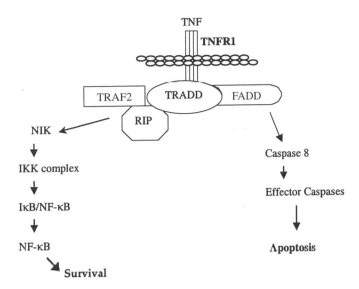

Fig. 1. Signaling events downstream of the type 1 tumor necrosis factor (TNF) receptor. Signals emanating from TNFR1 couple the receptor to cascades that promote apoptosis or cell survival and immunity. The balance between these cascades determines whether cells live or die.

kinases through its SH2 domain. Receptor binding brings the 110-kDa catalytic subunit of PI 3-kinase into proximity with the cell membrane, where it catalyzes phosphorylation of inositol phospholipids at the D-3 position, producing phosphatidylinositol 3,4,5 phosphate (PIP3). PIP3 is a lipid mediator that recruits pleckstrin homology-domain-containing proteins, such as Akt and the kinases that activate Akt, the PIP3-dependent kinases (PDKs), to the plasma membrane. Recruitment of these proteins to the same cellular domain permits phosphorylation and activation of Akt by the PDKs *(7)*.

Activation of PI 3-kinase and Akt by cytokines or growth factors promotes the survival of cells subjected to various insults *(7)*. Apoptosis in neurons deprived of growth factor and in fibroblasts exposed to ultraviolet (UV) irradiation is inhibited by insulin-like growth factor 1, and these protective effects are suppressed by inhibition of PI 3-kinase activity or expression of dominant-negative Akt. Conversely, constitutively active forms of PI 3-kinase or Akt can bypass the need for initiation of the survival signal by insulin-like growth factor (IGF)-1. These studies show that Akt activation can be necessary and sufficient for cell survival.

Akt promotes survival by phosphorylating substrates that decrease the activity of pro-apoptotic or increase the activity of anti-apoptotic proteins *(7)*. Phosphorylation of Bad by Akt/PKB promotes survival by preventing Bad from binding and inhibiting anti-apoptotic Bcl-x$_L$, and altering mitochondrial membrane potential. Akt phosphorylates a member of the forkhead family of transcription factors, FKHRL1, promoting its association with 14-3-3 proteins. This leads to retention of FKHRL1 in the cytoplasm, which silences its transcriptional activity and suppresses the expression of genes that promote apoptosis, including the gene that encodes the Fas ligand. Akt affects cell-cycle progression by regulating cyclin D function. This is accomplished by restricting p27^{Kip1} and p21^{WAF1} to the cytoplasm, thereby segregating these cell-cycle inhibitors from cyclin-dependent kinase (CDK)/cyclin. Akt phosphorylates and inhibits the activity of human caspase 9, which can initiate an enzyme cascade that promotes cell death. Additionally, Akt phosphorylates the Mdm2 oncoprotein, thus inducing its translocation from the cytoplasm into the nucleus *(8)*. Once this change of cellular localization is effected, Mdm2 can inhibit the function of the p53 tumor-suppressor protein and thereby promote

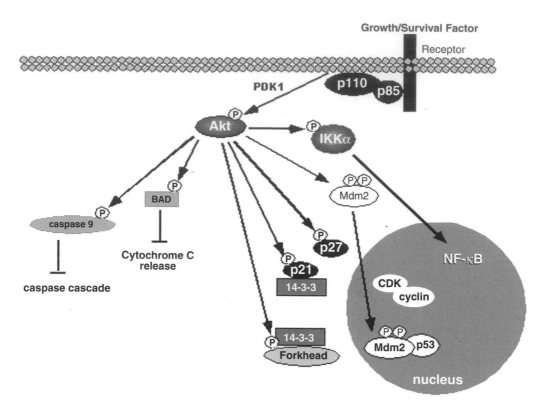

Fig. 2. The Akt serine-threonine kinase acts on a diverse group of substrates. Akt is a pleiotropic kinase that suppresses apoptosis by inhibiting the actions of proteins that promote cell death or promoting the actions of proteins that favor cell survival.

cell survival. **Figure 2** illustrates that Akt is a pleiotropic enzyme that promotes cell survival through actions on diverse substrates.

We identified a putative Akt phosphorylation site at amino acids 18–23 in IKKα, which led us to speculate that Akt might promote cell survival through activation of NF-κB *(9)*. As Akt is a downstream target for activated PI 3-kinase, we tested whether stimulation of cells with TNF would activate PI 3-kinase and subsequently Akt. We found that by acting through TNFR1, TNF induces the tyrosine phosphorylation of the p85 subunit of PI 3-kinase *(10)*. In embryonic kidney 293 cells and ME-180 human cervical carcinoma cells, TNF also increased the lipid kinase activity of PI 3-kinase; this effect was readily detectable within 5 min, and maximal sevenfold stimulation occurred after 20 min *(9)*. TNF also induced a time-dependent increase of Akt phosphorylation (activation) that correlated temporally with PI 3-kinase activation. Activation of Akt by TNF in various cell types was inhibited by wortmannin, a pharmacological inhibitor of PI 3-kinase, or by transient expression of cells with dominant-negative PI 3-kinase.

The demonstration that TNF activates Akt in a PI 3-kinase-dependent manner led to experiments using electrophoretic mobility shift assays (EMSAs), aimed at determining whether PI 3-kinase/Akt signaling would influence NF-κB DNA-binding activity. TNF induced NF-κB DNA binding activity in 293, HeLa, and ME-180 cells, and wortmannin inhibited this effect. NF-κB DNA binding was enhanced by transient transfection of cells with constitutively active PI 3-kinase (CA PI 3-kinase), constitutively active Akt (CA Akt), or NIK. Furthermore, co-transfection of NIK with CA PI-3-kinase or CA Akt produced an additive increase of NF-κB DNA binding. In contrast, transient ex-

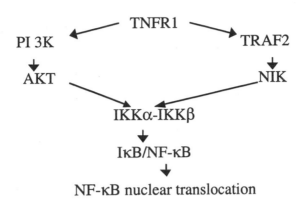

Fig. 3. A model for activation of nuclear factor (NF)-κB by tumor necrosis factor (TNF). TNF activates PI 3-kinase/Akt signaling and a second pathway that may include TNF receptor-associated factor-2 (TRAF2) and NF-κB-inducing kinase (NIK). The activities of these pathways converge on the IκB kinase (IKK) complex, which plays an obligate and complex role in activation of NF-κB.

pression of a dominant-negative PI 3-kinase (DN PI 3-kinase) inhibited TNF- or NIK-induced NF-κB DNA binding, whereas dominant-negative NIK (DN NIK) or wortmannin abrogated DNA binding induced by PI 3-kinase. These observations show that PI 3-kinase and Akt are components of a TNF-induced signaling pathway that modulates NF-κB DNA binding.

Kinase dead Akt (KD Akt) inhibited TNF-induced NF-κB DNA binding, and CA Akt by itself induced such binding, establishing that Akt is essential in this process. The ability of CA Akt to induce NF-κB DNA binding was inhibited by DN-NIK, and NF-κB DNA binding induced by NIK was inhibited by KD Akt. NF-κB reporter assays confirmed the results from EMSA, showing that CA Akt or TNF increased NF-κB-dependent gene activity, whereas the effect of TNF on this process was blocked by KD Akt. These observations show that Akt and NIK are both necessary for NF-κB DNA binding and transactivation.

The demonstration that TNF activates a PI 3-kinase signaling pathway, together with the identification of a putative Akt phosphorylation site in IKKα, suggested that IKKα might be a substrate for Akt (9). To test this supposition, it was first demonstrated that endogenous Akt and IKKα co-immunoprecipitate from cells and that treatment of cells with TNF increased the activity of Akt in purified Akt/IKKα complexes. In vitro kinase assays then demonstrated that elevation of Akt activity in IKKα immunocomplexes was accompanied by increased IKKα kinase activity. Wortmannin inhibited the activity of Akt in IKKα/Akt immunocomplexes, and this resulted in a corresponding decrement in the kinase activity of IKKα. Further support for the conclusion that IKKα is a substrate for Akt comes from experiments conducted in vitro that tested the ability of Akt to phosphorylate IKKα or an IKKα mutant in which threonine 23, an amino acid in the Akt phosphorylation site, was mutated to alanine. These experiments demonstrated that Akt can directly phosphorylate IKKα, but that this capacity is lost with mutation of the Akt phosphorylation site (threonine 23).

Activation of NF-κB by TNF is accompanied by rapid loss of IκBα, an event that permits cytoplasmic NF-κB to enter the nucleus, where it can act on target genes (5). Treatment of cells with wortmannin or transient expression of the mutant form of IKKα into cells blocked the ability of TNF to induce IκBα degradation. This result is yet another means of demonstrating that Akt plays a significant role in activation of NF-κB by TNF. **Figure 3** shows a model in which the respective parallel roles of TRAF2/NIK and PI 3-kinase/Akt pathways are illustrated. NIK and Akt both phosphorylate IKKα, albeit at different sites, and it would appear that both phosphorylation events play a significant role in modulating NF-κB function. Finally, it should be noted that Akt also appears to have the capacity to act, probably indirectly, on the p65 subunit of NF-κB, thereby directly increasing its transactivation activity. In combination, these observations demonstrate that Akt plays a role in suppressing TNF-initiated apoptotic signaling through activation of NF-κB.

PTEN (phosphatase and tensin homolog deleted on chromosome 10) is a dual-specificity phosphatase that dephosphorylates inositol lipids at the D3 position of the inositol ring, suggesting that PTEN antagonizes PI 3-kinase and PIP3 signaling *(11)*. The PTEN gene is mutated in 40–50% of high-grade gliomas, and in prostate, endometrial, breast, and lung cancers, as well as in other tumor types. In addition, PTEN is mutated in several rare autosomal-dominant cancer predisposition syndromes, including Cowden disease, Lhermitte–Duclos disease, and Bannayan–Zonana syndrome. The phenotype of knockout mice demonstrates a requirement for PTEN in normal development and confirms its role as a tumor suppressor. Ectopic expression of PTEN in tumor cells that carry mutations in the PTEN gene establish that it regulates the PI 3-kinase-dependent activation of Akt.

Additional support for a role for Akt in TNF induction of NF-κB activation comes from experiments demonstrating that PTEN inhibits the capacity of TNF to activate NF-κB *(12)*. Studies with PC-3 prostate cancer cells that do not express PTEN and DU145 prostate cancer cells that express PTEN showed that TNF activated Akt in the former, but not the latter cell line, and the ability of TNF to activate NF-κB was blocked by pharmacological inhibition of PI 3-kinase activity in the former, but not the latter, cells. Expression of PTEN in PC-3 cells, to a level comparable to that endogenously present in DU145 cells, inhibited TNF activation of NF-κB. The cell-type-specific ability of PTEN to negatively regulate the PI 3-kinase/AKT/NF-κB pathway may be important to its tumor suppressor activity.

The ability of PTEN to suppress that component of NF-κB activation mediated by PI 3-kinase/Akt signaling is important. NF-κB activation renders cells resistant to the cytotoxic activity of TNF and chemotherapy by inducing the expression of survival genes *(13–15)*. NF-κB activity also suppresses MyoD expression *(16)* and may thereby promote the muscle wasting associated with cancer, AIDS, and other chronic diseases. The demonstration that PTEN can suppress NF-κB activation by TNF suggests that its tumor-suppressor activity derives, in part, from its capacity to inhibit expression of genes that suppress the function of the cellular apoptotic machinery. Furthermore, PTEN may impair the ability of cytokines, such as TNF, to produce metabolic alterations, such as cachexia, that often lead to host mortality.

In addition to mediating survival signaling downstream of TNF receptors, Akt can be implicated in metabolic derangements induced by TNF. Elaboration of TNF is associated with insulin resistance that accompanies endotoxemia, cancer, trauma, and obesity *(17)*. The correlation between TNF production and insulin resistance is supported by the demonstration that administration of TNF to rats and humans reduces sensitivity to insulin. TNF-induced insulin resistance observed in animals has been replicated in adipocytes, hepatoma cells, fibroblasts, and myeloid and muscle cells *(17)*. TNF mediates its inhibitory action by targeting insulin receptor substrate-1 (IRS-1) *(18)*, a substrate for the insulin receptor tyrosine kinase *(19)*. Tyrosine phosphorylation of IRS-1 by the activated insulin receptor promotes interaction of IRS-1 with signaling proteins that promote insulin action *(19)*. Treatment of adipocytes or hepatocytes with TNF induces serine phosphorylation of IRS-1, which prevents its tyrosine phosphorylation by the insulin receptor and impairs the ability of the insulin receptor to transmit signals to downstream elements in the insulin signal transduction pathway *(18)*. For this reason, there has been great interest in identifying kinases that can effect the serine phosphorylation of IRS-1.

The demonstration that a TNF-induced PI 3-kinase/Akt signaling cascade plays a role in activating NF-κB led to experiments aimed at testing whether Akt might also be a mediator of TNF-induced insulin resistance *(20)*. Treatment of NIH 3T3 cells and myotubes with insulin increased insulin-promoted tyrosine phosphorylation of IRS-1. Pretreatment of these cells with TNF impaired the ability of subsequently applied insulin to promote the tyrosine phosphorylation of IRS-1. TNF activated

Akt in NIH 3T3 cells, making it a candidate serine-threonine kinase that might mediate the ability of TNF to impair signaling through IRS-1. This possibility was supported experimentally by the ability of inhibitors of PI 3-kinase to block the ability of TNF to impair insulin-induced tyrosine phosphorylation of IRS-1.

The PTEN tumor-suppressor protein is a dual-specificity phosphatase that inhibits PI 3-kinase function *(11)*. As the results described above implicated activation of PI 3-kinase signaling in TNF-induced insulin resistance, experiments were conducted to determine whether PTEN would have the opposite effect *(20)*. To accomplish this, readily transfectable 293 cells were transiently transfected with PTEN. Expression of PTEN increased insulin-induced tyrosine phosphorylation of IRS-1 two-fold and attenuated the ability of TNF to impair this process. Thus, PI 3-kinase promotes and PTEN antagonizes TNF-induced insulin resistance.

To determine whether Akt downstream of PI 3-kinase impairs insulin-induced tyrosine phosphorylation of IRS-1, this process was compared in NIH 3T3 cells and NIH 3T3 cells stably expressing CA Akt *(20)*. Insulin-induced tyrosine phosphorylation of IRS-1 was reduced by greater than 80% in cells expressing CA Akt, relative to tyrosine phosphorylation of IRS-1 induced by insulin in the parental NIH 3T3 cell line. The ability of TNF to impair insulin-induced tyrosine phosphorylation of IRS-1 in 293 cells was blocked by expression of KD Akt.

The observations described to this point implicate Akt in a lesion in insulin signaling through IRS-1. They do not demonstrate whether IRS-1 is a direct target for Akt or whether other kinases mediate the effect of Akt. Immunoprecipitations failed to demonstrate association of Akt with IRS-1. However, a target of Akt that has the potential to act on IRS-1 is the mammalian target of rapamycin (mTOR), also known as FRAP *(21)*. Three lines of experimental evidence support a role for mTOR in TNF-induced insulin resistance *(20)*: mTOR and IRS-1 associate with one another; TNF-induced insulin resistance is blocked by treatment of cells with rapamycin, a pharmacological inhibitor of mTOR; and mTOR induces the serine phosphorylation of IRS-1 on a consensus mTOR phosphorylation site.

TNF induces insulin resistance through multiple mechanisms. Tyrosine phosphatase inhibitors impair the ability of TNF to block insulin receptor autophosphorylation *(22)*. Among the tyrosine phosphatases that dephosphorylate the activated insulin receptor is SHP1 *(22)*. It is interesting that TNF promotes SHP1 association with the KDR receptor tyrosine kinase, thereby blocking its activation *(23)*. These observations suggest that tyrosine phosphatases are used by TNF to block the function of receptor tyrosine kinases, including the insulin receptor. TNF may also affect IRS-1 through activation of a PI 3-kinase/Akt/mTOR pathway that is antagonized by PTEN *(20)*. This pathway promotes serine phosphorylations that can uncouple IRS-1 from the insulin receptor, and blocks the ability of the receptor to tyrosine phosphorylate IRS-1 *(18,20)*. Non-tyrosine-phosphorylated IRS-1 cannot bind signaling proteins such as PI 3-kinase. The demonstration that IRS-1 and mTOR associate, and the ability of TNF to promote modification of IRS-1 on consensus mTOR phosphorylation sites, therefore provides a mechanism through which TNF may impair IRS-1 function in insulin signal transduction. It remains possible that a phosphatase, such as protein phosphatase 2A, which is inhibited by mTOR *(24)*, and another kinase, culminate and effect the final function of the PI 3-kinase/Akt/mTOR pathway, through which TNF impairs insulin-promoted tyrosine phosphorylation of IRS-1.

The relationship of our observations to the interplay between TNF and insulin action must be defined based on which cellular effects of insulin require tyrosine phosphorylation of IRS-1. Insofar as glucose transport is concerned, expression of IRS proteins in primary rat adipocytes enhances GLUT4 translocation and mutation of the insulin receptor, such that it cannot tyrosine phosphorylate IRS proteins abrogates insulin-induced glucose uptake *(25,26)*. In addition, ablation of both the IRS-1 and IRS-2 genes in mice supports a role for these adaptors in insulin-promoted glucose uptake *(27)*. However, IRS-1-independent signaling may also play a role in this component of insulin action. This

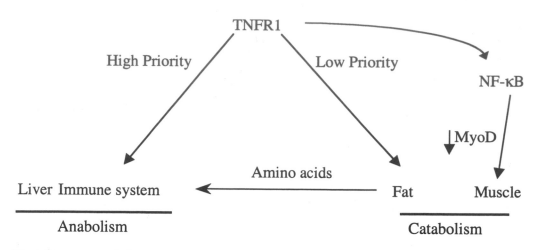

Fig. 4. Tumor necrosis factor (TNF) coordinates the systemic response to infections. During the acute-phase response, TNF is a component of a complex network of factors that induce a catabolic state in low-priority tissues, such as peripheral muscle and fat. This is coordinated with redistribution of the energy reserves thus liberated into high-priority tissues for wound repair and expansion of the immune system.

conclusion is supported by observations showing that expression of dominant inhibitory PTB or SAIN domains, which promote interaction of IRS-1 with the insulin receptor, fails to block insulin stimulation of glucose transport in adipocytes *(28)*. Furthermore, recruitment of PI 3-kinase to the platelet-derived growth-factor receptor in adipocytes, or recruitment of PI 3-kinase to IRS-1 proteins induced by interleukin-4 or cell-surface integrin crosslinking, fail to induce GLUT4 mobilization *(29–31)*. Also, a cell-permeable analog of the PI 3-kinase lipid mediator, PIP3, did not induce glucose uptake by itself, but in the presence of insulin and wortmannin, it caused GLUT4 translocation *(32)*. These observations suggest that insulin may be able to uniquely initiate IRS-1-independent signals that collaborate with IRS-1/PI 3-kinase-dependent signals to effect GLUT4 translocation. Thus, while IRS-1/PI 3-kinase/Akt signaling by itself is insufficient to mediate insulin stimulation of glucose transport, this pathway plays a more direct role in the anabolic actions of insulin, such as mitogenesis and protein synthesis *(33)*.

TNF is a component of a complex network of cytokines and other factors that are important to the host response to various insults that disturb homeostasis. In evaluating the significance of the observations described here to the systemic actions of TNF, it is useful to consider the integrative role that TNF plays in promoting the acute-phase response to infections and invasive stimuli, such as cancers *(34,35)*. During the acute-phase response, accelerated net breakdown of skeletal muscle and fat occurs with a concomitant shift to anabolic metabolism in the liver, to support the synthesis of acute-phase reactant proteins, as well as to bone marrow and wounds, for cellular proliferation within the immune system and for healing of injured tissue. These metabolic alterations represent a reprioritization of carbon and energy utilization in the injured or septic animal for survival (illustrated in **Fig. 4**). TNF activation of PI 3-kinase/Akt signaling may play a role in promoting the acute-phase response, at least in part through activation of NF-κB. NF-κB upregulates immune and cell-survival genes and suppresses MyoD expression in muscle, thereby contributing to the wasting of this tissue *(15,16)*. As shown here, PI 3-kinase/Akt signaling also inhibits insulin signaling through IRS-1 in muscle and fat, and inhibition of such anabolic activity in these peripheral tissues would likely be of benefit to a host organism mobilizing energy reserves in support of immunity and repair.

ACKNOWLEDGMENTS

Supported by grant CA67891 from the National Cancer Institute, NIH (DBD). The Indiana University Diabetes Graduate Training Program supported J. A. G.

REFERENCES

1. Vassalli, P. (1992) The pathophysiology of tumor necrosis factors. *Annu. Rev. Immunol.* **10**, 411–452.
2. Wallach, D., Varfolomeev, E. E., Malinin, N. L., Goltsev, Y. V., Kovalenko, A. V., and Boldin, M. P. (1999) Tumor necrosis factor receptor and Fas signaling mechanisms. *Annu. Rev. Immunol.* **17**, 331–367.
3. Smith, C.A. Farrah, T., and Goodwin, R. G. (1994) The TNF receptor superfamily of cellular and viral proteins: activation, costimulation, and death. *Cell* **76**, 959–962.
4. Ashkenazi, A. and Dixit, V. M. (1998) Death receptors: signaling and modulation. *Science* **281**, 1305–1308.
5. Karin, M. and Ben-Neriah, Y. (2000) Phosphorylation meets ubiquitination: the control of NF-kappaB activity. *Annu. Rev. Immunol.* **18**, 621–663.
6. Toker, A. and Cantley, L. C. (1997) Signalling through the lipid products of phosphoinositide-3-OH kinase. *Nature* **387**, 673–676.
7. Brazil, D. P. and Hemmings, B. A. (2001) Ten years of protein kinase B signalling: a hard Akt to follow. *Trends Biochem. Sci.* **26**, 657–664.
8. Mayo, L. D. and Donner, D. B. (2001) A phosphatidylinositol 3-kinase/Akt pathway promotes translocation of Mdm2 from the cytoplasm to the nucleus. *Proc. Natl. Acad. Sci. USA* **98**, 11,598–11,603.
9. Ozes, O. N., Mayo, L. D., Gustin, J. A., Pfeffer, S. R., Pfeffer, L. M., and Donner, D. B. (1999) NF-kappaB activation by tumour necrosis factor requires the Akt serine- threonine kinase. *Nature* **401**, 82–85.
10. Guo, D. and Donner, D. B. (1996) Tumor necrosis factor promotes phosphorylation and binding of insulin receptor substrate 1 to phosphatidylinositol 3-kinase in 3T3-L1 adipocytes. *J. Biol. Chem.* **271**, 615–618.
11. Maehama, T. and Dixon, J. E. (1999) PTEN: a tumour suppressor that functions as a phospholipid phosphatase. *Trends Cell. Biol.* **9**, 125–128.
12. Gustin, J. A., Maehama, T., Dixon, J. E., and Donner, D. B. (2001) The PTEN tumor suppressor protein inhibits tumor necrosis factor- induced nuclear factor kappa B activity. *J. Biol. Chem.* **276**, 27,740–27,744.
13. Van Antwerp, D. J., Martin, S. J., Kafri, T., Green, D. R., and Verma, I. M. (1996) Suppression of TNF-alpha-induced apoptosis by NF-kappaB. *Science* **274**, 787–789.
14. Wang, C. Y., Mayo, M. W., and Baldwin, A. S., Jr. (1996) TNF- and cancer therapy-induced apoptosis: potentiation by inhibition of NF-kappaB. *Science* **274**, 784–787.
15. Wang, C. Y., Mayo, M. W., Korneluk, R. G., Goeddel, D. V., and Baldwin, A. S., Jr. (1998) NF-kappaB antiapoptosis: induction of TRAF1 and TRAF2 and c-IAP1 and c- IAP2 to suppress caspase-8 activation. *Science* **281**, 1680–1683.
16. Guttridge, D. C., Mayo, M. W., Madrid, L. V., Wang, C. Y., and Baldwin, A. S., Jr. (2000) NF-kappaB-induced loss of MyoD messenger RNA: possible role in muscle decay and cachexia. *Science* **289**, 2363–2366.
17. Peraldi, P. and Spiegelman, B. (1998) TNF-alpha and insulin resistance: summary and future prospects. *Mol. Cell Biochem.* **182**, 169–175.
18. Hotamisligil, G. S., Peraldi, P., Budavari, A., Ellis, R., White, M. F., and Spiegelman, B. M. (1996) IRS-1-mediated inhibition of insulin receptor tyrosine kinase activity in TNF-alpha- and obesity-induced insulin resistance. *Science* **271**, 665–668.
19. Virkamaki, A., Ueki, K., and Kahn, C. R. (1999) Protein-protein interaction in insulin signaling and the molecular mechanisms of insulin resistance. *J. Clin. Invest.* **103**, 931–943.
20. Ozes, O. N., Akca, H., Mayo, L. D., et al. (2001) A phosphatidylinositol 3-kinase/Akt/mTOR pathway mediates and PTEN antagonizes tumor necrosis factor inhibition of insulin signaling through insulin receptor substrate-1. *Proc. Natl. Acad. Sci. USA* **98**, 4640–4645.
21. Sekulic, A., Hudson, C. C., Homme, J. L., et al. (2000) A direct linkage between the phosphoinositide 3-kinase-AKT signaling pathway and the mammalian target of rapamycin in mitogen-stimulated and transformed cells. *Cancer Res.* **60**, 3504–3513.
22. Kellerer, M., Lammers, R., and Haring, H. U. (1999) Insulin signal transduction: possible mechanisms for insulin resistance. *Exp. Clin. Endocrinol. Diabetes* **107**, 97–106.
23. Guo, D. Q., Wu, L. W., Dunbar, J. D., et al. (2000) Tumor necrosis factor employs a protein-tyrosine phosphatase to inhibit activation of KDR and vascular endothelial cell growth factor-induced endothelial cell proliferation. *J. Biol. Chem.* **275**, 11,216–11,221.
24. Peterson, R. T., Desai, B. N., Hardwick, J. S., and Schreiber, S. L. (1999) Protein phosphatase 2A interacts with the 70-kDa S6 kinase and is activated by inhibition of FKBP12-rapamycinassociated protein. *Proc. Natl. Acad. Sci. USA* **96**, 4438–4442.
25. Quon, M. J., Butte, A. J., Zarnowski, M. J., Sesti, G., Cushman, S. W., and Taylor, S. I. (1994) Insulin receptor substrate 1 mediates the stimulatory effect of insulin on GLUT4 translocation in transfected rat adipose cells. *J. Biol. Chem.* **269**, 27,920–27,924.

26. White, M. F., Livingston, J. N., Backer, J. M., et al. (1988) Mutation of the insulin receptor at tyrosine 960 inhibits signal transmission but does not affect its tyrosine kinase activity. *Cell* **54,** 641–649.
27. Bruning, J. C., Winnay, J., Bonner-Weir, S., Taylor, S. I., Accili, D., and Kahn, C. R. (1997) Development of a novel polygenic model of NIDDM in mice heterozygous for IR and IRS-1 null alleles. *Cell* **88,** 561–572.
28. Sharma, P. M., Egawa, K., Gustafson, T. A., Martin, J. L., and Olefsky, J. M. (1997) Adenovirus-mediated overexpression of IRS-1 interacting domains abolishes insulin-stimulated mitogenesis without affecting glucose transport in 3T3-L1 adipocytes. *Mol. Cell Biol.* **17,** 7386–7397.
29. Nave, B. T., Haigh, R. J., Hayward, A. C., Siddle, K., and Shepherd, P. R. (1996) Compartment-specific regulation of phosphoinositide 3-kinase by platelet-derived growth factor and insulin in 3T3-L1 adipocytes. *Biochem. J.* **318,** 55–60.
30. Isakoff, S. J., Taha, C., Rose, E., Marcusohn, J., Klip, A., and Skolnik, E. Y. (1995) The inability of phosphatidylinositol 3-kinase activation to stimulate GLUT4 translocation indicates additional signaling pathways are required for insulin-stimulated glucose uptake. *Proc. Natl. Acad. Sci. USA* **92,** 10,247–10,251.
31. Guilherme, A. and Czech, M. P. (1998) Stimulation of IRS-1-associated phosphatidylinositol 3-kinase and Akt/protein kinase B but not glucose transport by beta1-integrin signaling in rat adipocytes. *J. Biol. Chem.* **273,** 33,119–33,122.
32. Jiang, T., Sweeney, G., Rudolf, M. T., Klip, A., Traynor-Kaplan, A., and Tsien, R. Y. (1998) Membrane-permeant esters of phosphatidylinositol 3,4,5-trisphosphate. *J. Biol. Chem.* **273,** 11,017–11,024.
33. Kitamura, T., Ogawa, W., Sakaue, H., et al. (1998) Requirement for activation of the serine-threonine kinase Akt (protein kinase B) in insulin stimulation of protein synthesis but not of glucose transport. *Mol. Cell Biol.* **18,** 3708–3717.
34. Kushner, I., Ganapathi, M., and Schultz, D. (1989) The acute phase response is mediated by heterogeneous mechanisms. *Ann. NY Acad. Sci.* **557,** 19–29.
35. Warren, R. S., Donner, D. B., Starnes, H. F., Jr., and Brennan, M. F. (1987) Modulation of endogenous hormone action by recombinant human tumor necrosis factor. *Proc. Natl. Acad. Sci. USA* **84,** 8619–8622.

3

Protein Modifications by Nitric Oxide and Reactive Nitrogen Species

Harry Ischiropoulos

SUMMARY

Nitric oxide mediates a number of different physiological functions within every major organ system. Nitric oxide is a simple diatomic molecule that possesses a wide range of chemical reactivity and multiple potential reactive targets. Three basic biochemical pathways—interaction with metal centers, reaction with reduced thiols, and production of nitrogen oxides—will be considered and discussed in terms of modulating the biological function of proteins by nitric oxide.

Key Words: Nitrosylation; nitrosation; nitration; nitrogen dioxide; peroxynitrite; nitrosothiols; nitrotyrosine.

1. NITRIC OXIDE AND NITROGEN OXIDES

Nitric oxide is formed by the five-electron oxidation of one of the guanidino groups of L-arginine by nitric oxide synthases, and it is released in response to activation of endothelial cells by a variety of stimuli, such as shear stress, ATP, acetylcholine, bradykinin, and other vasodilators (1). As a small lipophilic molecule, nitric oxide can diffuse through membranes to reach its potential targets, such as soluble guanylate cyclase. In addition to its principal function in smooth-muscle relaxation, nitric oxide has been implicated in a number of important pathophysiological functions, such as the regulation of apoptosis, ion channel activity, and mitochondrial function (2–13). The selective reaction of nitric oxide with proteins, which regulates protein function in a reversible manner, provides a reasonable biochemical explanation for the ability of nitric oxide to regulate different aspects of cell biology. In addition, nitric oxide, via secondary reactions with oxygen and reactive oxygen species, can form reactive nitrogen species, such as nitrogen dioxide, dinitrogen trioxide, and peroxynitrite, which also react with proteins and cause covalent structural modifications (14). Three major posttranslational modifications of proteins that are mediated by nitric oxide and reactive nitrogen species have been described and studied extensively (a schematic representation of the principal reactions is depicted in **Fig. 1**):

1. Binding to iron-heme proteins, resulting in the nitrosylation of iron-heme center.
2. Reaction with reduced cysteine residues to form S-nitrosocysteine.
3. Reaction with tyrosine residues to form 3-nitrotyrosine.

The soluble guanylate cyclase and cytochrome oxidase of the complex IV in the mitochondrial electron transport systems are two of the well-recognized targets of nitric oxide (9,15,16). Whereas the reaction of nitric oxide with soluble guanylate cyclase constitutes the foundation for the principal biological function of nitric oxide, the biological consequences for the reaction with cytochrome

From: *Cell Signaling in Vascular Inflammation*
Edited by: J. Bhattacharya © Humana Press Inc., Totowa, NJ

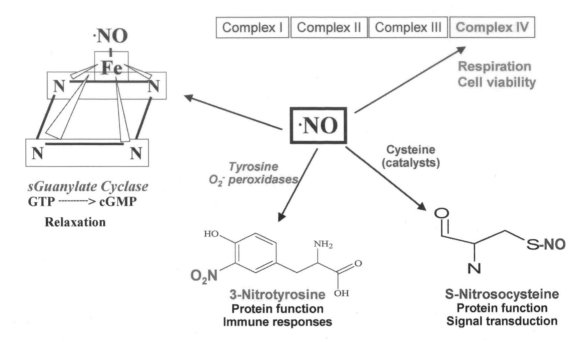

Fig. 1. Protein modifications by nitric oxide and reactive nitrogen species.

oxidase are still under investigation *(9)*. Furthermore, while the binding of nitric oxide to soluble guanylate cyclase results in activation of the enzyme, the interaction of nitric oxide with cytochrome oxidase results in an inhibitory process *(9,15,16)*.

Glyceraldehyde-3-phosphate dehydrogenase, ryanodine receptor, p21ras, hemoglobin, and caspase 3 are a few examples of more than 100 proteins that have been modified by *S*-nitrosation of cysteine residues in vivo *(2–13)*. Under certain conditions, enzymes facilitate both the formation and release or transfer of nitric oxide from *S*-nitrosocysteine, which implies that this process is regulated by selectively targeting specific proteins for modification *(9–13)*. Therefore *S*-nitrosation of the cysteine residues provides a selective and reversible covalent modification that regulates protein function and explains the ability of nitric oxide to regulate different cellular pathways simultaneously *(9–13)*.

Similar to *S*-nitrosocysteine, formation of nitrated tyrosine residues in proteins is under the regulation of enzymes, but unlike *S*-nitrosocysteine, the enzymatic removal of the nitro group from the aromatic ring of tyrosine residues has not been discovered, despite evidence for its existence *(17–23)*. Proteins modified by nitration include Mn superoxide dismutase, prostacyclin synthase, Ca^{2+}-ATPase, α-synuclein, actin, histones and the plasma proteins, ceruloplasmin, transferrin, anti-chymotrypsin, α1-protease inhibitor, and fibrinogen *(24–29)*. Nitration of tyrosine residues in these proteins has been found to inhibit, have no effect on, or in one case selectively enhance protein function.

2. SPECIFICITY OF CYSTEINE AND TYROSINE MODIFICATION BY NITRIC OXIDE AND NITRATING AGENTS

Both cysteine *S*-nitrosation and tyrosine nitration appear to be specific: only selective proteins and specific residues within these proteins are modified by *S*-nitrosation or tyrosine nitration. A number of the factors listed below provide a biochemical and biophysical rationale for this apparent selectivity. The selectivity can be derived mainly by the proximity of certain proteins to sites of nitric oxide generation, and by the biophysical properties of the target protein.

Compartmentalization and proximity to the target. Stamler et al. provided discussion of and several examples indicating that the proximity of a protein to the source of nitric oxide generation is an important factor in predicting the proteins modified by cysteine *S*-nitrosation *(9)*. We have reasoned that the biological reactivity of nitrating agents is closely associated with the sites of superoxide formation and peroxidases *(14)*. The superoxide dismutases maintain a low steady-state level of superoxide and thus prevent reactions between superoxide and iron-sulfur proteins or nitric oxide. However, in local environments where the superoxide dismutase is not efficient in removing superoxide, and under conditions where higher levels of superoxide are generated, peroxynitrite will be formed, and protein nitration will ensue. This may be the case with mitochondria, as Poderoso and co-workers have recently reported a superoxide-dependent nitration of mitochondrial proteins *(30)*. Similarly, the presence of peroxidases and hydrogen peroxide may be instrumental in forming nitrating agents at local sites *(31)*.

Biophysical properties of the target protein. The probability of a Cys-Glu or Asp motif, which likely contains a polar amino acid (Gly, Ser, The, Cys, Tyr, Asn, Gln) in the -2 position and either acidic (Glu, Asp) or basic amino acid (Lys, Arg) in the -1 position, may predict the site of *S*-nitrosation *(12)*. A sequence analysis failed to determine a similar sequence for tyrosine nitration, but several structural requirements may determine the sites of tyrosine nitration. These factors include the degree of surface exposure of the tyrosine, the folding of the protein, the absence of steric hindrances, the paucity of cysteine residues, and the proximity of the tyrosine residue to negatively charged residues *(32)*. Overall, the information that targets a tyrosine residue in a specific protein for modification appears to be embedded in the structure and local environment of the tyrosine residue in the protein. We should also note that other factors, such as the abundance of a protein, the abundance of cysteine and tyrosine residues, and the second-order rate constants for the reaction of the nitrogen species with the protein, do not appear to play any significant role in the selectivity of protein modification. It is clear that proteins found to be modified by S-nitrosation of cysteine and nitration of tyrosine residues in vivo are not the most abundantly expressed proteins. Moreover, *S*-nitrosation of selective cysteine residues of proteins takes place in the presence of several m*M* cytosolic glutathione levels. Similarly, the fact that nitration of protein tyrosine residues takes place even in the presence of reduced thiols and other peroxynitrite and nitrogen dioxide scavengers *(33)* indicates that simple rate constants are not the only factors determining the biological reactivity of nitric oxide and reactive nitrogen species.

In summary, the selective modification of cysteine and tyrosine residues may have a profound effect in the biological function of proteins in living organisms. *S*-nitrosation of cysteine residues is a reversible process, and thus it does not have a long-lasting effect on biological function; but it is sufficient to induce allosteric and signal transduction events. Similarly, tyrosine nitration can induce alterations in protein function. The removal of the nitro group or proteolytic degradation of the protein prevents any long-term effect on protein function. The failure to repair modified proteins could result in a sustained disturbance in protein function that could lead to the development of a pathogenic phenotype.

REFERENCES

1. Furchgott, R. F. (1996) The discovery of EDRF and its importance in the identification of nitric oxide. *JAMA* **276,** 1186–1188.
2. Molina y Vedia, L., McDonald, B., Reep, B., et al. (1992) Nitric oxide-induced S-nitrosylation of glyceraldehyde-3-phosphate dehydrogenase inhibits enzymatic activity and increases endogenous ADP-ribosylation. *J. Biol. Chem.* **267,** 24,929–24,932.
3. Lander, H. M., Milbank, A. J., Tauras, J. M., et al. (1996) Redox regulation of cell signaling. *Nature* **381,** 380–381.
4. Xu, L., Eu, J. P., Msissner, G., and Stamler, J. S. (1998) Activation of the cardiac calcium release channel (ryanodine receptor) by poly-S-nitrosylation. *Science* **279,** 234–237.
5. Gow, A. and Stamler, J. (1998) Reactions between nitric oxide and haemoglobin under physiological conditions. *Nature* **391,** 169–173.

6. Kim, Y. M., Talanian, R. V., and Billiar, T. R. (1997) Nitric oxide inhibits apoptosis by preventing increases in caspase-3-like activity via two distinct mechanisms. *J. Biol. Chem.* **272,** 31,138–31,148.
7. Mannick, J. B., Hausladen, A., Liu, L., et al. (1999) Fas-induced caspase denitrosylation. *Science* **284,** 651–654.
8. Lipton, A. J., Johnson, M. A., Macdonald, T., Lieberman, M. W., Gozal, D., and Gaston, B. (2001) S-nitrosothiols signal the ventilatory response to hypoxia. *Nature* **413,** 171–174.
9. Cooper, C. E. (2002) Nitric oxide and cytochrome oxidase: substrate, inhibitor or effector? *Trends Biochem. Sci.* **27,** 33–39.
10. Stamler, J. S., Lamas, S., and Fang, F. C. (2001) Nitrosylation: the prototypic redox-based signaling mechanism. *Cell* **106,** 675–683.
11. Simon, D. I., Mullins, M. E., Jia, L., Gaston, B., Singel, D. J., and Stamler, J. S. (1996) Polynitrosylated proteins: characterization, bioactivity, and functional consequences. *Proc. Natl. Acad. Sci. USA* **93,** 4736–4741.
12. Stamler, J. S., Toone, E. J., Lipton, S. A., and Sucher, N. J. (1997) (S)NO signals: translocation, regulation and a consensus motif. *Neuron* **18,** 691–696.
13. Liu, L., Hausladen, A., Zeng, M., Que, L., Heitman, J., and Stamler, J. S. (2001) A metabolic enzyme for S-nitrosothiol conserved from bacteria to humans. *Nature* **410,** 490–494.
14. Ischiropoulos, H. (1998) Biological tyrosine nitration: a pathophysiological function of nitric oxide and reactive oxygen species. *Arch. Biochem. Biophys.* **356,** 1–11.
15. Ballou, D. P., Zhao, Y., Brandish, P. E., and Marletta, M. A. (2002) Revisiting the kinetics of nitric oxide (NO) binding to soluble guanylate cyclase: the simple NO-binding model is incorrect. *Proc. Natl. Acad. Sci. USA* **99,** 12,097–12,101.
16. Bellamy, T. C., Wood, J., and Garthwaite, J. (2002) On the activation of soluble guanylyl cyclase by nitric oxide. *Proc. Natl. Acad. Sci. USA* **99,** 507–510.
17. Greenacre, S. A. B. and Ischiropoulos, H. (2001) Tyrosine Nitration: Localization, quantification, consequences for protein function and signal transduction. *Free Rad. Res.* **34,** 541–581.
18. Turko, I. V. and Murad, F. (2002) Protein nitration in cardiovascular diseases. *Pharmacol. Rev.* **54,** 619–634.
19. Brennan, M. L., Wu, W., Fu, X., et al. (2002) A tale of two controversies: defining both the role of peroxidases in nitrotyrosine formation in vivo using eosinophil peroxidase and myeloperoxidase-deficient mice, and the nature of peroxidase-generated reactive nitrogen species. *J. Biol. Chem.* **277,** 17,415–17,427.
20. Gow, A. J., Duran, D., Malcolm, S., and Ischiropoulos, H. (1996) Effects of peroxynitrite-induced protein modifications on tyrosine phosphorylation and degradation. *FEBS Lett.* **385,** 63–66.
21. Kamisaki, Y., Wada, K., Bian, K., et al. (1998) An activity in rat tissues that modifies nitrotyrosine-containing proteins. *Proc. Natl. Acad. Sci. USA* 95, 11,584–11,589.
22. Irie, Y., Saeki, M., Kamisaki, Y., Martin, E., and Murad, F. (2003) Histone H1.2 is a substrate for denitrase, an activity that reduces nitrotyrosine immunoreactivity in proteins. *Proc. Natl. Acad. Sci. USA* **100,** 5634–5639.
23. Souza, J. M., Choi, I., Chen, Q., et al. (2000) Proteolytic degradation of tyrosine nitrated proteins. *Arch. Biochem. Biophys.* **380,** 360–366.
24. MacMillan-Crow, L. A., Crow, J. P., Kerby, J. D., Beckman, J. S., and Thompson, J. A. (1996) Nitration and inactivation of Mn superoxide dismutase in chronic rejection of human renal allografts. *Proc Natl Acad Sci USA* **93,** 11,853–11,858.
25. Viner, R. I., Ferrington, D. A., Huhmer, A. F. R., Bigelow, D. J., and Schoneich, C. (1996) Accumulation of nitrotyrosine on the SERCA2a isoform of SR Ca-ATPase of rat skeletal muscle during aging: a peroxynitrite-mediated process? *FEBS Lett.* **379,** 286–290.
26. Giasson, B. I., Duda, J. E., Murray, I. V., et al. (2000) Oxidative damage linked to neurodegeneration by selective alpha-synuclein nitration in synucleinopathy lesions. *Science* **290,** 985–989.
27. Schmidt, P., Youhnovski, N., Daiber, A., et al. (2003) Specific nitration at tyrosine 430 revealed by high resolution mass spectrometry as basis for redox regulation of bovine prostacyclin synthase. *J. Biol. Chem.* **278,** 12,813–12,819.
28. Gole, M. D., Souza, J. M., Choi, I., et al. (2000) Plasma proteins modified by tyrosine nitration in acute respiratory distress syndrome. *Am. J. Physiol.* **278,** L961–967.
29. Aulak, K. S., Miyagi, M., Yan, L., et al. (2001) Proteomic method identifies proteins nitrated in vivo during inflammatory challenge. *Proc. Natl. Acad. Sci. USA* **98,** 12,056–12,061.
30. Schopfer, F., Riobo, N., Carreras, M. C., et al. (2000) Oxidation of ubiquinol by peroxynitrite: implications for protection of mitochondria against nitrosative damage. *Biochem. J.* **349,** 35–42.
31. Baldus, S., Eiserich, J. P., Mani, A., et al. (2001) Endothelial transcytosis of myeloperoxidase confers specificity to vascular ECM proteins as targets of tyrosine nitration. *J. Clin. Invest.* **108,** 1759–1770.
32. Souza, J. M., Daikhin, E., Yudkoff, M., Raman, C. S., and Ischiropoulos, H. (1999) Factors determining the selectivity of protein tyrosine nitration. *Arch. Biochem. Biophys.* **371,** 169–178.
33. Alvarez, B., Ferrer-Sueta, G., Freeman, B. A., and Radi, R.. (1998) Kinetics of peroxynitrite reaction with amino acids and human serum albumin. *J. Biol. Chem.* **274,** 842–848.

4

Redox Signaling in Hypoxic Pulmonary Vasoconstriction

E. Kenneth Weir, Zhigang Hong, Anthony Varghese, Daniel P. Nelson, and Andrea Olschewski

SUMMARY

Changes in oxygen tension are sensed by a variety of tissues, such as the carotid body, *ductus arteriosus* (DA), and pulmonary vasculature. In the fetus, hypoxia keeps the DA open and the pulmonary vessels constricted. After birth, hypoxic pulmonary vasoconstriction (HPV) helps to match ventilation and perfusion. HPV is induced by three general mechanisms—influx of calcium into the smooth muscle cells through

L-type channels and store-operated channels, release of calcium from the sarcoplasmic reticulum, and sensitization of actin/myosin to a given level of calcium. We show that reducing agents mimic the effects of hypoxia by reducing potassium current, causing membrane depolarization and increasing calcium influx in pulmonary artery smooth muscle cells (PASMCs), while doing exactly the opposite in the DA. On the other hand, oxidizing agents mimic normoxia by increasing potassium current, causing membrane hyperpolarization and reducing cytosolic calcium in PASMCs. They again do the opposite in the DA. As these redox agents elicit the same responses as shifts in oxygen tension, we consider that changes in oxygen may be signaled by changes in redox status.

Key Words: Oxygen; hypoxia; redox; potassium channels; pulmonary hypertension; *ductus arteriosus*.

1. INTRODUCTION

The ambient oxygen tension is sensed by many different cells in the body for different purposes. The type I cell of the carotid body monitors the oxygen tension in the systemic arterial blood and, if the tension falls, increases activity in the carotid sinus nerve to stimulate respiration *(1)*.

Adrenomedullary chromaffin cells and their related cell lines (PC 12, derived from pheochromocytoma *[2]* tissue, and MAH from embryonic rat adrenomedulla) *(3)* release catecholamines in response to hypoxia. Similarly, neuroepithelial bodies (NEB) in the lung *(4)* and the associated H-146 small-cell lung carcinoma line secrete neurotransmitters under hypoxic conditions *(5)*.

In the fetus, constriction of the small, resistance pulmonary arteries, as a result of hypoxia, reduces blood flow through the nonventilated lungs and diverts blood through the *ductus arteriosus*. At birth, in conjunction with ventilation of the lungs and a big rise in the arterial oxygen tension, the *ductus arteriosus* closes and the small, resistance pulmonary arteries dilate. The opposite effects of an increase in oxygen on the tone in these two vessels has fascinated researchers for many years.

The ability of animals to alter blood flow to maximize oxygen uptake is phylogenetically old, occurring in fish, amphibia, reptiles, and birds, as well as mammals. In the mammalian lung, hypoxia-induced vasoconstriction of small pulmonary arteries (about 200 to 400 μm in diameter in the cat) *(6)* in the vicinity of areas of atelectasis or consolidation, serves the useful purpose of diverting desaturated mixed venous blood away from these areas to others that are better ventilated. Hypoxic pulmonary vasoconstriction (HPV) occurs within 7 s of the start of hypoxic ventilation *(7)*.

From: *Cell Signaling in Vascular Inflammation*
Edited by: J. Bhattacharya © Humana Press Inc., Totowa, NJ

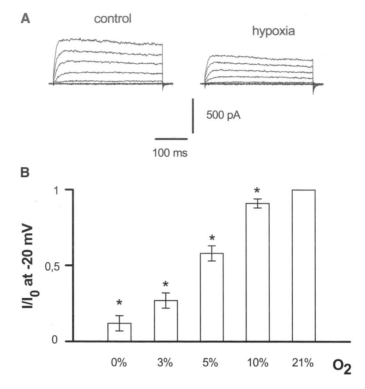

Fig. 1. Effect of hypoxia on whole-cell outward potassium current of pulmonary artery smooth muscle cells (PASMCs). **(A)** Representative 300-ms traces demonstrate potassium currents from PASMCs under normoxic conditions (left) and after 4-min exposure to low oxygen tension (right). Currents were evoked from a holding potential of –70 mV to +50 mV in incremental depolarizing 10-mV steps. **(B)** Hypoxia modulation of whole-cell potassium current at –20 mV. Currents were normalized relative to each cell's control current under normoxic conditions at –20 mV. Values are mean ± SEM. Five cells in each group. *$p < 0.05$ for difference from control (21% O_2).

Contraction in response to hypoxia can be seen in single pulmonary artery smooth-muscle cells (PASMCs), but can be enhanced or diminished by substances in the blood or released from the endothelium. One example of this is the observation that HPV can be ablated by a minute dose of endotoxin *(8)*. This effect can be mimicked by the intravenous infusion of plasma activated with zymosan to stimulate the formation of C5a *(9)*. A consequence of the C5a administration might be neutrophil adhesion, activation, and the production of reactive oxygen species (ROS).

2. SIGNALING OF HPV: ION CHANNELS

In PASCMCs, as in the type I cell of the carotid body, PC12 and MAH cells, NEBs, and H-146 cells, hypoxia causes inhibition of an outward potassium current (I_k), membrane depolarization, and entry of calcium though L-type voltage-gated calcium channels. It is likely that there is also hypoxia-induced release of intracellular calcium *(10)*. The inhibition of I_k, membrane depolarization, and increase in cytosolic calcium have a dose-response relationship to the severity of hypoxia *(11)*.

In **Fig. 1** it can be seen that at –20 mV, a membrane potential relatively close to the resting potential of the PASMC, the more severe the hypoxia, the greater the inhibition of I_k. Inhibition of I_k would not be meaningful in relation to cytosolic calcium levels if it did not cause significant membrane depolarization. In **Fig. 2** it is apparent that increasing severity of hypoxia leads to greater depolarization. This in turn is associated with higher calcium levels *(11)*.

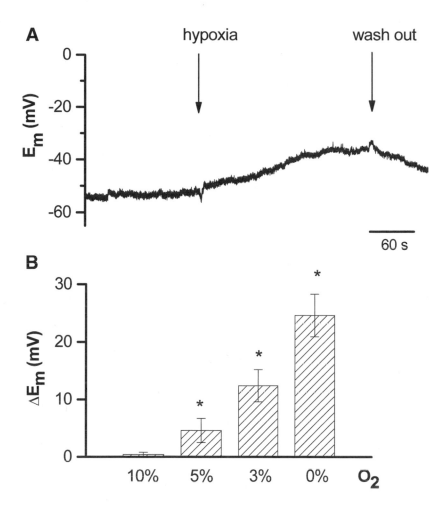

Fig. 2. Effects of hypoxia on resting membrane otential (E_m) measured with current-clamp in pulmonary artery smooth muscle cells (PASMCs). (**A**) Original recording shows the change in E_m during exposure to hypoxia (3% O_2). (**B**) Change in E_m (ΔE_m) was measured after 4-min exposure to 10% ($n = 7$), 5% ($n = 7$), 3% ($n = 5$), and 0% ($n = 7$) O_2. Values are mean ± SEM. *$p < 0.05$ for difference from control (21% O_2).

At least some of the oxygen-sensitive channels in PASMCs are voltage-sensitive potassium (K_v) channels. K_v channels are inhibited by 4-aminopyridine (4-AP). Applications of 4-AP to PASMCs results in an increase in cytosolic calcium (**Fig. 3**), presumably as a result of membrane depolarization and calcium influx. **Figure 3** also illustrates that hypoxia, in the absence of extracellular calcium around the PASMCs, increases cytosolic calcium. This calcium is likely to be released from the sarcoplasmic reticulum. These two components, influx and release, account for the total increase in calcium stimulated by hypoxia, with influx playing the greater part.

In the PASMCs, hypoxia results in a decrease in I_k and leads to vasoconstriction; but in the case of smooth muscle cells dissected from the *ductus arteriosus* (DASMCs), hypoxia increases I_K and leads to dilatation *(12)*. Consequently, it is apparent that either hypoxia gives rise to different signals or signaling cascades in PASMCs and DASMCs, which control potassium channels and the release of calcium within the cell, or the same signal elicited by hypoxia has opposite effects on the gating of some potassium channels, calcium channels, and/or calcium release mechanisms in the SMCs from

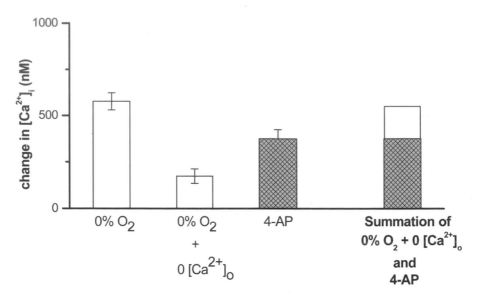

Fig. 3. Two independent mechanisms contribute to the hypoxia-induced cytosolic [Ca2+] increase in pulmonary artery smooth muscle cells. The release of internal [Ca2+] (0% O_2 + O [Ca2+] and the influx of external [Ca2+] mimicked by 4-AP-induced inhibition of I_k.

these vessels. Normoxic constriction of the DA occurs even in the absence of cyclo-oxygenase or nitric oxide synthase products, and after blockade of ET-A receptors *(13)*. This again makes it seem that the opposite responses to oxygen are not based on the release of endothelial factors.

3. SIGNALING OF HPV: REDOX

In 1986 we proposed that the tone, and possibly the structure, of the pulmonary vasculature is regulated by the redox status (GSH/GSSG, NADPH/NADP) of the pulmonary vascular smooth-muscle cell *(14)*. Subsequent work has supported the concept that changes in the sulfhydryl redox status transduce the effect of changing oxygen tension, although it is still unclear whether the primary shift is in the production of ROS, or in redox couples in the cytosol or the cell membrane. Hypoxia and metabolic inhibitors, such as rotenone and antimycin A, cause pulmonary vasoconstriction in the isolated rat lung and reduce whole-lung ROS production as measured by enhanced chemiluminescence *(15)*. Initially this provided support for a role for ROS, but subsequently normal HPV was demonstrated in the lungs of mice that lacked the 91 phox subunit of NADPH oxidase and had virtually no whole-lung chemiluminescence even during normoxia *(16)*.

It is clear that oxidants, such as diamide, can cause pulmonary vasodilatation, can rapidly reverse HPV, and can increase potassium current in PASMCs *(9,17,18)*. *N*-acetyl cysteine in the perfusate can decrease I_k in PASMCs *(17)*. Similarly, reduced glutathione can decrease I_k and cause membrane depolarization *(19)*. Likewise, reduced glutathione in the patch pipet can decrease potassium current, while oxidized glutathione increases it *(20)*. The reducing agents dithiothreitol (DTT), GSH, and NADH applied to the internal face of a PASMC patch decrease l_K but do not alter l_k in ear artery smooth-muscle cells (EASMCs) *(21)*. However, although oxidizing agents such as dithiobisnitrobenzoic acid (DTNB), GSSG, and NAD increase l_k in inside-out patches of PASMC, this effect is not specific, as it also occurs in EASMCs. Park et al. suggested that the basal state of the ESMCs, being more hypoxic than PASMCs, would also be more reduced and thus less affected by reducing agents. This would be in keeping with the increased levels of GSH measured in the lung after both acute and chronic hypoxia *(22)*.

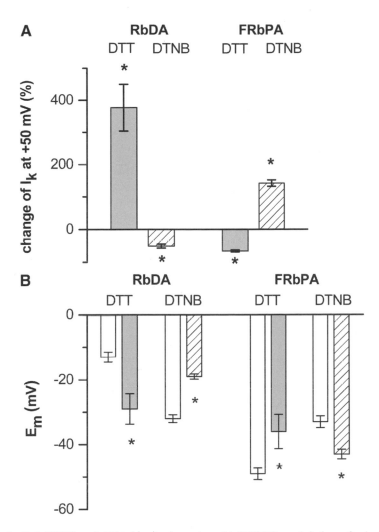

Fig. 4. Dithiothreitol (DTT) and dithiobisnitrobenzoic acid (DTNB) modulation of whole-cell potassium current resting membrane potential (E_m) of smooth muscle cells from fetal pulmonary arteries (FrbPA) and from ductus arteriosus (RbDA). (**A**) Effect of DTT and DTNB on whole-cell potassium current at +50 mV. Currents were normalized relative to each cell's control current under normoxic (DTT) or hypoxic (DTNB) conditions at +50 mV. Five cells in each group. Values are mean ± SEM. *$p < 0.05$ for difference from control.

Recently we examined the effects of the same reducing agent (DTT) and oxidizing agent (DTNB) on vascular ring tension in the PA and *ductus arteriosus* and on I_k, membrane potential (E_m), and cytosolic calcium (Ca^{2+}) in PASMCs and DASMCs *(23)*. Under normoxic conditions, DTT constricted fetal resistance PA rings, while in DA rings DTT acted as a potent dilator. In the PASMCs, DTT decreased I_k, and caused membrane depolarization and an increase in Ca^{2+}. However, in the DASMCs, DTT did exactly the opposite. In the case of the oxidizing agent DTNB, given under hypoxic conditions, fetal PA rings dilated and DA rings constricted. In the PASMCs, DTNB increased I_k and caused hyperpolarization, while in the DASMCs it did the opposite. These changes in I_k and E_m are illustrated in **Fig. 4**. The ability of these redox agents to elicit opposite responses in the PA and DA is consistent with a role for redox changes in their contrary responses to hypoxia and to normoxia. We are not aware of other interventions that can mimic the effects of oxygen by having opposite actions in the two vessels.

If redox changes were to signal changes in oxygen tension, how might they occur? Hypoxia might be signaled by a decrease in ROS, such as superoxide anion or hydrogen peroxide, generated by mitochondria or NADPH oxidase. Alternatively, hypoxia might be signaled by an increase in redox couples such as NAD(P)H/NAD(P) and GSH/GSSG. It is still controversial whether ROS go up or down during hypoxia (for review, *see 29*). Two examples related to oxygen sensing suggest that they may go down. In the neuroepithelial bodies of the lung, hypoxia inhibits I_k and hydrogen peroxide increases I_k *(24,25)*. Thus, if hydrogen peroxide is involved in the oxygen sensing, it should be reduced by hypoxia. In rat PA rings, hypoxia reduces ROS production as measured by lucigenin-enhanced chemiluminescence. Diphenyleneiodonium (DPI), an inhibitor of ROS production by NADPH oxidase, also reduces chemiluminescence, again suggesting that hypoxia reduces ROS *(16)*.

We consider that in both the PA and DA, during normoxia there are higher levels of ROS *(15,26,13)*. In the DASMCs, when catalase is included in the patch pipet solution, I_k is enhanced *(26)*. This indicates that endogenous hydrogen peroxide, generated during normoxia, inhibits I_k, leading to membrane depolarization and calcium entry. It is not clear whether ROS act directly on the oxygen-sensitive K^+ channel(s) or whether they alter the redox couples mentioned earlier. Hypoxia is known to increase the ratios of the reduced to the oxidized forms of cytosolic redox couples in the lung *(27,28)*. From the evidence discussed above, we consider that changes in oxygen levels are reflected in changes in the redox status of the cytoplasm of the smooth muscle cells. This in turn determines the gating of sarcolemmal K^+ channels, the influx of external calcium, and probably the release of calcium from the sarcoplasmic reticulum.

ACKNOWLEDGMENTS

Andrea Olschewski is supported by the Deutsche Forschungsgemeinschaft (01 127/1-1). E. K. Weir is supported by VA Merit Reviews funding and National Heart, Lung, and Blood Institute Grant ROI-HL-65322-01A1.

REFERENCES

1. Lopez-Barneo, J., Lopez-Lopez, J., Urena, J., et al. (1988) Chemotransduction in the carotid body: K^+ current modulated by Po2 in type I chemoreceptor cells. *Science* **242**, 580–582.
2. Zhu, W., Conforti, L., Czyzyk-Krzeska, M., et al. (1996) Membrane depolarization in PC12 cells during hypoxia is regulated by an O_2-sensitive K^+ current. *Am. J. Physiol.* **40**, C568–C665.
3. Fearon, I., Thompson, R., Samjoo, I., et al. (2002) O_2-sensitive K^+ channels in immortalised rat chromaffin-cell-derived MAH cells. *J. Physiol.* **545.3**, 807–818.
4. Youngson, C., Nurse, C., Yeger, H., et al. (1993) Oxygen sensing in airway chemoreceptors. *Nature* **365**, 153–155.
5. O'Kelly, I., Lewis, A., Peers, C., et al. (2000) O_2 sensing by airway chemoreceptor-derived cells. *J. Biol. Chem.* **275**, 7684–7692.
6. Shirai, M., Sada, K., and Niromiya, I. (1986) Effects of regional alveodar hypoxia and hypercapnia on small pulmonary vessels in cats. *J. Appl. Physiol.* **61**, 440–448.
7. Jensen, K., Mico, A., Czartolomna, J., et al. (1992) Rapid onset of hypoxic vasoconstriction in isolated lings. *J. Appl. Physiol.* **72**, 2018–2033.
8. Reeves, J. and Grover, R. (1974) Blockade of acute hypoxic pulmonary hypertension by endotoxin. *J. Appl. Physiol.* **36**, 328–332.
9. Weir, E., Tierney, J., Chesler, E., et al. (1983) Zymosan activation of plasma reduces hypoxic pulmonary vasoconstriction. *Resp. Physiol.* **53**, 295–306.
10. Salvaterra, C. and Goldman, W. (1993) Acute hypoxia increases cytosolic calcium in cultured pulmonary srterial myocytes. *Am. J. Physiol.* **264**, L323–L328.
11. Olschewski, A., Hong, Z., Nelson, D., et al. (2002) Graded response of K^+ current, membrane potential and [Ca^{2+}]i to hypoxia in pulmonary arterial smooth muscle. *Am. J. Physiol. Lung Cell Mol. Physiol.* **283**, L1143–L1150.
12. Tristani-Firouzi, M., Reeve, H., Tolarova, S., et al. (1996) Oxygen-induced constriction of rabbit ductus arteriosus occurs via inhibition of a 4-aminopyridine-, voltage-sensitive potassium channel. *J. Clin. Invest.* **98**, 1959–1965.
13. Michelakis, E., Rebeyka, I., Wu, X., et al. (2002) O_2 sensing in the human *ductus arteriosus*. *Circ. Res.* **91**, 478–486.
14. Archer, S., Will, J., and Weir, E. (1986) Redox status in the control of pulmonary vascular tone. *Herz* **11**, 127–141.
15. Archer, S., Huang, J., Henry, T., et al. (1993) A redox-based O_2 sensor in rat pulmonary vasculature. *Circ. Res.* **73**, 1100–1112.
16. Archer, S., Reeve, H., Michelakis, E., et al. (1999) O_2 sensing is preserved in mice lacking the gp91 phox subunit of NADPH oxidase. *Proc. Natl. Acad. Sci. USA* **96**, 7944–7949.

17. Post, J., Weir, E., Archer, S., et al. (1993) Redox regulation of K⁺ channels and hypoxic pulmonary vasoconstriction. In: Weir, E. K., Hume, J. R., and Reeves, J. T. (eds), *Ion Flux in Pulmonary Vascular Control*. Plenum, New York, pp. 189–204.

18. Reeve, H., Weir, E., Nelson, D., et al. (1995) Opposing effects of oxidants and antioxidants on K⁺ channel activity and tone in rat vascular tissue. *Exp. Physiol.* **80,** 825–834.

19. Yuan, X-J., Tod, M., Rubin, L., et al. (1994) Deoxyglucose and reduced glutathione mimic effects of hypoxia on K⁺ and Ca²⁺ conductances in pulmonary artery cells. *Am. J. Physiol.* **2994,** L52–L63.

20. Weir, E. and Archer, S. (1995) The mechanism of acute hypoxic pulmonary vasoconstriction: the tale of two channels. *FASEB J.* **9,** 183–189.

21. Park, M., Lee, S., Lee, S., et al. (1995) Different modulation of Ca-activated K channels by the intracellular redox potential in pulmonary and ear arterial smooth muscle cells of the rabbit. *Eur. J. Physiol.* **430,** 308–314.

22. Reeve, H., Michelakis, E., Nelson, D., et al. (2001) Alterations in a redox oxygen sensing mechanism in chronic hypoxia. *J. Appl. Physiol.* **90,** 2249–5226.

23. Olschewski, A., Hong, Z., Peterson, D., et al. (2004) Opposite effects of redox status on membrane potential, cytosolic calcium, and tone in pulmonary arteries and *ductus arteriosus*. *Am. J. Physiol. Lung Cell Mol. Physiol.* **286,** L15–L22.

24. Wang, D., Youngson, C., Wong, V., et al. (1996) NADPH-oxidase and a hydrogen peroxide-sensitive K⁺ channel may function as an oxygen sensor complex in airway chemoreceptors and small cell lung carcinoma cell lines. *Proc. Natl. Acad. Sci. USA* **93,** 13182–13187.

25. Fu, X., Nurse, C., and Wang, Y. (1999) Selective modulation of membrane currents by hypoxia in intact airway chemoreceptors from neonatal rabbit. *J. Physiol.* **514,** 139–150.

26. Reeve, H., Tolarova, S., Nelson, D., et al. (2001) Redox control of oxygen sensing in the rabbit *ductus arteriosus*. *J. Physiol.* **533.1,** 253–261.

27. Chander, A., Dhariwal, K., and Viswanathan, R. (1980) Pyridine nucleotides in lung and liver of hypoxic rats. *Life Sci.* **26,** 1935–1945.

28. Baxter, L., Snetkov, V., Aaronson, P., et al. (2002) Pulmonary and systemic vascular smooth muscle demonstrate differential sensitivity to hypoxia in terms of the rise in mitochondrial NAD(P)H. *J. Physiol.* **544P,** S030.

29. Weir, E. K., Hong, Z., Porter, V., and Reeve, E. (2002) Redox signaling in oxygen sensing by vessels. *Resp. Physiol. Neurobiol.* **132,** 121–130.

cGMP-Dependent Protein Kinase in Regulation of the Perinatal Pulmonary Circulation

Usha Raj, Yuansheng Gao, Srinivas Dhanakoti, and Fred Sander

SUMMARY

At birth, the increase in oxygen tension results in upregulation of the nitric oxide-cGMP pathway in the pulmonary vasculature and facilitates vasodilation and a fall in pulmonary vascular resistance. In the perinatal period, both cAMP and cyclic guanosine monophosphate (cGMP) act via cGMP-dependent protein kinase (PKG) in mediating relaxation of the pulmonary circulation, with cGMP working predominantly via PKG. Oxygen exposure results in an increase in PKG activity, PKG protein content, and mRNA expression in fetal pulmonary vascular smooth muscle. The increased production of reactive oxygen species in pulmonary vascular smooth muscle that occurs during hypoxia in the fetus is responsible for downregulation of PKG activity and the PKG protein levels in pulmonary vascular smooth muscle in the fetus, which is reversed on exposure to increased oxygen tension at birth. PKG mRNA expression also appears to be regulated by nitric oxide and cGMP, such that chronic exposure of pulmonary vascular smooth muscle to nitric oxide and cGMP results in downregulation of PKG mRNA levels. This might be one mechanism by which chronic inhalation therapy with nitric oxide in neonates with persistent pulmonary hypertension of the newborn results in development of resistance to nitric oxide-mediated vasodilation in the pulmonary circulation.

Key Words: Nitric oxide-cGMP-cGMP dependent pathway; fetal pulmonary circulation; oxygen-dependent signaling; pulmonary vascular smooth muscle.

1. INTRODUCTION

In the fetus, pulmonary vasomotor tone is maintained at a high level by the action of a variety of constrictor pathways. The low oxygen tension in the fetal environment is thought to be the primary trigger for upregulation of constrictor mechanisms as well as the downregulation of vasodilator mechanisms. In the transition from fetal to neonatal life at birth, there is a dramatic fall in pulmonary vascular resistance, which is brought about by a host of events. The sudden increase in oxygen tension following the first breath is thought to be the primary stimulus for upregulation of dilator mechanisms. Other stimuli for the vasodilatory pathways are an increase in shear stress on vascular endothelium induced by the increase in pulmonary blood flow after birth, and the increase in stretch that the blood vessels are subjected to by the larger breathing movements postnatally. These stimuli result in an increase in vasodilator mediators, such as endothelium-derived nitric oxide, prostaglandins I_2 and E_2, β-adrenergic agents, and bradykinin (1).

We have previously reported (2–6) that there is heterogeneity in relaxation responses of pulmonary arteries and veins of near-term fetal and newborn lambs to cGMP- and cAMP-elevating agents. We have also shown that fetal and neonatal intrapulmonary arteries and veins are much more sensi-

From: *Cell Signaling in Vascular Inflammation*
Edited by: J. Bhattacharya © Humana Press Inc., Totowa, NJ

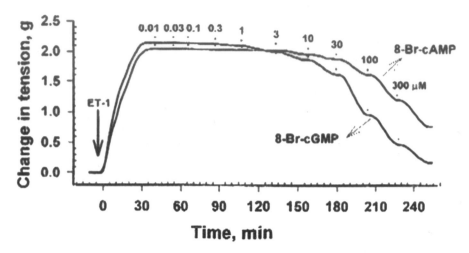

Fig. 1. Relaxation responses of intact pulmonary arteries of newborn lambs to 8-bromo-cGMP (8-BrcGMP) and 8-bromo-cAMP (8-BrcAMP). Active tension (g/dry wt of tissue) of the arteries was first raised by endothelin-1 (3 n*M*; ET-1), followed by exposure to increasing concentrations (0.01–300 µ*M*) of 8-BrcGMP or 8-BrcAMP, respectively. Changes in tension induced by both agents are recorded over a 4-h period. A representative trace is shown.

tive to cGMP-induced relaxation than cAMP. Based on our data, we believe that the nitric oxide (NO)-cGMP pathway of vasodilation is critically important in the perinatal period. A representative trace, shown in **Fig. 1**, depicts the change in tension (g) of pulmonary arteries, previously raised by endothelin-1 (ET-1) (3 n*M*), to increasing concentrations (10 n*M*–300 µ*M*) of 8-Br-cGMP or 8-Br-cAMP, observed over a 4-h period. The control tension raised by ET-1 was 1.12 ± 0.13 and 0.98 ± 0.10 g/mg tissue, for 8-Br-cGMP- and 8-Br-cAMP-treated vessels ($n = 5$ animals/group), respectively. Maximal relaxation responses were 92.1 ± 4.9 % and 59.1 ± 6.8 % for vessels treated with 300 µ*M* 8-Br-cGMP or 8-Br-cAMP, respectively. The calculated EC_{50} (µ*M*) values were 35.5 ± 5.2 and 120.2 ± 15.8 for 8-Br-cGMP and 8-Br-cAMP, respectively. **Figure 2** shows that the EC_{50} for cGMP is significantly lower in fetal and newborn ovine intrapulmonary arteries and veins, suggesting that perinatal pulmonary vessels are more sensitive to relaxation by cGMP than cAMP.

Cyclic guanosine monophosphate (cGMP) plays an important role in smooth-muscle relaxation and acts mainly by the cGMP-PKG pathway *(7,8)*. Action of cGMP in animal cells is mediated via three different receptors: (1) cGMP-dependent protein kinase (PKG), (2) cGMP-gated channel proteins, and (3) cGMP-regulated phosphodiesterase (PDEs). PKG was first described in animal tissues *(9)*, and Felbel et al. *(10)* first suggested that PKG might mediate smooth-muscle relaxation. PKG is a serine/threonine protein kinase, and its activity is modulated by autophosphorylation of its serine or threonine residues. The same residues are phosphorylated in its protein substrates. PKG exists in high concentrations in lung, smooth muscle, cerebellum, smooth-muscle-related cells such as pericytes and contractile mesangial cells, and platelets *(11)*.

The high level of PKG in organs is thought to be largely derived from the smooth muscle of blood vessels. PKG is found in both cytoplasmic and membranous fractions of tissue homogenate, and its distribution is tissue dependent. In lung and smooth muscle, PKG is predominantly cytoplasmic, while in intestinal epithelial cells or platelets, it is almost entirely membrane-bound *(11,12)*. PKG exists in animal cells in two forms—type I and type II. The type-I form, usually cytoplasmic, is a dimer of identical subunits (molecular mass approx 78 kDa each) and the type-II form, predominantly membrane-bound, is a monomer with a mass of approx 86 kDa. Type-I PKG is a mixture of two closely related isoforms (type Iα and Iβ), which have been purified from vascular tissues. cDNA encoding type-I forms have been cloned. Both isoforms are homodimers with blocked amino termini

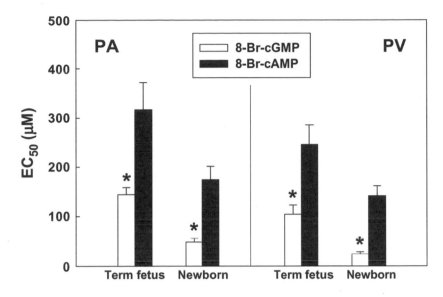

Fig. 2. Calculated EC_{50} (nM) for 8-BrcGMP and 8-BrcAMP in intrapulmonary arteries and veins of fetal and newborn lambs. Concentration of 8-BrcGMP required to induce 50% relaxation in all vessel types was lower than that of 8-BrcAMP. Newborn vessels were more sensitive than fetal vessels to 8-BrcGMP. In both fetal and newborn lambs, veins were more sensitive than arteries to relaxation responses mediated by the cyclic nucleotides. *Significant difference from vessels treated with 8-BrcAMP ($p < 0.05$)

(type-Iα acetylated) and both bind 2 moles of cGMP/mole of PKG. However, they may exhibit differences in activity *(11,13)*. In vascular smooth muscle (bovine coronary arteries, bovine and human aortas) type Iα and Iβ are present in approximately equal proportions. Cyclic GMP analog effects on tracheal and vascular smooth muscle show a strong relation between the potencies with which analogs activate purified type Iα PKG and the concentrations required to induce relaxation in these tissues *(11)*. The relative roles of type I and type II PKG in relaxing pulmonary vascular smooth muscle are not known.

Activation of PKG is the primary mechanism of vasodilation induced by agents that elevate intracellular cGMP. The mechanisms by which PKG acts are still not clearly elucidated. Studies suggest that PKG may cause smooth muscle to relax by reducing $[Ca^{++}]_I$ through the following mechanisms: (1) by stimulating a Ca^{++}-ATPase of sarcoplasmic reticulum and thus increasing sequestration of $[Ca^{++}]_I$ *(14)*, (2) by phosphorylating inositol 1,4,5-triphosphate receptor and subsequently reducing Ca^{++} release from sarcoplasmic reticulum *(15)*, (3) by stimulating Ca^{++}-activated K^+ channels and thus causing membrane hyperpolarization *(16)*, (4) by inhibiting Ca^{++} channels *(17)*, and (5) by stimulating smooth-muscle phosphatase activity, which causes dephosphorylation of the myosin light chain and thus relaxation *(18)* (*see* **Fig. 3**).

We have investigated the role of PKG in both cGMP- and cAMP-mediated pulmonary vasodilation by examining the relaxation responses of ovine pulmonary arteries to 8-Br-cGMP and 8-Br-cAMP, in the absence or presence of selective PKG inhibitor, Rp-8-Br-PET-cGMPs ($K_i = 0.03$ μM), or selective PKA inhibitor KT-5720 ($K_i = 0.056$ μM), and determined the activation of PKG by cGMP and cAMP in pulmonary arterial extracts.

Involvement of PKG or PKA in cGMP-induced relaxation of arteries: experiments were carried out in the presence of cell-permeable inhibitors of PKG and PKA. The inhibitors, Rp-8-Br-PET-cGMPS (a potent inhibitor of PKG, $K_i = 0.035$ μM) and KT-5720 (a potent inhibitor of PKA, $K_i = 0.056$ μM) did not significantly affect resting tension in the arteries. Pretreatment with Rp-8-Br-PET-cGMPS significantly inhibited 8-Br-cGMP-induced relaxation of arteries; only approx 40% relax-

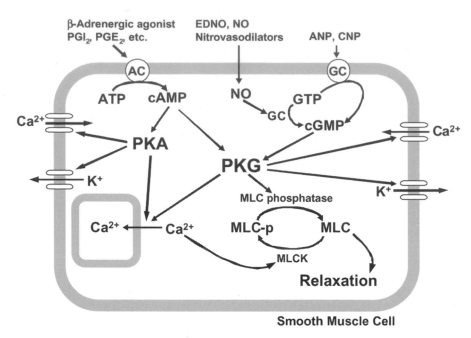

Fig. 3. Depiction of intracellular signaling pathways in pulmonary vascular smooth muscle. NO, nitric oxide; PKG, cGMP-dependent protein kinase; PKA, protein kinase A; EDNO, endothelium-derived nitric oxide;
ANF, atrial natriuretic factor; AC, adenylyl cyclase; GC, guanylyl cyclase; MLC, myosin light chain; MLC-p,
phosphorylated myosin light chain; MLCK, myosin light chain kinase.

ation was observed with 300 μM 8-Br-cGMP. In the presence of 8-Br-PET-cGMPS (**Fig. 4**), KT-
5720 did not have any effect.

Involvement of PKA or PKG in cAMP-induced relaxation of arteries: as shown in **Fig. 5**, the
maximal relaxation response of arteries was approx 59% with 300 μM 8-Br-cAMP, and this relaxation was inhibited by both KT-5720 (50 μM) and Rp-8-Br-PET-cGMPS (30 μM). There was no
significant difference ($P > 0.05$) between the two inhibitors in their inhibitory effect on relaxation
induced by 8-Br-cAMP. Our results indicate that ovine pulmonary arteries are more sensitive to
relaxation induced by cGMP than cAMP and that activation of PKG plays a major role in both cGMP-
and cAMP-induced relaxation.

Importance of PKG-1 in the normal fetal to neonatal transition: in animal models of neonatal
pulmonary hypertension, the NO-cGMP pathway has been shown to be impaired *(19–25)*. Furthermore, in some models of hypoxia-induced pulmonary hypertension in the neonatal*(26,27)* and adult
(28) animal, the vasodilator response of pulmonary vessels to cGMP is specifically impaired. Other
reports in the literature indicate that hypoxia attenuates cGMP-mediated effects in vascular smooth
muscle *(29,30)*. We were first to establish in the literature that PKG is a major pathway by which
cGMP mediates vasodilation in the developing pulmonary vasculature *(7,8)*. We hypothesize that the
impaired pulmonary vascular responses to cGMP in these animal models of neonatal pulmonary
hypertension may be explained by impaired PKG activity. Hofmann et al. have developed knockout
mice bearing homozygous PKG type-1 null mutations (in both α and β) to eliminate PKG type-1
gene expression and abolish NO/cGMP-dependent vascular relaxation *(31,32)*. Notably in this knockout, there is a very high amount of fetal loss, most of them dying immediately after birth. Only 20–
25% of the fetuses survive at birth (Dr. Pryzwansky, University of North Carolina, personal
communication), and of the survivors, several more die within days. This strongly supports our con-
tention that PKG is critical for fetal to neonatal transition. Surviving PKG deficient mice have sys-

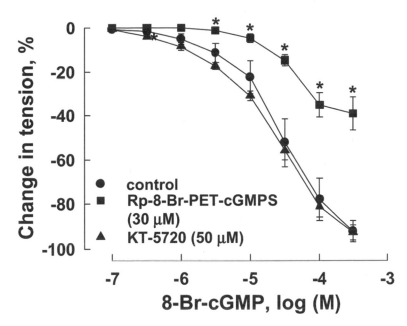

Fig. 4. Effects of Rp-8-β-phenyl-1, N^2-etheno-8-bromo-guanosine cyclic monophosphorothioate (Rp-8-Br-PET-cGMPS) and KT-5720 on 8-Br-cGMP-induced relaxation of pulmonary arteries of newborn lambs. Experiments were performed during contraction to endothelin-1 (3 nM). Values are means ± SE ($n = 5$ animals for all groups except KT-5720, where $n = 4$). Control tensions (g/mg dry wt of tissue) raised by endothelin-1 were 1.12 ± 0.13 for untreated tissue (control), 1.05 ± 0.11 for tissue treated with Rp-8-Br-PET-cGMPs, and 1.03 ± 0.06 for tissue treated with KT-5720. Changes in tension are expressed as percent contraction to endothelin-1. *Significant difference ($p < 0.05$) from control.

temic hypertension. Hofmann did not study the pulmonary vessels but did report that PKG activity was absent in lung homogenates. Aortic rings showed a 90-fold increase in cGMP production but did not relax in response to cGMP analog (100 μM). Thus, in survivors, other mechanisms of vasodilation must be in play.

Oxygen effect on cGMP-PKG-mediated pulmonary vasodilation: because at birth, an increase in oxygen tension is an important biological stimulus, the role of oxygen in upregulating the cGMP-PKG pathway in fetal pulmonary vascular smooth muscle cells (PVSMC) is being actively investigated. Gao et al. have found that fetal pulmonary vessels exposed to oxygen have an augmented relaxation response to cGMP when preconstricted, compared to fetal vessels that have not been exposed to oxygen **(Fig. 6)**. This augmented relaxation response to cGMP is mostly abolished if PKG kinase activity is blocked, suggesting that the effect of oxygen is predominantly on PKG activity. Oxygen can increase PKG activity by affecting (a) the catalytic rate/amount of cGMP binding, (b) the dissociation rate of bound cGMP, (c) autophosphorylation of PKG, (d) its intracellular location, (e) oxidation of thiol groups in PKG protein via generation of oxygen radicals, (f) inhibition of substrate binding, (g) the proteolytic rate of PKG, (h) conformational change, (i) kinetics of ATP binding, (j) activation of an inhibitor of PKG, (k) binding of other regulatory factors to allosteric site(s), and (l) complexing with other protein factors. These mechanisms need to be investigated.

Oxygen effect on pulmonary vasoactivity via reactive oxygen and nitrogen species (ROS/RNS). biologically relevant reactive oxygen species (ROS) include superoxide anion (O_2^-), hydrogen peroxide (H_2O_2), and hydroxy radical (·OH). Approximately 1–3% of all tissue oxygen consumption occurs through the partial reduction of oxygen to O_2^-, with this species present at a steady-state concentration of approx 10 pM, increasing to 0.01–0.1 μM in pathological states *(33)*. Under physi-

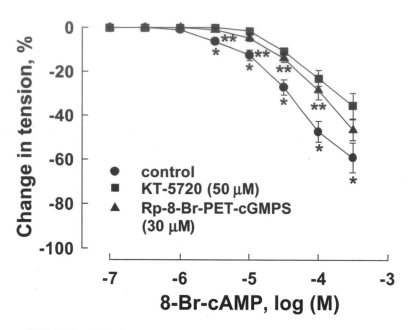

Fig. 5. Effects of KT-5720 and Rp-8-Br-PET-cGMPS on 8-BrcAMP-induced relaxation of pulmonary arteries of newborn lambs. Experiments were performed during contraction to endothelin-1 (3 nM). Values are means ± SE (n = 5). Control tensions (g/mg dry wt of tissue) raised by endothelin-1 were 0.98 ± 0.10 for untreated tissue (control), 1.01 ± 0.06 for tissue treated with Rp-8-Br-PET-cGMPS, and 0.98 ± 0.09 for tissue treated with KT-5720. Changes in tension are expressed as percent contraction to endothelin-1. *Significant difference (p < 0.05) from vessels treated with KT-5720; **significant difference between control and vessels treated with Rp-8-Br-PET-cGMPS.

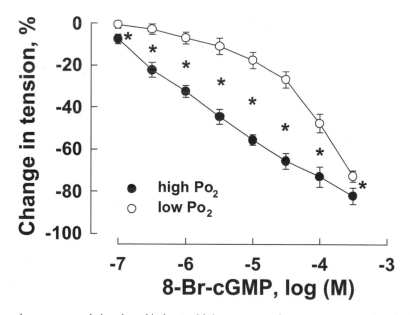

Fig. 6. Intrapulmonary vessels incubated in low or high oxygen tensions were preconstricted with endothelin-1 and then exposed to increasing concentrations of cGMP, as described for Fig. 4. The responsiveness to cGMP was significantly augmented by exposure of the vessels to a high oxygen tension, indicating that signaling mechanisms downstream from cGMP were augmented by oxygen. *Significant difference (p < 0.05) between high and low oxygen tension.

ological conditions, antioxidant enzymes such as superoxide dismutase (SOD), glutathione peroxidase, and catalase modulate ambient steady-state levels of ROS *(34)*. In vascular SMC, recent studies show that the majority of O_2^- produced is attributable to NAD(P)H oxidases. The cardiovascular NAD(P)H oxidases are low-output, slow-release enzymes with biochemical characteristics that differ considerably from those of neutrophil NADPH oxidase. Also, the vascular enzymes appear to have a moderate constitutive activity that is absent in phagocytes. The kinetics of activation on cellular stimulation are also unique; O_2^- is produced in minutes to hours in endothelial cells, vascular SMC, and fibroblasts, in contrast to the almost instantaneous release seen in neutrophils *(35)*. In lungs, O_2^- inhibits cGMP-mediated vasodilation; in contrast, H_2O_2 augments vasodilation via activation of soluble guanylyl cyclase *(36)*.

Reactive oxygen and nitrogen species in pulmonary vascular smooth muscle: biologically relevant nitrogen species include nitric oxide (NO) and peroxynitrite. Endothelial and vascular SMC produce both NO and O_2^- *(35–37)*. These two radicals can recombine to form peroxynitrite. NO reacts more rapidly with O_2^- than SOD and can scavenge O_2^- very efficiently.

Although SOD concentration in cells is 1–10 μM, the rapid reaction of NO with O_2^- assures that peroxynitrite is always formed *(33)*. Normally in the cell, peroxynitrite is converted to nitrosoglutathione mainly by reduced glutathione. These thiol intermediates may subsequently regenerate NO and cause vasodilation *(38)*. When cellular glutathione levels are low, as in hypoxia, peroxynitrite is likely to accumulate. Peroxynitrite is a powerful one- and two-electron oxidant, which can cause DNA damage. Protein tyrosine nitration by peroxynitrite may interfere with phosphorylation/dephosphorylation-signaling pathways or alter protein function *(39)*. In pulmonary arterial SMC, production of ROS and NOS may dramatically increase during hypoxia *(40,41)*. Recent studies identify a novel mitochondrial nitric oxide synthase *(42)*. A drop in cellular pO_2 may stimulate NO production by this enzyme or lead to liberation of NO from heme-binding sites in cytoplasm and mitochondrial matrix *(42)*, and this NO may readily react with O_2^- to form peroxynitrite. Increased production of ROS in hypoxia may decrease intracellular glutathione levels and lead to further peroxynitrite accumulation, due to reduced conversion of peroxynitrite by glutathione into thiol intermediates *(43)*. The net effect might be that during hypoxia, there is greater accumulation of peroxynitrite than under normoxic conditions.

Previously, ROS have been viewed as toxic, leading to DNA damage and lipid oxidation. Recent data suggest that this concept may be incorrect. It is believed that ROS are produced in a controlled fashion and have critical cellular functions as second messengers. Activation of signaling cascades and redox-sensitive transcription factors leads to induction of many genes in vascular cells *(35,44,45)*. No one has studied the role of ROS and/or RNS in modulating PKG activity, protein levels, and gene expression. Preliminary data have been presented to show that in fetal PVSMC, increased levels of peroxynitrite are produced during hypoxia, which decrease PKG protein levels. Additionally, data have also been presented to show that exogenous peroxynitrite (1 p*M*) decreased PKG protein level in fetal PVSMC by approx 30%, suggesting that peroxynitrite is involved in regulation of PKG protein level during hypoxia.

Regulation of PKG type-1 gene expression: PKG type 1 is the major intracellular substrate for cGMP in vascular SMC *(46)*. In humans, PKG-1 gene expression is highest in aorta, heart, kidneys, and adrenals, and lowest in lung, thymus, and liver *(47)*. PKG-1 isoforms α and β are differentially expressed, being equally expressed in aorta, with 90% α isoform in lung and predominately β isoform in uterus *(47)*. The mechanisms by which PKG-1 gene expression and the expression of the specific isoforms are regulated remain elusive *(48,49)*. Agents that can regulate PKG-1 gene expression levels in vivo include angiotensin II, transforming growth factor (TGF)-β, and tumor necrosis factor (TNF)-α, all of which decreased PKG mRNA levels to approx 40%, 6 h after their addition to cultured rat aortic SMC, followed by recovery to normal levels after 24 h *(47)*. Lincoln et al. showed that in rat aortic SMC, PKG-1 gene expression increased with increasing cell density and decreased with repetitive passage of cells, and that this effect was not due to serum-derived factors *(48)*. In human vascular SMC, PKG-1 mRNA levels could not be increased by agents that elevate cGMP, or growth factors such as platelet-derived growth factor (PDGF), TGF-β, or angiotensin. Lincoln also showed that in bovine and rat aorta SMC, PKG-1 mRNA levels progressively decrease during 5–48 h of incubation with the nitrovasodilators SNAP and SNP, and that this is due to decreasing gene transcription and not due to mRNA destabilization.

Downregulation of PKG following chronic exposure to nitric oxide and cGMP: inhaled NO is used as a selective pulmonary vasodilator for a number of pulmonary vasculature diseases, such as persistent pulmonary hypertension of the newborn and congenital heart disease with pulmonary hypertension *(50,51)*. However, a life-threatening increase in pulmonary vascular resistance may occur with acute withdrawal of inhaled NO. There are numerous reports that an acute and potentially life-threatening increase in pulmonary vascular resistance can occur upon acute withdrawal of inhaled NO *(50–54)*. In newborns with persistent pulmonary hypertension, this can result in a sudden decrease in systemic arterial oxygen saturation. In children with congenital heart disease, an increase in PVR may compromise cardiac output. This rebound pulmonary hypertension can occur after only hours of therapy and is independent of the initial response; patients with no initial pulmonary vasodilatory response can have life-threatening pulmonary vasoconstriction upon withdrawal. The underlying mechanism is not clear *(52,53)*. In juvenile lambs, endothelial nitric oxide synthase (eNOS) activity of pulmonary arteries is reduced after inhaled NO therapy. The development of NO tolerance is alleviated by endothelin A (ETA) receptor antagonists and superoxide scavengers, suggesting the involvement of endothelin and superoxide production*(54)*. NO tolerance during NO inhalation therapy may share some mechanisms with the NO tolerance that develops during nitrovasodilator treatment. In systemic blood vessels, continuous exposure to nitric oxide (NO) or nitrovasodilators induces NO tolerance. Multiple factors may be involved in the development of NO tolerance, such as downregulation of aortic eNOS protein expression *(55)*, induction of phosphodiesterase 1A1 *(56)*, and a decrease in sGC protein levels *(57)*. In the aortas of transgenic mice (Tg) overexpressing eNOS in the endothelium, relaxations to acetylcholine, sodium nitroprusside, atrial natriuretic peptide, and 8-bromo-cGMP were also significantly reduced. Furthermore, soluble guanylyl cyclase (sGC) activity, PKG protein levels, and PKG enzyme activity are decreased in Tg vessels *(58)*. In rats and rabbits that are tolerant to nitroglycerin, as well as in patients who have developed tolerance to nitroglycerin, a marked decrease of P-VASP, a surrogate parameter for in vivo PKG activity, was observed *(59,60)*. In bovine aortic SMC, continuous exposure to nitrovasodilators results in marked suppression of PKG I mRNA *(49)*. Recently, Sellak et al. have reported that chronic exposure to NO, cAMP, and cGMP downregulates PKGIα expression in bovine and rat aortic smooth-muscle cells through transcription factor Sp1 *(61)*. We have data to show that exposure of pulmonary vessels and PVSMC to nitric oxide and cGMP for as short a period as 20 h results in downregulation of PKG.

Regulation of gene transcription by cyclic GMP: cGMP is a known modulator of transcription factor binding and gene transcription. Idriss et al. have shown that cGMP analogs can increase reporter gene activity by acting through the serum response element (SRE), AP-1 binding site, and cAMP response element (CRE) of the human fos promoter, and that this activity is dependent upon PKG activity *(62)*. cGMP treatment can increase or decrease transcription-factor binding and reporter gene activity in a tissue-specific manner. For example, Gertzberg et al. showed that AP-1 binding to DNA in pulmonary endothelial cells is increased by 8-Br-cGMP. This binding is dependent upon PKG activity, and is not affected by incubation with 8-Br-cAMP or increases in PKA activity *(63)*. Thus, activation of AP-1 binding in the pulmonary endothelial model studied by Gertzberg is not due to "cross-talk" between the cGMP-PKG and cAMP-PKA pathways, although an indirect effect whereby increased cGMP levels might suppress PKA activity via cGMP stimulation of PDEII is discussed. On the other hand, binding of AP-1 as well as nuclear factor (NF)-κB decreases in rat livers perfused with 8-Br-cGMP *(64)*, while in cat hearts perfused with 8-Br-cGMP, AP-1 activity is unaffected and that of NF-κB is increased *(65)*. In perfused heart, NF-κB binding was demonstrated to require PKG activity, which was shown to directly phosphorylate the NF-κB inhibitor IκBα, leading to activation of NF-κB *(65)*. The activity of AP-1 may be modulated by PKG phosphorylation of the AP-1 subcomponents cFOS and cJUN *(63)*. The cAMP-regulated transcription factor CREB can be phosphorylated indirectly by 8-Br-cGMP acting through PKG, which activates adenylyl cyclase, ultimately leading to increased binding to CRE *(66)*. There is just one study to date of transcription-factor regulation of the PKG1 promoter. Lincoln et al. demonstrated SP1 binding at two sites within the first 47 bp of the PKG1α promoter *(61)*. Incubation with 8pCTP-cGMP caused decreased binding and decreased reported gene expression, primarily via activation of PKA.

2. CONCLUSIONS

In the newly born infant, the immediate fall in pulmonary vascular resistance is mediated mainly via the nitric oxide-cGMP-PKG pathway. Fetal pulmonary vessels appear to be exquisitely sensitive to the vasodilator actions of cGMP as compared to cAMP. We have shown that cGMP acts primarily by activation of PKG and that oxygen upregulates PKG-dependent pulmonary vasodilation. In the fetus, the hypoxic environment results in downregulation of this pathway, and exposure to oxygen results in augmentation of cGMP-mediated vasodilation by upregulation of PKG. Hypoxia results in increased reactive oxygen species being generated in the vascular smooth-muscle cells that appear to be responsible for downregulation of PKG protein. This unique oxygen-sensitive mechanism of regulation of the pulmonary circulation is present in the perinatal pulmonary circulation.

ACKNOWLEDGMENTS

We thank Nik Phou for excellent secretarial assistance. This work was supported in part by grants from National Heart Lung Blood Institute, HL 59435 and HL 75187.

REFERENCES

1. Fineman, J. R., Soifer, S. J., and Heymann, M. A. (1995) Regulation of pulmonary vascular tone in the perinatal period. *Annu. Rev. Physiol.* **57,** 115–134.
2. Gao, Y., Tolsa, J. F., and Raj, J. U. (1998) Heterogeneity in endothelium-derived nitric oxide-mediated relaxation of different sized pulmonary arteries of newborn lambs. *Pediatr. Res.* **44,** 723–729.
3. Gao, Y., Tolsa, J. F., Shen, H., and Raj, J. U. (1998) Effect of selective phosphodiesterase inhibitors on response of ovine pulmonary arteries to prostaglandin E2. *J. Appl. Physiol.* **84,** 13–18.
4. Gao, Y., Zhou, H., Ibe, B. O., and Raj, J. U. (1996) Prostaglandins E_2 and I_2 cause greater relaxations in pulmonary veins than in arteries of newborn lambs. *J. Appl. Physiol.* **81,** 2534–2539.
5. Gao, Y., Zhou, H., and Raj, J. U. (1995) Heterogeneity in role of endothelium-derived NO in pulmonary arteries and veins of full-term fetal lambs. *Am. J. Physiol.* **268,** H1586–H1592.
6. Gao, Y., Zhou, H., and Raj, J. U. (1995) Endothelium-derived nitric oxide plays a larger role in pulmonary veins than in arteries of newborn lambs. *Circ. Res.* **76,** 559–565.
7. Gao, Y., Dhanakoti, S., Tolsa, J. F., and Raj, J. U. (1999) Role of protein kinase G in nitric oxide- and cGMP-induced relaxation of newborn ovine pulmonary veins. *J. Appl. Physiol.* **87,** 993–998.
8. Dhanakoti, S. N., Gao, Y., Nguyen, M. Q., and Raj, J. U. (2000) Involvement of cGMP-dependent protein kinase in the relaxation of ovine pulmonary arteries to cGMP and cAMP. *J. Appl. Physiol.* **88,** 1637–1642.
9. Kuo, J. F. and Greengard, P. (1970) Cyclic nucleotide-dependent protein kinases. VI. Isolation and partial purification of a protein kinase activated by guanosine 3′,5′-monophosphate. *J. Biol. Chem.* **245,** 2493–2498.
10. Felbel, J., Trockur, B., Ecker, T., Landgraf, W., and Hofmann, F. (1988) Regulation of cytosolic calcium by cAMP and cGMP in freshly isolated smooth muscle cells from bovine trachea. *J. Biol. Chem.* **263,** 16,764–16,771.
11. Francis, S. H. and Corbin, J. D. (1994) Structure and function of cyclic nucleotide-dependent protein kinases. *Annu. Rev. Physiol.* **56,** 237–272.
12. Lincoln, T. M., Komalavilas, P., Boerth, N. J., MacMillan Crow, L. A., and Cornwell, T. L. (1995) cGMP signaling through cAMP- and cGMP-dependent protein kinases. *Adv. Pharmacol.* **34,** 305–322.
13. Lincoln, T. M. and Cornwell, T. L. (1993) Intracellular cyclic GMP receptor proteins. *FASEB J.* **7,** 328–38.
14. Rashatwar, S. S., Cornwell, T. L., and Lincoln, T. M. (1987) Effects of 8-bromo-cGMP on Ca^{++} levels in vascular smooth muscle cells: possible regulation of CA^{++} ATPase by cGMP-dependent protein kinase. *Proc. Natl. Acad. Sci. USA* **84,** 5685–5689.
15. Komalavilas, P. and Lincoln, T. M. (1996) Phosphorylation of the inositol 1,4,5-trisphosphate receptor. Cyclic GMP-dependent protein kinase mediates cAMP and cGMP dependent phosphorylation in the intact rat aorta. *J. Biol. Chem.* **271,** 21,933–21,938.
16. Alioua, A., Huggins, J. P., and Rousseau, E. (1995) PKG-I alpha phosphorylates the alpha-subunit and upregulates reconstituted GKCa channels from tracheal smooth muscle. *Am. J. Physiol.* **268,** L1057–L1063.

17. Xiong, Z. and Sperelakis, N. (1995) Regulation of L-type calcium channels of vascular smooth muscle cells. *J. Mol. Cell Cardiol.* **27**, 75–91.
18. Wu, X., Somlyo, A. V., and Somlyo, A. P. (1996) Cyclic GMP-dependent stimulation reverses G-protein-coupled inhibition of smooth muscle myosin light chain phosphate. *Biochem. Biophys. Res. Commun.* **220**, 658–663.
19. Durmowicz, A. G., Orton, E. C., and Stenmark, K. R. (1993) Progressive loss of vasodilator responsive component of pulmonary hypertension in neonatal calves exposed to 4,570 m. *Am. J. Physiol.* **265**, H2175–H2183.
20. Fike, C. D. and Kaplowitz, M. R. (1996) Chronic hypoxia alters nitric oxide-dependent pulmonary vascular responses in lungs of newborn pigs. *J. Appl. Physiol.* **81**, 2078–2087.
21. Fike, C. D., Kaplowitz, M. R., Thomas, C. J., and Nelin, L. D. (1998) Chronic hypoxia decreases nitric oxide production and endothelial nitric oxide synthase in newborn pig lungs. *Am. J. Physiol.* **274**, L517–L526.
22. North, A. J., Moya, F. R., Mysore, M. R., et al. (1995) Pulmonary endothelial nitric oxide synthase gene expression is decreased in a rat model of congenital diaphragmatic hernia. *Am. J. Respir. Cell Mol. Biol.* **13**, 676–682.
23. Steinhorn, R. H., Russell, J. A., and Morin, F. C., III. (1995) Disruption of cGMP production in pulmonary arteries isolated from fetal lambs with pulmonary hypertension. *Am. J. Physiol.* **268**, H1483–H1489.
24. Shaul, P. W., Yuhanna, I. S., German, Z., Chen, Z., Steinhorn, R. H., and Morin, F. C., III. (1997) Pulmonary endothelial NO synthase gene expression is decreased in fetal lambs with pulmonary hypertension. *Am. J. Physiol.* **272**, L1005–L1012.
25. Villamor, E., Le Cras, T. D., Horan, M. P., Halbower, A. C., Tuder, R. M., and Abman, S. H. (1997) Chronic intrauterine pulmonary hypertension impairs endothelial nitric oxide synthase in the ovine fetus. *Am. J. Physiol.* **272**, L1013–L1020.
26. Tulloh, R. M., Hislop, A. A., Boels, P. J., Deutsch, J., and Haworth, S. G. (1997) Chronic hypoxia inhibits postnatal maturation of porcine intrapulmonary artery relaxation. *Am. J. Physiol.* **272**, H2436–H2445.
27. Berkenbosch, J. W., Baribeau, J., and Perreault, T. (2000) Decreased synthesis and vasodilation to nitric oxide in piglets with hypoxia-induced pulmonary hypertension. *Am. J. Physiol. Lung Cell Mol. Physiol.* **278**, L276–L283.
28. Jernigan, N. L. and Resta, T. C. (2002) Chronic hypoxia attenuates cGMP-dependent pulmonary vasodilation. *Am. J. Physiol. Lung Cell Mol. Physiol.* **282**, L1366–L1375.
29. Tamaoki, J., Tagaya, E., Yamawaki, I., and Konno, K. (1996) Hypoxia impairs nitrovasodilator-induced pulmonary vasodilation: role of Na-K-ATPase activity. *Am. J. Physiol.* **271**, L172–L177.
30. Peng, W., Hoidal, J. R., Karwande, S. V., and Farrukh, I. S. (1997) Effect of chronic hypoxia on K+ channels: regulation in human pulmonary vascular smooth muscle cells. *Am. J. Physiol.* **272**, C1271–C1278.
31. Pfeifer, A., Klatt, P., Massberg, S., et al. (1998) Defective smooth muscle regulation in cGMP kinase I-deficient mice. *EMBO J.* **17**, 3045–3051.
32. Sausbier, M., Schubert, R., Voigt, V., et al. (2000) Mechanisms of NO/cGMP-dependent vasorelaxation. *Circ. Res.* **87**, 825–830.
33. Freeman, B. A., Gutierrez, H., and Rubbo, H. (1995) Nitric oxide: a central regulatory species in pulmonary oxidant reactions. *Am. J. Physiol.* **268**, L697–L698.
34. Pryor, W. A. (1986) Oxy-radicals and related species: their formation, lifetimes, and reactions. *Annu. Rev. Physiol.* **48**, 657–667.
35. Griendling, K. K., Sorescu, D., and Ushio-Fukai, M. (2000) NAD(P)H oxidase: role in cardiovascular biology and disease. *Circ. Res.* **86**, 494–501.
36. Cherry, P. D., Omar, H. A., Farrell, K. A., Stuart, J. S., and Wolin, M. S. (1990) Superoxide anion inhibits cGMP-associated bovine pulmonary arterial relaxation. *Am. J. Physiol.* **259**, H1056–H1062.
37. Heitsch, H., Brovkovych, S., Malinski, T., and Wiemer, G. (2001) Angiotensin-(1-7)-stimulated nitric oxide and superoxide release from endothelial cells. *Hypertension* **37**, 72–76.
38. Iesaki, T., Gupte, S. A., Kaminski, P. M., and Wolin, M. S. (1999) Inhibition of guanylate cyclase stimulation by NO and bovine arterial relaxation to peroxynitrite and H_2O_2. *Am. J. Physiol.* **277**, H978–H985.
39. Cuzzocrea, S., Riley, D. P., Caputi, A. P., and Salvemini, D. (2001) Antioxidant therapy: a new pharmacological approach in shock, inflammation, and ischemia/reperfusion injury. *Pharmacol. Rev.* **53**, 135–159.
40. Marshall, C., Mamary, A. J., Verhoeven, A. J., and Marshall, B. E. (1996) Pulmonary artery NADPH-oxidase is activated in hypoxic pulmonary vasoconstriction. *Am. J. Respir. Cell Mol. Biol.* **15**, 633–644.
41. Killilea, D. W., Hester, R., Balczon, R., Babal, P., and Gillespie, M. N. (2000) Free radical production in hypoxic pulmonary artery smooth muscle cells. *Am. J. Physiol. Lung Cell Mol. Physiol.* **279**, L408–L412.
42. Giulivi, C. (1998) Functional implications of nitric oxide produced by mitochondria in mitochondrial metabolism. *Biochem. J.* **332 (Pt 3)**, 673–679.
43. Deneke, S. M. and Fanburg, B. L. (1989) Regulation of cellular glutathione. *Am. J. Physiol.* **257**, L163–L173.
44. Kietzmann, T., Fandrey, J., and Acker, H. (2000) Oxygen radicals as messengers in oxygen-dependent gene expression. *News Physiol. Sci.* **15**, 202–208.
45. Thannickal, V. J. and Fanburg, B. L. (2000) Reactive oxygen species in cell signaling. *Am. J. Physiol. Lung Cell Mol. Physiol.* **279**, L1005–L1028.
46. Carvajal, J. A., Germain, A. M., Huidobro-Toro, J. P., and Weiner, C. P. (2000) Molecular mechanism of cGMP-mediated smooth muscle relaxation. *J. Cell Physiol.* **184**, 409–420.
47. Tamura, N., Itoh, H., Ogawa, Y., et al. (1996) cDNA cloning and gene expression of human type Ialpha cGMP-dependent protein kinase. *Hypertension* **27**, 552–557.
48. Cornwell, T. L., Soff, G. A., Traynor, A. E., and Lincoln, T. M. (1994) Regulation of the expression of cyclic GMP-dependent protein kinase by cell density in vascular smooth muscle cells. *J. Vasc. Res.* **31**, 330–337.

49. Soff, G. A., Cornwell, T. L., Cundiff, D. L., Gately, S., and Lincoln, T. M. (1997) Smooth muscle cell expression of type I cyclic GMP-dependent protein kinase is suppressed by continuous exposure to nitrovasodilators, theophylline, cyclic GMP, and cyclic AMP. *J. Clin. Invest.* **100,** 2580–2587.
50. Rich, G. F., Lowson, S. M., Johns, R. A., Daugherty, M. O., and Uncles, D. R. (1994) Inhaled nitric oxide selectively decreases pulmonary vascular resistance without impairing oxygenation during one-lung ventilation in patients undergoing cardiac surgery. *Anesthesiology* **80,** 57–62.
51. Roberts, J. D., Jr., Fineman, J. R., Morin, F. C., III, et al. (1997) Inhaled nitric oxide and persistent pulmonary hypertension of the newborn. The Inhaled Nitric Oxide Study Group. *N. Engl. J. Med.* **336,** 605–610.
52. Miller, O. I., Tang, S. F., Keech, A., and Celermajer, D. S. (1995) Rebound pulmonary hypertension on withdrawal from inhaled nitric oxide. *Lancet* **346,** 51–52.
53. Lavoie, A., Hall, J. B., Olson, D. M., and Wylam, M. E. (1996) Life-threatening effects of discontinuing inhaled nitric oxide in severe respiratory failure. *Am. J. Respir. Crit. Care Med.* **153,** 1985–1987.
54. Wedgwood, S., McMullan, D. M., Bekker, J. M., Fineman, J. R., and Black, S. M. (2001) Role for endothelin-1-induced superoxide and peroxynitrite production in rebound pulmonary hypertension associated with inhaled nitric oxide therapy. *Circ. Res.* **89,** 357–364.
55. Vaziri, N. D. and Wang, X. Q. (1999) cGMP-mediated negative-feedback regulation of endothelial nitric oxide synthase expression by nitric oxide. *Hypertension* **34,** 1237–1241.
56. Kim, D., Rybalkin, S. D., Pi, X., et al. (2001) Upregulation of phosphodiesterase 1A1 expression is associated with the development of nitrate tolerance. *Circulation* **104,** 2338–2343.
57. Papapetropoulos, A., Go, C. Y., Murad, F., and Catravas, J. D. (1996) Mechanisms of tolerance to sodium nitroprusside in rat cultured aortic smooth muscle cells. *Br. J. Pharmacol.* **117,** 147–155.
58. Yamashita, T., Kawashima, S., Ohashi, Y., et al. (2000) Mechanisms of reduced nitric oxide/cGMP-mediated vasorelaxation in transgenic mice overexpressing endothelial nitric oxide synthase. *Hypertension* **36,** 97–102.
59. Schulz, E., Tsilimingas, N., Rinze, R., et al. (2002) Functional and biochemical analysis of endothelial (dys)function and NO/cGMP signaling in human blood vessels with and without nitroglycerin pretreatment. *Circulation* **105,** 1170–1175.
60. Mulsch, A., Oelze, M., Kloss, S., et al. (2001) Effects of in vivo nitroglycerin treatment on activity and expression of the guanylyl cyclase and cGMP-dependent protein kinase and their downstream target vasodilator-stimulated phosphoprotein in aorta. *Circulation* **103,** 2188–2194.
61. Sellak, H., Yang, X., Cao, X., Cornwell, T., Soff, G. A., and Lincoln, T. (2002) Sp1 transcription factor as a molecular target for nitric oxide– and cyclic nucleotide–mediated suppression of cGMP-dependent protein kinase-Ialpha expression in vascular smooth muscle cells. *Circ. Res.* **90,** 405–412.
62. Idriss, S. D., Gudi, T., Casteel, D. E., Kharitonov, V. G., Pilz, R. B., and Boss, G. R. (1999) Nitric oxide regulation of gene transcription via soluble guanylate cyclase and type I cGMP-dependent protein kinase. *J. Biol. Chem.* **274,** 9489–9493.
63. Gertzberg, N., Clements, R., Jaspers, I., et al. (2000) Tumor necrosis factor-alpha-induced activating protein-1 activity is modulated by nitric oxide-mediated protein kinase G activation. *Am. J. Respir. Cell Mol Biol.* **22,** 105–115.
64. Kiemer, A. K., Vollmar, A. M., Bilzer, M., Gerwig, T., and Gerbes, A. L. (2000) Atrial natriuretic peptide reduces expression of TNF-alpha mRNA during reperfusion of the rat liver upon decreased activation of NF-kappaB and AP-1. *J. Hepatol.* **33,** 236–246.
65. Kalra, D., Baumgarten, G., Dibbs, Z., Seta, Y., Sivasubramanian, N., and Mann, D. L. (2000) Nitric oxide provokes tumor necrosis factor-alpha expression in adult feline myocardium through a cGMP- dependent pathway. *Circulation* **102,** 1302–1307.
66. Moon, C., Sung, Y. K., Reddy, R., and Ronnett, G. V. (1999) Odorants induce the phosphorylation of the cAMP response element binding protein in olfactory receptor neurons. *Proc. Natl. Acad. Sci. USA* **96,** 14,605–14,610.

6

Glutamate Receptor Activation in the Pathogenesis of Acute Lung Injury

Sami I. Said

SUMMARY

The excitatory amino acids glutamate and aspartate, acting on glutamate receptors, exert important physiological functions in the central nervous system. But overactivation of these receptors can produce neuronal cell injury and death. Recent studies show that the glutamate agonist N-methyl-D-aspartate (NMDA) can trigger acute lung injury (ALI), manifested by high-permeability pulmonary edema, and that NMDA receptor subtypes are expressed in normal rat lung. These findings suggest that glutamate signaling may be involved in the pathogenesis of ALI and, as such, may be a novel target for the prevention or attenuation of this condition.

Key Words: Glutamate receptors; lung injury; NMDA; excitotoxicity; excitatory amino acids.

1. GLUTAMATE IS A PHYSIOLOGICAL NEUROTRANSMITTER

The amino acids glutamate and aspartate, abundantly present in the mammalian central nervous system (CNS), are the major excitatory neurotransmitters. These excitatory amino acids (EAAs), acting on glutamate receptors, play an important role in many physiological functions, including learning, memory, development, and other forms of synaptic plasticity *(1)*. More recently, glutamate has received some recognition as a neurotransmitter in the peripheral nervous system, and glutamate receptors have been detected in several sites outside the CNS *(2,3)*.

2. GLUTAMATE IS POTENTIALLY TOXIC TO NEURONS: EXCITOTOXICITY

Despite its physiological role as a neurotransmitter, glutamate can be lethal to neurons upon intense exposure *(4)*. Overactivation of glutamate receptors has been implicated in neuronal degeneration and loss in such acute conditions as hypoxia-ischemia, hypoglycemia, head injury, stroke, and prolonged epileptic seizures, as well as in chronic neurodegenerative diseases, including Alzheimer's disease, Huntington's disease, Parkinson's disease, amyotrophic lateral sclerosis, and acquired immunodeficiency syndrome (AIDS) dementia *(4)*. In most instances, neuronal cell loss is attributable to *excitotoxicity*, a term derived from its mediation by excitatory amino acid receptors.

3. GLUTAMATE RECEPTORS

Several classes of glutamate receptors, widely distributed throughout the CNS, have been identified *(5)*. Already cloned and characterized are three subtypes of ionotropic receptors, classified according to their activation by specific agonists: N-methyl-D-aspartate (NMDA), AMPA (α-amino-3-hydroxy-5-methyl-4-isoxazole-propinate) and kainate receptors, and a family of het-

From: *Cell Signaling in Vascular Inflammation*
Edited by: J. Bhattacharya © Humana Press Inc., Totowa, NJ

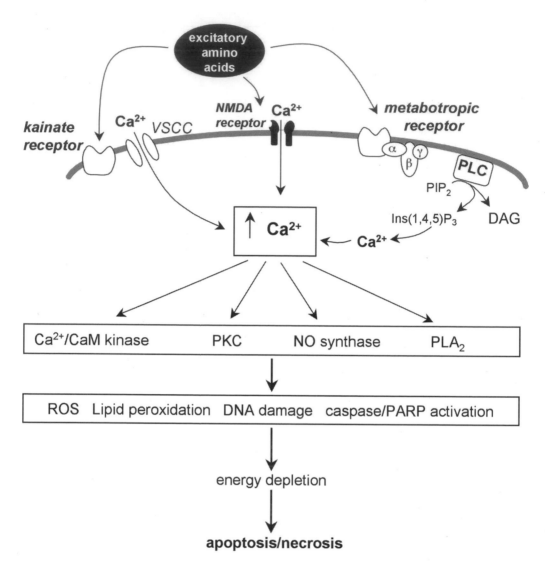

Fig. 1. Schematic representation of signaling pathways and enzymatic reactions triggered by glutamate receptor activation that lead to cell death. CaM, calmodulin; DAG, diacylglycerol; Ins(1,4,5)P_3, inositol 1,4,5 trisphosphate; NMDA, *N*-methyl-D-aspartate; NO, nitric oxide; PARP, poly(ADP-ribose) polymerase; PKC, protein kinase C; PLA$_2$ and PLC, phospholipase A$_2$ and C, respectively; ROS, reactive oxygen species; VSCC, voltage-sensitive Ca^{2+} channels. (Reproduced with permission from ref. *17*.)

erogeneous, G protein-coupled metabotropic receptors. These receptors regulate the activity of membrane enzymes and ion channels, and act through different second-messenger systems (**Fig. 1**). The NMDA receptor has been the focus of much attention because of its implication in excitotoxic *(4)*, as well as neuroexcitatory, events.

4. THE NMDA RECEPTOR

The NMDA receptor forms an ion channel whose permeability to Ca^{2+} is increased upon ligand binding *(6)*. Calcium permeability can be blocked by Mg^{2+}. Functional NMDA receptors in the brain are formed by combinations of two subunits: NR1 and NR2. NR1 exists as a family of eight isoforms formed by alternative splicing at three exons (N1, C1, C2), and contains a binding site for the cofactor glycine. The NR2 subfamily consists of four individual isoforms: NR2A, NR2B, NR2C, NR2D, and contains the glutamate (NMDA) binding site. NMDA receptor isoforms are differentially expressed in different regions of the brain, where they presumably mediate site-specific functions *(5)*.

5. GLUTAMATE TOXICITY IN THE LUNG: EXCITOTOXICITY AS A MECHANISM OF LUNG INJURY

As mentioned above, other investigators have reported the presence of NMDA-type glutamate receptors in nonneuronal tissues, such as pancreatic-islet β-cells, megakaryocytes *(2,3)*, and cerebral microvasculature. Our interest in the potential occurrence of glutamate toxicity in the lung, and its pathophysiological significance, began with the demonstration that the excitotoxin NMDA caused acute lung injury in the rat *(7)*. The injury was in the form of high-permeability edema, marked by increased lung weight, increased protein content in bronchoalveolar lavage (BAL) fluid, and elevated airway and pulmonary artery pressures. The injury was prevented by NMDA receptor blockade and was nitric oxide (NO) dependent *(7)*.

These observations raised the possibility that glutamate (NMDA) toxicity could be a novel mechanism in the pathogenesis of acute lung injury, as seen in the acute respiratory distress syndrome (ARDS) *(8)*. To validate this hypothesis, at least two criteria need to be fulfilled. First, NMDA toxicity must be shown to be involved in lung injury induced by other than the application of NMDA itself. Secondly, NMDA receptors should be expressed in the lung. To test the first requirement, we demonstrated that the NMDA receptor antagonist MK-801 reduced acute pulmonary injury due not only to NMDA itself, but also to the oxidants paraquat and xanthine + xanthine oxidase *(9)*. These findings suggested that endogenous activation of NMDA receptors, probably by glutamate released from damaged cells, could play a role in oxidant lung injury. Data from neuroscience have shown that intracellular glutamate levels are a thousand-fold greater than extracellular levels, and that glutamate released from injured neurons acts as a source of excitotoxic injury of other cells *(10)*. The significance of this mechanism, by which glutamate toxicity can be perpetuated and amplified, has yet to be explored in the lung.

6. NMDA RECEPTORS ARE EXPRESSED IN TIIE LUNG

The observation that high concentrations of the glutamate agonist NMDA induced high- permeability pulmonary edema implied the presence of NMDA receptors in the lung, particularly in the alveolar-capillary area. For direct evidence, we used a variety of experimental approaches to identify the subtypes of NMDA receptors expressed in the lung, and to localize them to specific regions of the lungs and airways. First, with the help of immunhistochemical techniques, we demonstrated the presence of NMDAR 2B in airway neurons *(11)*. We then showed by autoradiography the localization of specific binding of NMDA receptor antagonist MK-801 to alveolar walls and bronchial smooth-muscle and epithelial cells *(12)*. More recently, the use of RT-PCR revealed the constitutive expression of the NR1 and four NMDAR2 receptor subunits in rat lung. mRNA for the NR1 and NMDAR 2D subunits were constitutively expressed in the peripheral lung, mid-lung, and central-lung regions, as well as in alveolar macrophages. NMDAR 2A and 2B expression was not detectable in any of the lung regions examined, while NMDAR 2C was present in peripheral and mid-lung regions. Western blot analysis confirmed the presence of NR1 isoforms with C2 sites in peripheral rat lung. It is likely that the localization of these receptor subunits in the lung is largely nonneuronal, particularly in peripheral lung, which is devoid of neurons *(13)*.

7. HOW DOES GLUTAMATE KILL CELLS?

As stated before, activation of the NMDA receptor opens up a receptor-gated Ca^{2+} channel, causing the rapid influx of Ca^{2+} into the cell. In neurons, the sharp elevation of Ca^{2+} concentration induces the activation of several enzyme pathways and signaling cascades, including various protein kinases, phospholipases, lipoxygenase, cyclooxygenase, proteases and NOS, and the generation of reactive oxygen species (ROS, oxygen free radicals) and peroxynitrite, a toxic reaction product of NO and superoxide. These reaction cascades culminate in lipid peroxidation, DNA strand breaks, and activation of caspases and poly (ADP-ribose) polymerase (PARP). As a result of these events, the affected cells die, through both apoptosis and necrosis (**Fig. 1**) *(14,15)*. In the lung, we have shown that acute NMDA exposure increases NO production and activates caspase-3 *(15)*. Furthermore, both NO synthase (NOS) inhibitors and PARP inhibitors block the development of high-permeability pulmonary edema in response to NMDA, and injury is attenuated or delayed in both neuronal NOS- and PARP-knockout mice compared to wild-type *(16)*.

8. CONCLUSIONS

Glutamate, an excitatory neurotransmitter that can be lethal to neurons upon hyperactivation of NMDA receptors, can also induce acute lung injury when added directly to perfused rat lungs. In addition, we have provided evidence that NMDA-type glutamate receptors are present in the lungs, and that activation of these receptors plays a major role in the pathogenesis of oxidant lung injury. We postulate that signaling via NMDA receptors may be a pathogenetic factor in the acute lung injury of ARDS (and may also be causally related to bronchial asthma *[17]*). Recognition of the potential significance of glutamate toxicity could lead to the introduction of novel therapeutic approaches. The physiological role(s) of glutamate signaling in the lung remains to be determined.

REFERENCES

1. Mayer, M. L., and Westbrook, G. L. (1987) The physiology of excitatory amino acids in the vertebrate central nervous system. *Prog. Neurobiol.* **28**, 197–276.
2. Erdö, S. L. (1991) Excitatory amino acid receptors in the mammalian periphery. *Trends Pharmacol. Sci.* **12**, 426–429.
3. Skerry, T. M. and Genever, P. G. (2001) Glutamate signaling in non-neuronal tissues. *Trends Pharmacol. Sci.* **22**, 174–181.
4. Olney, J. W. (1990) Excitotoxic amino acids and neuropsychiatric disorders. *Annu. Rev. Pharmacol. Toxicol.* **30**, 47–71.
5. Nicoletti, F., Bruno, V., Copani, A., et al. (1996) Metabotropic glutamate receptors: a new target for the therapy of neurodegenerative disorders? *Trends Neurosci.* **19**, 267–271.
6. Choi, D. W. (1992) Excitotoxic cell death. *J. Neurobiol.* **23**, 1261–1276.
7. Said, S. I., Berisha, H. I., and Pakbaz, H. (1996) Excitotoxicity in the lung: N-methyl-D-asparate-induced, nitric oxide-dependent, pulmonary edema is attenuated by vasoactive intestinal peptide and by inhibitors of poly (ADP-ribose) polymerase. *Proc. Natl. Acad. Sci. USA* **93**, 4688–4692.
8. Ware, L. B. and Matthay, M. A. (2000) The acute respiratory distress syndrome. *New Engl. J. Med.* **342**, 1334–1349.
9. Said, S. I., Pakbaz, H., Berisha, H. I., et al. (2000) NMDA receptor activation: critical role in oxidant tissue injury. *Free Radical Biol. Med.* **28**, 1300–1302.
10. Gegelashvili, G. and Schousboe, A. (1997) High affinity glutamate transporters: regulation of expression and activity. *Mol. Pharmacol.* **52**, 6–15.
11. Robertson, B. S., Satterfield, B. E., Said, S. I., et al. (1998) N-methyl-D-asparate receptors are expressed by intrinsic neurons of rat larynx and esophagus. *Neurosci. Letts.* **244**, 77–80.
12. Said, S. I., Dey, R. D., and Dickman, K. Glutamate signaling in the lung. *Trends Pharmacol. Sci.* (2001) **22**, 344–345.
13. Youssef, J., Dickman, K., Mathew, S., et al. (2001) Ionotropic glutamate receptors in lungs: functional basis for excitotoxic injury. *Am. J. Resp. Crit. Care* **163**, A460.
14. Ankarcrona, M., Dypbukt, J. M., Bonfoco, E., et al. (1995) Glutamate-induced neuronal death: a succession of necrosis or apoptosis depending on mitochondrial function. *Neuron* **15**, 961–973.
15. Said, S. I., Pakbaz, H., Berisha, H. I., et al. (1997) Apoptosis is a major component of excitotoxic lung injury. *Am. J. Respir. Crit. Care Med.* **154**, A95.
16. Akaza, H., Pakbaz, H., Berisha, H. I., et al. (1997) Critical role of neuronal nitric oxide synthase (nNOS) in excitotoxic lung injury: evidence from nNOS-knockout mice. *Am. Respir. Crit. Care Med.* **154**, A95.
17. Said, S. I. (1999) Glutamate receptors and asthmatic airway disease. *Trends Pharmacol. Sci.* **20**, 132–134.

7

Carboxyl Methylation of Small GTPases and Endothelial Cell Function

Sharon Rounds, Elizabeth O. Harrington, and Qing Lu

SUMMARY

Posttranslational modifications of small GTPases regulate enzyme activity and subcellular localization, resulting in altered cellular functions. The role of small-GTPase carboxyl methylation in modulating endothelial functions is not well understood. In our study, we have used cultured endothelial cells to assess the effects of inhibition of carboxyl methylation on endothelial cell function. We have found that isoprenylcysteine carboxyl methyltransferase (ICMT) inhibitors cause relocalization of focal adhesion complexes and apoptosis of endothelial cells. This is accompanied by decreased carboxyl methylation and decreased activation of Ras GTPase. Furthermore, overexpression of Ras prevents apoptosis caused by the ICMT inhibitor adenosine/homocysteine. Thus, we conclude that inhibition of Ras carboxyl methylation causes endothelial cell apoptosis. We have also found that ICMT inhibitors decrease endothelial cell migration and monolayer permeability, an effect that may be related to impaired RhoA carboxyl methylation and activation. Thus, it is evident that altered small-GTPase methylation has multiple effects on endothelial cell functions.

Key Words: Small GTPases; Ras; RhoA; carboxyl methylation; endothelium; apoptosis; cell migration; monolayer permeability.

1. INTRODUCTION

Endothelial cell injury is a hallmark of vascular injury caused by sepsis or associated with trauma. Apoptosis is a form of endothelial cell injury that controls the removal of cells during development and in response to injury. Evidence for apoptosis has been reported in lungs of patients with acute respiratory distress syndrome (ARDS) (1), in atherosclerosis (2), in hyperoxia-induced lung injury (3), and in allograft rejection of heart transplants (4). Furthermore, apoptosis is the mechanism by which angiogenesis is inhibited by angiostatin, a peptide inhibitor of neovascularization (5). Thus, the balance between endothelial cell apoptosis and proliferation is crucial in vascular injury and repair and in angiogenesis.

Angiogenesis plays a role in repair from lung injury and in conditions of abnormal lung repair, such as idopathic pulmonary fibrosis. Endothelial cell migration is an important step in angiogenesis. Changes in microvascular permeability are a hallmark of acute lung injuries such as ARDS. Thus, it is important to understand the regulation of endothelial cell apoptosis, migration, and monolayer permeability.

2. SMALL GTPASES AND THEIR POSTTRANSLATIONAL MODIFICATIONS

2.1. Small GTPases

The small GTPases are a superfamily of monomeric regulatory guanosine 5'-triphosphate (GTP)-binding proteins. The Ras protein was the first characterized of this superfamily, which is now known

From: *Cell Signaling in Vascular Inflammation*
Edited by: J. Bhattacharya © Humana Press Inc., Totowa, NJ

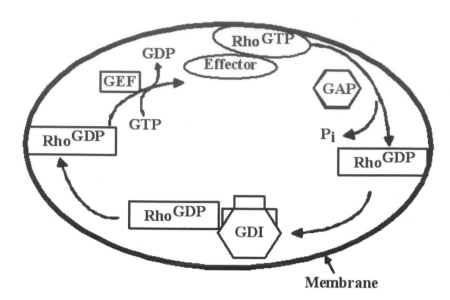

Fig. 1. Small GTPase activation cycle. GEF = guanine nucleotide exchange factor; GAP = GTPase activating protein; GDI = guanine nucleotide dissociation inhibitor.

to consist of five major classes—Ras, Rho, Rab, Arf, and RAN. In our recent work we have focused on effects of carboxyl methylation on Ras and Rho GTPases.

Mammalian small GTPases are 20- to 25-kDa GTP-binding proteins that regulate a variety of cellular functions and are ubiquitously expressed *(6,7)*. These proteins act as "molecular switches" and control cell processes by shuttling between active and inactive GTP-bound states *(6)*.

As an example, a simplified model of the Rho family GTPase cycle is displayed in **Fig. 1**. GTP binding and Rho activation are modulated by guanine exchange factors (GEFs), by GTPase-activating proteins (GAPs), and by guanine nucleotide dissociation inhibitors (GDIs) *(7)*.

The pathway(s) by which small GTPases regulate the organization of the actin cytoskeleton and associated functions is complex and the subject of intense investigation. For example, among the downstream mammalian targets of Rho identified to date are phosphatidylinositol-4-phosphate 5-kinase (PIP 5-kinase), which converts PIP to PIP2 *(8,9)*, the serine/threonine kinases ROKα/Rho kinase and p160ROCK *(8)*, and p140mDia *(10)*. Upstream regulation of Rho activity includes factors regulating cell localization and GTP binding, as noted above. In this monograph, we focus on carboxyl methylation as a means of modulating small-GTPase activation, recognizing that there are other possible modulators of GTPase action, both upstream and downstream.

Among the effects of Rho activation are changes in cell contractile properties *(11)*, such as induction of stress fibers, regulation of cell motility, enhancement of smooth-muscle contractility, and changes in myosin light chain (MLC) phosphorylation resulting in altered endothelial barrier function *(12,13)*. In addition, RhoA GTPase activation modulates integrin-mediated cell-matrix interactions via regulation of formation of focal adhesion complexes *(9)*.

2.2. Posttranslational Processing Alters Small-GTPase Function and Localization

Reversible posttranslational modifications of proteins are important mechanisms of intracellular communication. Phosphorylation is a well-studied means of modulating enzyme activity in cell signaling pathways. Methylation is analogous to phosphorylation in modulating the activity and/or location of signaling proteins, but is not as well studied. Four types of methylation reactions have been described *(14)*: (1) carboxylmethylation of glutamate side chains of cytoplasmic domains of bacterial

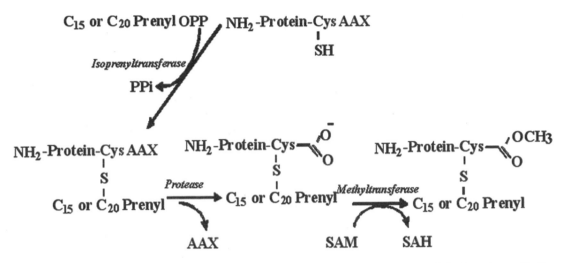

Fig. 2. Posttranslational processing of the C-terminal CAAX (C = cysteine, A = aliphatic amino acid, X = any amino acid) motif in small GTPases.

chemotaxis receptors; (2) methylation of α-carboxyl groups of terminal leucine in phosphatase 2A; (3) N^G,N^G-dimethylation of arginines in hetergeneous nuclear ribonucleoproteins; and (4) α-carboxyl methylation of cysteines in isoprenylated proteins that terminate in the CAAX motif (C = cysteine, A = aliphatic amino acid, X = any amino acid). Carboxyl methylation is reversible and thus is capable of regulating protein activity and/or location *(14)*.

Ras and Rho GTPases display a cysteine located four amino acids from the C-terminus (CAAX motif) and are subjected to a sequence of posttranslational processing (**Fig. 2**), which first involves prenylation of the cysteine with either a farnesyl (C15) or geranylgeranyl (C20) group. Prenylation is followed by proteolysis, which removes the terminal AAX amino acids. The final step is methyl esterification of the carboxyl of the prenylated cysteine by isoprenylcysteine-*O*-carboxyl methyltransferase (ICMT, EC 2.1.1.100) which utilizes *S*-adenosylmethionine (SAM) as the methyl donor, producing *S*-adenosylhomocysteine (SAH). Prenylcysteine methyl transferases have been shown to be localized in the endoplasmic reticulum membrane in *Saccharomyces cerevisiae (15)* and in mammalian cells *(16)*.

Prenylation of the CAAX motif targets proteins to the endomembrane, where they are proteolyzed and methylated. Targeting of RhoA GTPase to the cytosol is also modulated by binding to Rho guanine nucleotide dissociation inhibitor (RhoGDI) *(17)*.

Less is known about the role of methylation in regulating membrane trafficking of small GTPases. Methylation may facilitate membrane localization by enhancing hydrophobicity *(14)*, but may also regulate protein–protein interactions in a reversible manner *(18)*. In the case of RhoA GTPase, carboxyl methylation increases the half-life of the protein by decreasing degradation *(19)*. In the case of Ras GTPase, the CAAX motif is necessary for efficient tracking of Ras from the cytosol through the endomembrane system and out to the plasma membrane *(18)*. In support of the importance of isoprenylcysteine carboxyl methyltransferase (ICMT), Bergo and associates have also found that ICMT-deficient mice die by mid-gestation and lack ability to methylate Ras *(20)*.

The tools available to assess the effects of ICMT on endothelial cell functions are limited by lack of availability of an ICMT dominant negative plasmid. However, in vitro studies have demonstrated that *S*-adenosylhomocysteine (SAH) exerts product inhibition of ICMT (**Fig. 3**) *(21)*. Accumulation of SAH occurs when the action of SAH hydrolase is reversed by increased intracellular concentrations of the products adenosine and homocysteine. We have utilized adenosine and homocysteine to assess the effects of ICMT inhibition on endothelial cell function. We have studied a model of endot-

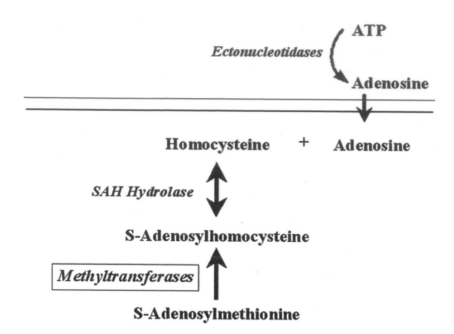

Fig. 3. Intracellular adenosine metabolism. This cartoon illustrates cellular uptake of adenosine and the effects of increased intracellular adenosine on reversal of *S*-adenosylhomocysteine (SAH) hydrolase. Increased cell concentrations of SAH, in turn, exert product inhibition of methyltransferases.

helial cell apoptosis caused by extracellular ATP and adenosine, which is dependent upon cellular uptake of adenosine, derived by ectonucleotidase action on ATP *(22)*. The effect of adenosine was potentiated by homocysteine and mimicked by inhibitors of SAH hydrolase *(23)*. We have found that adenosine increases endothelial-cell SAH and decreases the ratio of *S*-adenosylmethionine (SAM) to SAH, a condition favoring inhibition of ICMT *(23)*. This model of endothelial cell injury has been a useful tool to assess the effects of inhibition of methyltransferases on small-GTPase methylation, activation, and function.

In addition, chemical inhibitors of ICMT are available, such as *N*-acetyl-*S*-geranylgeranyl-L-cysteine (AGGC) and *N*-acetyl-*S*-farnesyl-L-cysteine (AFC). These agents compete with endogenous substrates for methylation. We found that the chemical inhibitors of ICMT, AGGC and AFC, also caused endothelial cell apoptosis. The inactive analog, *N*-acetyl-geranyl-L-cysteine (AGC), had no effect *(24,25)*.

3. CARBOXYL METHYLATION OF RAS GTPASE AND ENDOTHELIAL CELL APOPTOSIS

3.1. Inhibition of ICMT Causes Disruption of Focal Adhesion Complexes and Endothelial Cell Apoptosis

Focal adhesion complexes are critical in maintaining cell–extracellular matrix interactions. Disruption of cell–substratum association causes apoptosis of anchorage-dependent cells, such as endothelial cells. This process has been termed *anoikis* or *homelessness (26)*.

Focal adhesion complexes are protein aggregates that link cytoskeletal actin filaments to the cytoplasmic domain of extracellular matrix receptors (integrins) and mediate intracellular signal transduction (**Fig. 4**) *(11)*. Among the components of focal adhesion complexes are cytoplasmic domains of α and β integrin subunits; intracellular signaling proteins, such as the tyrosine kinases, Src, and

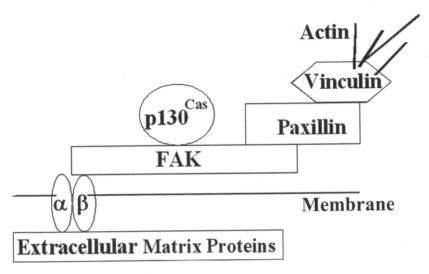

Fig. 4. Components of focal adhesion complexes.

focal adhesion kinase (FAK); actin-binding structural proteins, such as vinculin, talin, and α-actinin; and adaptor proteins, such as paxillin and p130[Cas], which mediate protein–protein interactions.

We found that disruption of focal adhesion complexes occurred after only a few hours of incubation with adenosine/homocysteine (**Fig. 5**) *(27)*. This was followed by caspase-dependent degradation of FAK, paxillin, and p130[Cas], and apoptosis *(27)*. However, caspase inhibition did not alter relocalization of focal adhesion complex components. These studies indicate that disruption of focal adhesion complexes, independent of caspase activation, is an important early event in adenosine/homocysteine-induced apoptosis. As further evidence of the central importance of focal adhesion complexes in endothelial apoptosis, we have reported that overexpression of focal adhesion kinase blunts endothelial apoptosis resulting from adenosine/homocysteine *(28)*.

3.2. Ras Carboxyl Methylation Is Involved in Endothelial Cell Apoptosis

Ras GTPases are signaling proteins important in many cellular functions, including the organization of cytoskeletal proteins necessary for cell motility, adhesion, and proliferation *(10)*. It is possible that ICMT modulates apoptosis through effects on carboxyl methylation of small GTPases. Indeed, the absence of ICMT caused mislocalization of K-Ras from the plasma membrane to cytoplasm in cells derived from ICMT knockout embryos *(29)*, suggesting that carboxyl methylation of C-terminal isoprenylcysteine is important in subcellular localization and possibly in normal enzymatic function of K-Ras GTPase. Wang et al. demonstrated that coincubation of endothelial cells with homocysteine and the adenosine deaminase inhibitor erythro-9-(2-hydroxy-3-nonyl)-adenosine (EHNA), a maneuver which inhibits carboxyl methyltransferase activity, decreased plasma membrane localization of Ras *(30)*. These data again suggest the importance for carboxyl methylation of Ras GTPase in protein subcellular localization. Yet, little is known about the effects of ICMT inhibition and the importance of alterations in posttranslational modification on small-GTPase function.

We assessed the effects of ICMT inhibitors on Ras carboxyl methylation and activation. We found that adenosine/homocysteine and AGGC decreased Ras activation, and that AGGC decreased Ras carboxyl methylation (**Fig. 6**) *(25)*. Furthermore, we found that overexpression of wild-type or dominant active Ras blunted adenosine/homocysteine-induced endothelial cell apoptosis *(25)*. These results indicate that inhibitors of ICMT cause endothelial cell apoptosis by interfering with carboxyl methylation and activation of Ras GTPase.

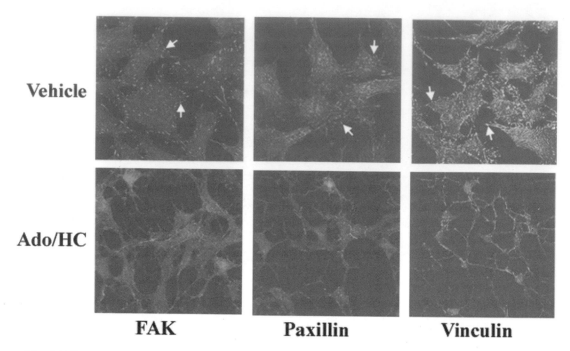

Fig. 5. Effects of adenosine/homocysteine on focal adhesion complexes. Cultured bovine pulmonary artery endothelial cells were incubated with medium alone (vehicle), or adenosine/homocysteine (100 μM) for 4 h. Cells were then assessed for localization of focal adhesion complexes (arrows) with antibodies directly against FAK, paxillin and vinculin by immunofluorescence microscopy.

4. CARBOXYL METHYLATION OF SMALL GTPASES AND CELL MIGRATION

Actomyosin stress fiber formation occurs in endothelial cells in response to a variety of stimuli, such as shear stress and thrombin. Cell migration is complex, involving a coordinated sequence of events, including cell extension, attachment of extended lamellipodia, contraction, release of focal adhesion complexes, and recycling of adhesive and signaling materials *(31)*. Inhibition of stress fiber formation inhibits endothelial cell motility.

Effects of small-GTPase activation on endothelial cell migration appear to be stimulus specific. Inhibition of RhoA prevented cell migration in response to wounding *(32)*. However, Liu et al. have reported that sphingosine-1-phosphate, but not vascular endothelial growth factor (VEGF), -induced endothelial cell chemotaxis is dependent on Rho activation *(33)*. Furthermore, Soga et al. have reported that VEGF- and collagen-stimulated endothelial cell chemotaxis were dependent on Rac, but not on RhoA GTPase activation *(34)*. Soga et al. point out that although overexpression of dominant active RhoA enhanced microvascular endothelial cell stress fiber and focal adhesion complex formation, there was no effect on chemotaxis *(34)*. Thus, it is possible that other small GTPases are more important than RhoA in regulating endothelial-cell motility, dependent upon the stimulus. Indeed, cell extension and lamellipodia formation are thought to involve the small GTPases Rac and Cdc42, while RhoA GTPase regulates stress fiber formation and focal adhesion complex formation *(31)*. Thus, the role of small GTPases in regulation of cell migration is complex.

We have found that ICMT inhibitors decrease lamellipodia formation stimulated by hepatocyte growth factor (HGF) *(35)*. In addition, adenosine/homocysteine decreases both baseline and HGF-stimulated endothelial cell migration *(35)*. Further studies will be necessary to determine which small GTPase(s) is (are) critical to endothelial cell migration.

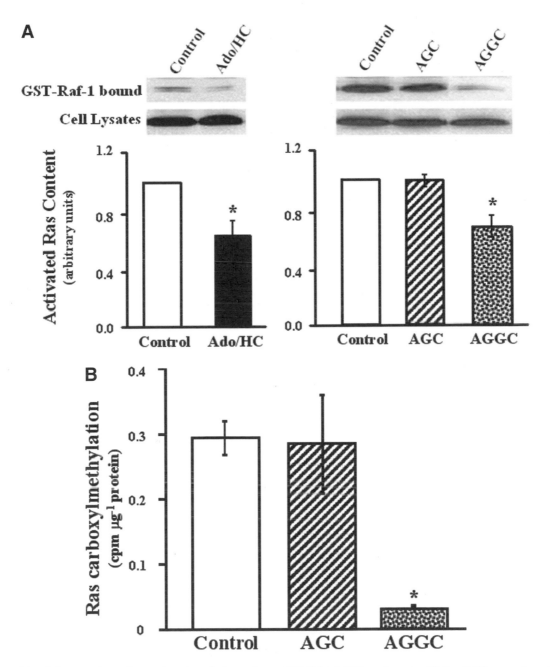

Fig. 6. Isoprenylcysteine carboxyl methyltransferase (ICMT) inhibition attenuates H-Ras GTPase carboxyl methylation and activity. porcine aortic endothelial cells were incubated in the absence or presence of 100 μM Ado/HC, 20 μM AGC, or 20 μM AGGC (**A** and **B**) for 4 h at 37°C. In **A**, cell lysates were harvested and active Ras GTPase was purified with glutathione-*S*-transferase (GST) fused Raf-1 protein bound to glutathione agarose beads. Parallel gels were run with corresponding crude lysates. All gels were immunoblotted for H-Ras GTPase. Immunoblot signals were quantitated by densitometry and are presented as the mean ± standard error of the ratio of GST-Raf-1-bound H-Ras GTPase to total H-Ras GTPase present in crude lysate. In **B**, H-Ras GTPase was immunoprecipitated, resolved on sodium dodecyl sulfate (SDS)-polyacrylamide gel electrophoresis (PAGE), and immunoblotted for H-Ras GTPase. Illuminated bands were excised, hydrolyzed, and the level of 3H-methyl incorporation was determined. $n = 4$. *$p < 0.05$.

5. CARBOXYL METHYLATION OF SMALL GTPASES AND MONOLAYER PERMEABILITY

The actomyosin cytoskeleton is also critical in modulating monolayer permeability. Cell activation by a variety of agents, including thrombin, tumor necrosis factor (TNF)-α, and reactive oxygen species, and stretch stimulates stress fiber formation, followed by the appearance of intercellular gaps and enhanced monolayer permeability *(36)*. The process of enhancement of monolayer permeability is complex, involving disruption of focal adhesion complexes, phosphorylation of MLC, stress fiber formation, and disruption of cell–cell junctions. Inhibition of stress fiber formation by inhibition of MLC kinase has been shown to prevent monolayer permeability caused by a variety of agents.

RhoA GTPase stimulation by lysophosphatidic acid or by overexpression of dominant active RhoA mutants enhances stress fiber formation in a number of cell types, while inhibition of RhoA GTPase, such as by C3 exotoxin and overexpression of dominant negative mutants, has the opposite effect *(37,38)*. In endothelial cells, inhibition of RhoA GTPase prevented stress fiber formation, MLC phosphorylation, and increased monolayer permeability caused by thrombin *(39–42)*, oxidized low-density lipoprotein *(43)*, bacterial lipopolysaccharide *(42)*, histamine *(13)*, and shear stress *(44)*. The mechanism of RhoA GTPase-induced increases in monolayer permeability may involve activation of the downsteam effector Rho kinase, resulting in phosphorylation of MLC. Alternatively, Rho kinase may inhibit MLC phosphatase (PP1M), indirectly increasing MLC phosphorylation *(36)*. Less well understood in endothelial cells are other mechanisms by which RhoA may modulate stress fiber formation, including effects on mDia, PIP 5-kinase, ERM proteins, Na^+/H^+ exchanger, adducin, and LIM kinase *(13)*. Finally, it is also possible that other small GTPases, Rac1 and Cdc42, modulate endothelial monolayer permeability by altering cell-cell junctions. We hypothesized that decreased carboxyl methylation and decreased activation of either RhoA or Rac1/Cdc42 might alter endothelial monolayer permeability. We have found that ICMT inhibitors decrease endothelial monolayer permeability *(35,45)*. This was concomitant with decreased carboxyl methylation and activation of RhoA GTPase. Further studies are needed to determine the identity of small GTPase(s) involved in regulation of monolayer permeability.

6. IN VIVO CORRELATION

The studies reported above were all performed using cultured bovine pulmonary artery endothelial cells. Recent studies suggest that increased concentrations of adenosine causes lung-cell apoptosis in the intact organism. Blackburn et al. have developed a very interesting model of lung injury in which the enzyme adenosine deaminase (ADA) is absent and lung adenosine levels are increased. In ADA-deficient mice, alveologenesis was lacking *(46)*. Subsequently these investigators have reported increased apoptosis in lungs from ADA-deficient animals *(47)*. These studies suggest that increased adenosine causes lung-cell apoptosis, perhaps through inhibition of ICMT.

In another recent study Cohen et al. assessed the effects of an adenosine deaminase inhibitor, 2'-deoxycoformycin, on vascular leakage in a mouse model of sepsis caused by cecal ligation and puncture *(48)*. These investigators found that the ADA inhibitor decreased vascular leakage and improved mortality in this model of multisystem organ failure. These results suggest that increased adenosine decreases vascular permeability in vivo, an effect potentially related to ICMT inhibition.

Clearly, further work is needed to determine the in vivo effects of changes in small-GTPase methylation and activation.

ACKNOWLEDGMENTS

The authors acknowledge the contributions of Robert Bellas, Julie Newton, Kerri-Lynn Sheahan, and Kristina Kramer to the work reported here. The authors also acknowledge funding from the VA (Merit Review), the VA/Department of Defense (Collaborative Research Award), and the NHLBI (HL 64936 and HL 67795).

REFERENCES

1. Polunovsky, V. A., Chen, B., Henke, C., et al. (1993) Role of mesenchymal cell death in lung remodeling after injury. *J. Clin. Invest.* **92**, 388–397.
2. Cai, W., Devaux, B., Schaper, W., and Schaper, J. (1997) The role of Fas/APO 1 and apoptosis in the development of human atherosclerotic lesions. *Atherosclerosis* **131**, 177–186.
3. Barazzone, C., Horowitz, S., Donati, Y. R., Rodriguez, I., and Piguet, P. F. (1998) Oxygen toxicity in mouse lung: pathways to cell death. *Am. J. Respir. Cell Mol. Biol.* **19**, 573–581.
4. Szabolcs, M., Michler, R. E., Yang, X., et al. (1996) Apoptosis of cardiac myocytes during cardiac allograft rejection. Relation to induction of nitric oxide synthase. *Circulation* **94**, 1665–1673.
5. Claesson-Welsh, L., Welsh, M., Ito, N., et al. (1998) Angiostatin induces endothelial cell apoptosis and activation of focal adhesion kinase independently of the integrin-binding motif RGD. *Proc. Natl. Acad. Sci. USA* **95**, 5579–5583.
6. Boivin, D., Bilodeau, D., and Beliveau, R. (1996) Regulation of cytoskeletal functions by Rho small GTP-binding proteins in normal and cancer cells. *Can. J. Pharmacol.* **74**, 801–810.
7. Ridley, A. (2000) Rho GTPases: integrating integrin signaling. *J. Cell Biol.* **150**, F107–F109.
8. Van Aelst, L. and D'Souza-Schorey, C. (1997) Rho GTPases and signaling networks. *Genes Dev.* **11**, 2295–2322.
9. Hall, A. (1998) Rho GTPases and the actin cytoskeleton. *Science* **279**, 509–514.
10. Mackay, D. and Hall, A. (1998) Rho GTPases. *J. Biol. Chem.* **273**, 20,685–20,688.
11. Burridge, K. and Chrzanowska-Wodnicka, M. (1996) Focal adhesions, contractility, and signaling. *Annu. Rev. Cell Dev. Biol.* **12**, 463 518.
12. Garcia, J. G., Verin, A. D., Schaphorst, K., et al. (1999) Regulation of endothelial cell myosin light chain kinase by Rho, cortactin, and p60(src). *Am. J. Physiol.* **276**, L989–L998.
13. van Nieuw Amerongen, G. P., Draijer, R., Vermeer, M. A., and van Hinsbergh, V. W. M. (1998) Transient and prolonged increase in endothelial permeability induced by histamine and thrombin. Role of protein kinases, calcium, and RhoA. *Circ. Res.* **83**, 1115 1123.
14. Djordjevic, S., Stock, A. M., Chen, Y., and Stock, J. B. (1999) Protein methyltransferases involved in signal transduction. In: Chen X. and Blumenthal, R. M.(eds.), *S-Adenosylmethionine-Dependent Methyltransferases: Structure and Functions.* World Scientific, Singapore: 149–183.
15. Romano, J. D., Schmidt, W. K., and Michaelis, S. (1998) The Saccharomyces cerevisiae prenylcysteine carboxyl methyltransferase Ste14p is in the endoplasmic reticulum membrane. *Mol. Biol. Cell* **9**, 2231–2247.
16. Dai, Q., Choy, E., Chiu, V., et al. (1998) Mammalian prenylcysteine carboxyl methyltransferase is in the endoplasmic reticulum. *J. Biol. Chem.* **273**, 15,030–15,034.
17. Michaelson, D. S. J., Murphy, G., D'Eustachio, P., Rush, M., and Philips, M. R. (2001) Differential localization of Rho GTPases in live cells: regulation by hypervariable regions and RhoGDI binding. *J. Cell Biol.* **152**, 111–126.
18. Choy, E., Chiu, V. K., Silletti, J., et al. (1999) Endomembrane trafficking of ras: the CAAX motif targets proteins to the ER and Golgi. *Cell* **98**, 69–80.
19. Backlund, P. S. J. (1997) Post-translational processing of RhoA. Carboxyl methylation of the carboxyl-terminal prenylcysteine increases the half-life of RhoA. *J. Biol. Chem.* **272**, 33,175–33,180.
20. Bergo, M. O., Leung, G. K., Ambroziak, P., et al. (2001) Isoprenylcysteine carboxyl methyltransferase deficiency in mice. *J. Biol. Chem.* **276**, 5841–5845.
21. Stephenson, R. and Clarke, S. (1990) Identification of a C-terminal carboxyl methyltransferase in rat liver membranes utilizing a synthetic farnesyl cysteine-containing peptide substrate. *J. Biol. Chem.* **265**, 16,248–16,254.
22. Dawicki, D. D., Chatterjee, D., Wyche, J., and Rounds, S. (1997) Extracellular ATP and adenosine cause apoptosis of pulmonary artery endothelial cells. *Am. J. Physiol.* **273**, L485–L494.
23. Rounds, S., Yee, W. L., Dawicki, D. D., Harrington, E., Parks, N., and Cutaia, M. V. (1998) Mechanism of extracellular ATP- and adenosine-induced apoptosis of cultured pulmonary artery endothelial cells. *Am. J. Physiol.* **275**, L379–L388.
24. Rounds, S., Harrington, E., Bellas, R., and Newton, J. (2002) Methylation and endothelial cell apoptosis. *Am. J. Resp. Crit. Care Med.* **165**, A102.
25. Kramer, K., Harrington, E., Lu, Q., et al. (2003) Isoprenylcysteine carboxyl methyltransferase activity modulates endothelial cell apoptosis. *Mol. Biol. Cell* **14**, 848–857.
26. Frisch, S. M., Vuori, K., Ruoslahti, E., and Chan-Hui, P-Y. (1996) Control of adhesion-dependent cell survival by focal adhesion kinase. *J. Cell Biol.* **134**, 793–799.
27. Harrington, E., Smeglin, A., Newton, J., Ballard, G., and Rounds, S. (2001) Adenosine/homocysteine-induced disruption of endothelial cell focal adhesion contacts requires protein tyrosine phosphatase and caspase activity. *Am. J. Physiol. Lung Cell Mol. Physiol.* **280**, L342–L353.
28. Bellas, R., Harrington, E., Sheahan, K. L., Newton, J., and Rounds, S. (2002) Over-Expression of focal adhesion kinase protects against adenosine/homocysteine-induced apoptosis. *Am. J. Physiol. Lung Cell Mol. Physiol.* **282**, L1135–L1142.
29. Bergo, M. O., Leung, G. K., Ambroziak, P., Otto, J. C., Casey, P. J., and Young, S. G. (2000) Targeted inactivation of the isoprenylcysteine carboxyl methyltransferase gene causes mislocalization of K-Ras in mammalian cells. *J. Biol. Chem.* **275**, 17,605–17,610.
30. Wang, H., Yoshizumi, M., Lai, K., et al. (1997) Inhibition of growth and p21ras methylation in vascular endothelial cells by homocysteine but not cysteine. *J. Biol. Chem.* **272**, 25,380–25,385.
31. Rousseau, S., Houle, F., and Huot, J. (2001) Integrating the VEGF signals leading to actin-based motility in vascular endothelial cells. *Trends Cardiovasc. Med.* **10**, 321–327.

32. Aepfelbacher, M., Essler, M., Huber, E., Sugai, M., and Weber, P. C. (1997) Bacterial toxins block endothelial wound repair. Evidence that RhoGTPases control cytoskeletal rearrangements in migrating endothelial cells. *Arterio. Thromb. Vasc. Biol.* **17,** 1623–1629.

33. Liu, F., Verin, A. D., Wang, P., et al. (2001) Differential regulation of sphingosine-1-phosphate- and VEGF-induced endothelial cell chemotaxis. *Am. J. Respir. Cell Mol. Biol.* **24,** 711–719.

34. Soga, N., Namba, N., McAllister, S., et al. (2001) Rho family GTPases regulate VEGF-stimulated endothelial cell motility. *Exp. Cell Res.* **269,** 73–87.

35. Harrington, E., Newton, J., and Rounds, S. (2002) Methyltransferase inhibition decreases endothelial cell migration and monolayer permeability. *FASEB J.* **16,** A209.

36. Dudek, S. M. and Garcia, J. G. N. (2001) Cytoskeletal regulation of pulmonary vascular permeability. *J. Appl. Physiol.* **91,** 1487–1500.

37. Amano, M., Chihara, K., Kimura, K., et al. (1997) Formation of actin stress fibers and focal adhesions enhanced by Rho-kinase. *Science* **275,** 1308–1311.

38. Kaibuchi, K., Kuroda, S., and Amano, M. (1999) Regulation of the cytoskeleton and cell adhesion by the Rho family GTPases in mammalian cells. *Annu. Rev. Biochem.* **68,** 459–486.

39. Wojciak-Slothard, B., Potempa, S., Eichholtz, T., and Ridley, A. J. (2001) Rho and Rac but not Cdc42 regulate endothelial cell permeability. *J. Cell Sci.* **114,** 1343–1355.

40. Carbajal, J. M. and Schaeffer, R. C., Jr. (1999) RhoA inactivation enhances endothelial barrier function. *Am. J. Physiol.* **277,** C955–C964.

41. Vouret-Craviari, V., Boquet, P., Pouyssegur, J., and van Obberghen-Schilling, E. (1998) Regulation of the actin cytoskeleton by thrombin in human endothelial cells: Role of Rho proteins in endothelial barrier function. *Mol. Biol. Cell.* **9,** 2639–2653.

42. Essler, M., Staddon, J. M., Wever, P. C., and Aepfelbacher, M. (2000) Cyclic AMP blocks bacterial liposaccharide-induced myosin light chain phosphorylation in endothelial cells through inhibition of Rho/Rho kinase signaling. *J. Immunol.* **164,** 6543–6549.

43. Essler, M., Retzer, M., Bauer, M., Heemskerk, J. W., Aepfelbacher, M., and Siess, W. (1999) Mildly oxidized low density lipoptotein induces contraction of human endothelial cells through activation of Rho/Rho kinase and inhibition of myosin light chain phosphatase. *J. Biol. Chem.* **274,** 30,361–30,364.

44. Li, S., Chen, B. P. C., Azuma, N., et al. (1999) Distinct roles for the small GTPases Cdc42 and Rho in endothelial responses to shear stress. *J. Clin. Invest.* **103,** 1141–1150.

45. Lu, Q., Harrington, E., Hai, C-M., et al. (2004) Isoprenylcysteine carboxyl methyltransferase (ICMT) modulates endothelial monolayer permeability: involvement of RhoA carboxyl methylation. *Circ. Res.* **94,** 306–315.

46. Blackburn, M., Volmer, J., Thrasher, J., et al. (2000) Metabolic consequences of adenosine deaminase deficiency in mice are associated with defects in alveologenesis, pulmonary inflammation, and airway obstruction. *J. Exp. Med.* **192,** 159–170.

47. Banerjee, S., Zhong, H., and Blackburn, M. (2002) Adenosine signaling in normal and abnormal alveologenesis. *Am. J. Resp. Crit. Care Med.* **165,** A641.

48. Cohen, E., Law, W., Easington, C., et al. (2002) Adenosine deaminase inhibition attenuates microvascular dysfunction and improves survival in sepsis. *Am. J. Resp. Crit. Care Med.* **166,** 16–20.

8

Pressure-Induced Inflammatory Signaling in Lung Endothelial Cells

Wolfgang M. Kuebler

SUMMARY

Elevation of lung capillary pressure is a frequent clinical consequence of left-sided heart disease and characteristically results in the formation not only of pulmonary edema, but also of inflammatory reactions in the lung. These processes are largely attributable to mechano-induced second-messenger responses in lung capillary endothelial cells. Pressure- and stretch-induced mobilization of intra- and extracellular calcium mediates an increase in capillary permeability, thus contributing to pulmonary edema formation. In addition, endothelial calcium signaling promotes the exocytosis of endothelial Weibel-Palade bodies and, in consequence, vascular expression of P-selectin, thus initiating the sequestration of circulating leukocytes.

Inflammatory effects of mechanical forces are not only evident in endothelial cell cultures, but are a prominent feature in intact lung capillaries, as demonstrated by *in situ* fluorescence imaging techniques. Clinical data support the notion of pressure-induced inflammatory signaling in the pulmonary microvasculature, which may play an important, yet commonly neglected role in the pathophysiology of acute and chronic pressure-induced lung disease.

Key Words: Lung edema; pulmonary venous hypertension; hydrostatic pressure; mechanotransduction; pulmonary endothelium; endothelial dysfunction; calcium signaling; exocytosis; P-selectin; leukocyte-endothelial interaction.

1. INTRODUCTION

In lung capillaries, endothelial cells serve numerous physiological functions, such as the maintenance of microvascular barrier properties, the establishment of a nonthrombogenic luminal surface, or the release of vasoactive factors such as nitric oxide (NO), prostacyclin (PGI$_2$), or cytochrome P450-derived arachidonic acid metabolites. Under inflammatory and/or thrombogenic conditions, the endothelium moreover releases pro-inflammatory cytokines and pro-coagulant factors and promotes the adhesion and emigration of leukocytes and the sequestration of platelets. These endothelial functions and reactions are regulated by complex intracellular second-messenger pathways, which are evoked not only by activation of receptors on the cell surface, but also by mechanical forces such as shear, stretch, or pressure stress. Here, we will focus specifically on endothelial signaling pathways in response to increased capillary pressure in the lung.

2. THE PATHOGENESIS OF HYDROSTATIC STRESS IN LUNG CAPILLARIES

By far the most common cause of increased hydrostatic pressure in lung capillaries is pulmonary congestion resulting from left-sided atrial, ventricular, or valvular heart disease. Lung capillary pres-

From: *Cell Signaling in Vascular Inflammation*
Edited by: J. Bhattacharya © Humana Press Inc., Totowa, NJ

sure (P_c) depends largely upon left atrial pressure (P_{LA}), which is markedly elevated under these pathological conditions. In healthy subjects, P_{LA} rarely exceeds 6 mmHg, but may rise above 20 mmHg during strenuous exercise *(1)*. Rare causes of increased hydrostatic stress in lung capillaries include extrinsic compression of central pulmonary veins due to fibrosing mediastinitis, adenopathies or tumors, or idiopathic disorders such as pulmonary veno-occlusive disease.

In addition, increased lung capillary pressure may also derive from downstream transmission of pulmonary arterial hypertension. This unique phenomenon may play a prominent role in the pathogenesis of high-altitude and neurogenic pulmonary edema. While arterial/arteriolar vasoconstriction is considered to be the predominant cause of pulmonary hypertension in both scenarios, edema formation correlates closely with pulmonary capillary, but not arterial, pressure *(2)*. The hemodynamic mechanisms underlying capillary hypertension in high-altitude pulmonary edema are still discussed, but three main hypotheses have been proposed:

1. Lung capillaries frequently branch off directly from large arterioles and form complex perivascular networks *(3)*. These capillary beds are less protected from arterial hypertension and co-localize with the site of initial fluid accumulation in diverse pathologic states, including high-altitude pulmonary edema.
2. Uneven distribution of arteriolar smooth-muscle cells may cause inhomogeneous hypoxic vasoconstriction and hence result in regional overperfusion *(4)*.
3. Finally, hypoxia induces pulmonary venoconstriction, which may account for up to 20% of the total increase in pulmonary vascular resistance *(5)*.

3. ENDOTHELIAL DYSFUNCTION IN LUNG CAPILLARY HYPERTENSION

The notion of pressure-induced pathology in lung capillaries was long determined by the basic concepts of transcapillary fluid dynamics, with little attention to active cellular responses. Elevated microvascular pressure increases lung fluid filtration, as described by the Starling equation, and thus promotes the formation of hydrostatic pulmonary edema. Since under physiological conditions, more than 80% of total transendothelial protein flux is attributable to convection, P_c determines not only the rate of passive fluid filtration but also that of protein transport. In addition, transmural pressures greater than 40 mmHg can cause capillary stress failure, which is characterized by ultrastructural disruptions of both the capillary endothelial and the alveolar epithelial layer, and may result in interstitial and alveolar extravasation of blood cells and plasma proteins *(6)*.

However, recent reports indicate that the lung microvascular response to high pressure may be more complex. P_{LA} elevation to 20–50 cmH$_2$O increases the lung capillary filtration coefficient (K_{fc}) *(7)* and enhances transvascular protein flow *(8)*. Bhattacharya et al. reported an exponential increase in lung wet weight at increased hydrostatic pressure, indicating a progressive deterioration of the microvascular barrier function *(9)*. In isolated perfused rat lungs exposed to pulmonary venous pressures of 24 mmHg, Parker and Ivey demonstrated an increase in K_{fc} that was largely inhibitable by isoproterenol *(7)*. The authors suggested that isoproterenol may inhibit the Ca^{2+}-dependent activation of endothelial myosin light chain kinase by increasing the intracellular concentration of cAMP, thus proposing an active endothelial response regulated by different second-messenger pathways.

More recently, increased hydrostatic pressure was shown to induce apoptosis in lung capillary endothelial cells *(10)* and impair active Na$^+$ transport in alveolar type II cells, as well as alveolar fluid absorption *(11)*. Although the latter phenomenon reflects an epithelial response, it requires signal communication across the endothelial layer and the alveolo-capillary membrane, which presumably involves activation of second-messenger pathways and/or intercellular signaling molecules *(12)*.

The notion of an active endothelial reaction to pressure stress is based on the principles of mechanotransduction, which mediates cellular responses to mechanical stress through activation and regulation of intracellular second-messenger pathways. Of relevance are not only endothelial responses to compressive effects of vascular pressure, but also to possible stretch-induced effects occurring secondary to vascular distension. Vessel distension may, in addition, alter capillary hemodynamics, and thus affect shear forces acting on the endothelial layer. Since the microvascular endothelium forms the front line exposed to hemodynamic alterations, microvascular endothelial cells are considered to direct pressure-dependent cellular responses. However, a traditional difficulty in the understanding of mechano-induced effects and underlying mechanotransduction pathways lies in the quantification of single cell responses in the complex, dynamic, and multicellular context of an intact microvascular bed.

4. *IN SITU* IMAGING OF ENDOTHELIAL RESPONSES TO HYDROSTATIC STRESS

We have addressed this issue through the application of fluorescence microscopy and digital imaging techniques in venular capillaries of the isolated, blood-perfused rat lung. This approach, which enables optical analyses of endothelial responses to elevated capillary pressure, is briefly described here. Experiments are performed in the previously described model of the isolated, blood-perfused rat lung *(13)*. Lungs are constantly inflated and continuously pump perfused with 14 mL/min autologous rat blood. At baseline, pulmonary artery pressure (P_{PA}) is adjusted to 10 cmH$_2$O and P_{LA} to 5 cmH$_2$O. For local delivery of fluorophores, a microcatheter is advanced through the left atrium into the pulmonary venous system and wedged in a small vein draining a capillary area on the lung surface. Via this microcatheter, fluorophores are loaded into subpleural lung capillaries and/or the capillary endothelium, depending on their membrane permeability. Fluorescence is excited by single-wavelength illumination generated either by a monochromator or a filter wheel. Fluorescence emission is collected through appropriate objectives and filters by a digital camera and subjected to digital image analysis.

5. ENDOTHELIAL CA^{2+} RESPONSE TO HYDROSTATIC STRESS IN LUNG CAPILLARIES

Specifically, we considered the possibility that hydrostatic stress may trigger changes in the cytosolic Ca^{2+} concentration ($[Ca^{2+}]_i$) in capillary endothelial cells. $[Ca^{2+}]_i$ is a ubiquitous second-messenger system mediating cellular responses to chemical, electrical, mechanical, or humoral stimuli. $[Ca^{2+}]_i$ transients play a central role in endothelial mechanotransduction and can be evoked in vitro by mechanical stretch *(14)* or direct pressure stress *(15)*. We therefore monitored endothelial $[Ca^{2+}]_i$ in lung capillaries *in situ* by use of the fura-2 ratio imaging technique *(13)*. Membrane-permeant fura-2/AM, which de-esterifies intracellularly to the impermeant Ca^{2+}-indicator fura-2, is loaded to capillary endothelial cells of the isolated rat lung using the venous microcatheter. From the ratio of endothelial fluorescence intensities determined at excitation wavelengths of 340 and 380 nm, respectively, endothelial $[Ca^{2+}]_i$ is calculated based on a K_d of 224 nmol/L and appropriate calibration parameters *(13)*.

In a first set of experiments, we studied the endothelial $[Ca^{2+}]_i$ response during a 30-min increase of P_{LA} from 5 to 20 cmH$_2$O. Corresponding P_{PA} rose from 10 to 24 cmH$_2$O. P_{LA} elevation results in a rapid dilation of lung venular capillaries and a progressive increase in mean endothelial $[Ca^{2+}]_i$. Concomitantly, $[Ca^{2+}]_i$ oscillations, which are absent in cultured endothelial cells in vitro but generated spontaneously in intact lung microvessels *in situ (13)*, increase in amplitude, but not in frequency *(16)*. These $[Ca^{2+}]_i$ transients demonstrate an active endothelial second-messenger response to elevated lung hydrostatic pressure. Both increases are initiated after a temporal lag of approx 5 min and continue progressively over the 30-min interval of P_{LA} elevation (**Fig. 1**). Returning P_{LA} to physiological values re-establishes the baseline $[Ca^{2+}]_i$ profile in less than 2 min. The approx 5-min lag in the onset of the observed $[Ca^{2+}]_i$ responses contrasts with reports from cultured endothelial cells, in which mechanical stretch mobilizes $[Ca^{2+}]_i$ within seconds *(14)*. In vivo, the lag may constitute a protective mechanism, since lung capillary endothelial cells are physiologically exposed to cyclic

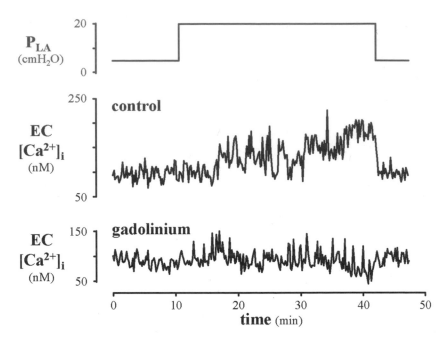

Fig. 1. Endothelial cell cytosolic Ca^{2+} concentration (EC $[Ca^{2+}]_i$) response to increased pulmonary left atrial pressure (P_{LA}, top graph). Tracings of $[Ca^{2+}]_i$ in representative, single endothelial cells of lung venular capillaries were obtained under control conditions (center graph) and during infusion of the cation channel blocker gadolinium (bottom graph). Note baseline $[Ca^{2+}]_i$ oscillations and pressure-induced $[Ca^{2+}]_i$ oscillations of increased amplitude in both tracings. Methods and experimental protocol have previously been described in detail *(16)*.

pressure pulsations transmitted from the arterial system and distortional stress during the breathing cycle. Since the lag interval exceeds the time course of these oscillatory distortions, it may act as a lowpass filter and prevent endothelial activation by these physiological cycles.

To determine the sensitivity of the endothelial $[Ca^{2+}]_i$ response to hydrostatic stress, we determined the effects of different levels of pressure elevation. The resulting increases in mean endothelial $[Ca^{2+}]_i$ and in the amplitude of $[Ca^{2+}]_i$ oscillations occur in linear proportion to the imposed pressure stress, and are evident at pressure increases of as little as 5 cmH$_2$O *(16)*. This finding indicates that in the lung, microvascular pressure elevations that were previously considered nonpathogenic suffice to activate endothelial second-messenger signaling.

In order to determine the origin of these pressure-induced endothelial $[Ca^{2+}]_i$ transients, we elevated P_{LA} while infusing capillaries with either gadolinium (GdCl$_3$) (an inhibitor of both stretch- and pressure-activated cell membrane cation channels) or a Ca^{2+}-free buffer. Both treatments inhibit the increase in mean endothelial $[Ca^{2+}]_i$ but not the increase in $[Ca^{2+}]_i$ oscillations (**Fig. 1**). Hence, the endothelial $[Ca^{2+}]_i$ response to hydrostatic stress is complex and involves at least two different mechanotransduction pathways:

1. Hydrostatic stress induces Ca^{2+} influx through mechanosensitive, gadolinium-inhibitable cation channels. This finding is consistent with previous reports in cultured endothelial cells exposed to uniaxial stretch *(14)*.
2. In addition, pressure elevation enhances $[Ca^{2+}]_i$ oscillations, which are independent from external Ca^{2+} and gadolinium-inhibitable cation channels, and thus result from mobilization of intracellular Ca^{2+} stores.

Since in cultured endothelial cells, cyclic stretch activates phospholipase C leading to the generation of inositol 1,4,5-trisphosphate (IP$_3$) and IP$_3$-mediated Ca^{2+} release from intracellular Ca^{2+} pools

(17), activation of the phospholipase C/IP_3-pathway may account for the pressure-induced generation of endothelial $[Ca^{2+}]_i$ oscillations *in situ*. Taken together, hydrostatic stress evokes complex $[Ca^{2+}]_i$ signaling in lung capillary endothelial cells that involves mobilization of both extra- and intracellular Ca^{2+}.

Sequential images and fast Fourier analysis revealed that both spontaneous and pressure-induced $[Ca^{2+}]_i$ oscillations are spatially heterogeneous, in that they originate from a specific subset of endothelial cells and are propagated for short distances along the capillary wall as intercellular Ca^{2+} waves *(13,16)*. Accordingly, the cells from which these Ca^{2+} waves originate are called "pacemaker cells." Pacemaker cells are preferentially located at the microvascular branch points and characterized by a 30% higher $[Ca^{2+}]_i$ as compared to adjacent nonpacemaker endothelial cells *(16)*. The unique ability of the pacemaker cells to generate $[Ca^{2+}]_i$ oscillations remains to be elucidated, but so far methods for isolating this specific subset of cells have not been established.

From pacemaker cells, $[Ca^{2+}]_i$ oscillations are propagated as intercellular Ca^{2+} waves to adjacent nonpacemaker endothelial cells with a velocity of approx 5 μm/s. The gap junctional uncoupler heptanol blocks wave propagation without impairing $[Ca^{2+}]_i$ oscillations in pacemaker cells *(13,16)*. Hence, intercellular Ca^{2+} waves are communicated through gap junctions, a mechanism previously attributed to the generation and intercellular communication of IP_3. In various cell types, such as tracheal epithelium or hepatocytes, intercellular Ca^{2+} waves have been reported to coordinate cellular functions like ciliary beat frequency or bile flow. Interestingly, intercellular Ca^{2+} waves are absent in capillaries of chronic hypertensive lungs, which are simultaneously characterized by an impaired control of the vascular lumen (unpublished observation). Hence, interendothelial Ca^{2+} waves may be relevant in the control of vessel diameters and microhemodynamics, and achieve functional homogeneity in lung capillaries.

6. PRO-INFLAMMATORY EFFECTS OF HYDROSTATIC STRESS

The question arises as to the pathophysiological relevance of pressure-induced endothelial $[Ca^{2+}]_i$ signaling in lung capillaries. Since intracellular $[Ca^{2+}]_i$ transients play a key role in the regulation of vesicular trafficking, pressure-induced increases of endothelial $[Ca^{2+}]_i$ may promote Ca^{2+} dependent exocytotic vesicle fusion events. In vesicular exocytosis, docking of cytosolic vesicles at the cell membrane is followed by the fusion of cell and vesicle membranes and the formation of a fusion pore, allowing for the secretion of vesicular storage products into the extracellular space *(18)*. $[Ca^{2+}]_i$ closely regulates the latter process by activating Ca^{2+}-binding proteins, such as calmodulin or annexin, which mediate membrane fusion. The hypothesis of pressure-induced, Ca^{2+}-dependent vesicular trafficking is testable *in situ* by the use of the styryl pryridinium dye FM1-43, which has been used extensively to monitor vesicular trafficking in neuronal *(19)* and nonneuronal cells *(20)*. FM1-43 is virtually nonfluorescent in aqueous solution, but yields a bright fluorescent signal once it interchelates with a lipid bilayer. Initiation of exocytosis increases fluorescence in FM1-43 treated cells as the dye attaches to new membrane at the fusion pore *(20)*. Subsequent removal of FM1-43 from the medium causes fluorescence decay as dye is lost from exocytic vesicles *(19)*.

When FM1-43 is infused over 5 min into a lung venular capillary, little fusion pore formation is detectable at baseline *(21)*. At elevated P_{LA} of 20 cmH_2O, however, a marked and progressive formation of fusion pores is evident at endothelial cell locations (**Fig. 2**). FM1-43 fluorescence is predominantly localized at microvascular branch points and appears as single spots of up to 4 μm in diameter, which presumably result from exocytosis of large endothelial vesicles such as Weibel-Palade bodies. The evoked fluorescent spots appear within as little as 3 μm of one another, indicating that a single endothelial cell can support exocytotic events at several locations on its apical plasma membrane. Pretreatment of lungs with the cell-membrane cation channel inhibitor gadolinium has no effect on capillary FM1-43 at baseline. However, gadolinium blocks the increase of FM1-43 fluorescence during P_{LA} elevation, indicating that the enhanced formation of fusion pores results from pressure-induced $[Ca^{2+}]_i$ signaling in lung capillary endothelial cells (**Fig. 2**).

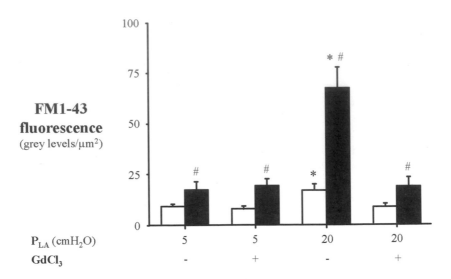

Fig. 2. Pressure-induced formation of exocytotic fusion pores in lung venular capillaries. After a 5-min infusion of the fusion pore marker FM1-43, capillary fluorescence was quantified in 5×5 μm^2 pixels at midsegmental (white bars) and branch point (black bars) locations. Data were obtained at P_{LA} of 5 cmH_2O and after 30 min of P_{LA} elevation to 20 cmH_2O in control and gadolinium-treated lungs. * $p < 0.05$ vs P_{LA} of 5 cmH_2O, # $p < 0.05$ vs mid-segmental locations. Methods and experimental protocol have previously been described in detail *(21)*.

   Potential candidates for vesicular exocytosis in endothelial cells are the Weibel-Palade bodies, which serve as storage pools for the pro-coagulant von Willebrand factor, the chemokine interleukin-8, and the leukocyte and platelet adhesion receptor P-selectin in resting endothelium. Upon activation by Ca^{2+}-mobilizing agents such as histamine or thrombin, Weibel-Palade bodies are exocytosed within minutes and P-selectin is expressed on the vascular surface, promoting the interaction of circulating leukocytes and platelets with the vascular wall. By use of *in situ* micropuncture techniques, we performed indirect immunofluorescence labeling for P-selectin in venular capillaries of the isolated perfused rat lung. Consistent with previous reports, P-selectin expression in lung capillaries is barely detectable at baseline *(22)*. In contrast, hydrostatic pressure increases the expression of P-selectin throughout the luminal vessel surface *(21)*. Increased P-selectin expression is clearly of endothelial, not of platelet origin, since simultaneously determined immunofluorescence attributable to the platelet-specific antigen CD41 is completely absent. The spatial continuity of P-selectin expression along the microvascular wall allows leukocytes to roll along the length of the microvessels *(23)*. However, P-selectin expression is particularly pronounced at the vascular branch points, and hence parallels the spatial distribution of exocytotic fusion pores. This similarity could be confirmed in pixel-to-pixel correlation analyses of fluorescence labelings by FM1-43 and P-selectin immunostaining, respectively *(21)*. Preferential exocytosis of P-selectin at microvascular branch points may facilitate tethering and initiate rolling of leukocytes emerging out of the capillary bed.
   Although gadolinium given under baseline conditions has no effect on P-selectin expression, the blocker abolishes the enhanced P-selectin expression at high pressure, indicating involvement of cation channels and $[Ca^{2+}]_i$ signaling in the P-selectin response to pressure stress. Hence, in endothelial cells of intact lung capillaries, hydrostatic pressure induces second-messenger pathways that promote exocytotic events and P-selectin expression on the vascular surface. Since P-selectin mediates leukocyte rolling as a substantial part of the early inflammatory response, its enhanced expression reflects a pro-inflammatory response to pressure stress. Moreover, P-selectin is implicated in the pathogenesis of various forms of neutrophil-dependent lung injury, including complement activation and ischemia/reperfusion injury *(24,25)*. To assess the effects of hydrostatic pressure on vascular

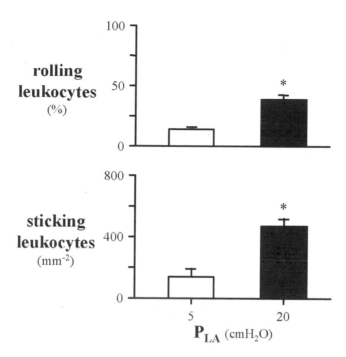

Fig. 3. Leukocyte/endothelial cell interaction in lung venular capillaries. The fraction of rolling leukocytes (top graph) and the number of sticking leukocytes (bottom) were determined at P_{LA} of 5 cmH_2O (white bars) and after 30 min of P_{LA} elevation to 20 cmH_2O (black bars). * $p < 0.05$ vs P_{LA} of 5 cmH_2O. Methods have previously been described in detail *(23)*.

inflammation and neutrophil accumulation in lung microvessels directly, we quantified *in situ* the kinetics of native white blood cells labeled with the mitochondrial dye rhodamin 6G *(26)*. At baseline, the majority of leukocytes pass lung venular capillaries without interacting with the endothelial layer. However at elevated P_{LA}, leukocyte/endothelial cell interaction becomes a prominent feature, thus confirming the pro-inflammatory effect of hydrostatic pressure. P_{LA} elevation increases not only the fraction of leukocytes rolling along the vascular wall, but also the number of leukocytes firmly adherent to the endothelium (**Fig. 3**). Adherent leukocytes are again predominantly localized in the vicinity of microvascular junctions. In addition, occasional extravasation of leukocytes can be observed. Pressure-dependent leukocyte/endothelial cell interaction is blocked in the presence of the cation channel blocker gadolinium, indicating that increased leukocyte sequestration does not result from altered hemodynamic shear forces, but from second-messenger responses in lung endothelial cells.

The spatial distribution of exocytotic events, P-selectin expression, and leukocyte/endothelial cell interaction is of striking similarity in that all phenomena occur primarily at microvascular branch points. A rheological explanation for this site dominance may be considered, since in large vessels, vascular bifurcations are characterized by changing gradients of shear force and increased turbulence. However, Reynolds number in lung capillaries is low, due to the relatively slow blood flow in the pulmonary microcirculation *(23)*, thus maintaining low shear rates and making turbulence an unlikely event. An alternative explanation for the site dominance may lie in the heterogeneity of lung capillary endothelial cells. Branch points are the preferential location for endothelial pacemaker cells, which are characterized by a higher $[Ca^{2+}]_i$ as compared to adjacent nonpacemaker endothelial cells *(16)*. Because endothelial $[Ca^{2+}]_i$ regulates the extent of exocytosis, P-selectin expression, and subsequent cell/cell interaction, pacemaker cells may be responsible for the spatial distribution of these phenomena, and thus play an important role in the onset of pressure-induced vascular inflammation.

These findings demonstrate that lung endothelial cells respond actively and rapidly to the challenge of high vascular pressure by initiating second-messenger signaling cascades that promote lung inflammatory responses. Pressure-induced leukocyte accumulation may be particularly relevant in the pulmonary microcirculation, since under physiological conditions the lung harbors a large reservoir of marginated leukocytes *(27)*, and neutrophils contribute importantly to various forms of lung injury.

7. EVIDENCE FROM CLINICAL STUDIES

The notion of a pressure-induced inititation of this pro-inflammatory cascade is supported by several clinical studies. Sakamaki and coworkers demonstrated elevated plasma concentrations of soluble P-selectin and von Willebrand factor not only in plasma from patients with pulmonary arterial hypertension, but also in those with pulmonary venous hypertension, indicating that capillary hydrostatic pressure promotes the exocytosis of endothelial Weibel-Palade bodies in the clinical situation *(28)*. In patients with cardiogenic respiratory failure, Geppert and coworkers detected reduced plasma concentrations of soluble L-selectin as compared to critically ill patients without respiratory failure *(29)*. L-selectin removal was predominantly confined to the pulmonary compartment, as determined by transpulmonary gradient calculation, suggesting that lung endothelial activation and expression of L-selectin counterligands may have occurred. Most importantly, inflammation and leukocyte infiltration are directly evident as increased numbers of white cells and elevated cytokine levels in bronchoalveolar lavage fluid of subjects with hydrostatic edema or high-altitude pulmonary edema *(30,31)*. These inflammatory processes may surpass the actual duration of pressure stress, which could account for the vulnerability of these patients to recurrent edema formation *(32)*.

8. INTERCOMPARTMENTAL COMMUNICATION

Despite considerable evidence for pressure-induced leukocyte sequestration in the lung, it remains unclear how leukocytes extravasate into the interstitial and alveolar space in the absence of an obvious chemotactic gradient. A possible explanation may lie in the recent observations that hydrostatic pressure not only induces active responses in capillary endothelial, but also in alveolar epithelial cells. At increased hydrostatic pressure, Ca^{2+}-dependent exocytosis of lamellar bodies is increased in alveolar type-II cells *(33)*, while active Na^+ transport is reduced *(11)*. Epithelial stimulation by hydrostatic pressure presumably results from second-messenger-mediated, intercellular communication between endothelial and epithelial cells across the alveolo-capillary barrier, which plays an important role in intercompartmental propagation of pro-inflammatory stimuli *(12)*. Stretch-induced endothelial generation of intra- and intercellular signaling molecules such as nitric oxide *(34)* or reactive oxygen species *(35)* may play an important role in the intercompartmental propagation of vascular pressure stress. Upon stimulation, alveolar type-II cells secrete a variety of chemokines, which may facilitate pressure-induced leukocyte migration in the lung. Further research is required to gain better insights into the complex signaling pathways across the alveolar membrane.

9. ENDOTHELIAL RESPONSES TO MECHANICAL STRESS IN VITRO

Here, we have focused specifically on endothelial $[Ca^{2+}]_i$ signaling in lung capillaries and its relevance for pressure-induced inflammatory responses. However, a large number of additional endothelial responses to mechanical stimulation by either direct pressure or stretch effects have been proposed in vitro. These include the secretion of vasoconstrictive *(36)* as well as vasodilatory mediators *(37)*, chemokines *(38)*, growth factors *(39)*, and tissue-type plasminogen activator *(40)*. In addition, mechanical factors regulate endothelial cell orientation, proliferation, and apoptosis *(41,42)*. These cellular responses involve the activation of transcription factors *(43)* and tyrosine kinases *(44)*, and may be mediated by second messengers such as reactive oxygen species *(45)* or cAMP *(46)*. However, the extent to which these responses are present and of physiological/pathophysiological relevance in the intact pulmonary microcirculation remains to be elucidated.

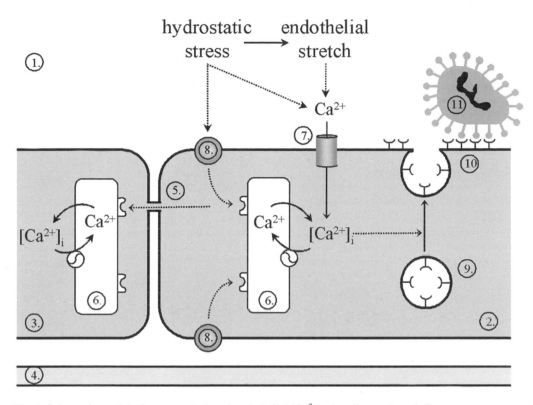

Fig. 4. Schematic model of pressure-induced endothelial $[Ca^{2+}]_i$ signaling and pro-inflammatory response in lung venular capillaries. (1) Vascular lumen. (2) Endothelial pacemaker cell. (3) Endothelial nonpacemaker cell. (4) Basement membrane. (5) Intercellular propagation of Ca^{2+} waves through gap junctions. (6) Intracellular Ca^{2+} pool with Ca^{2+}-ATPase. (7) Mechanosensitive, gadolinium-inhibitable cation channel. (8) Gadolinium-independent mechanosensor amplifying $[Ca^{2+}]_i$ oscillations. (9) Weibel-Palade body. (10) P-selectin expressed on the endothelial surface. (11) Leukocyte interacting with the vascular wall via P-selectin.

10. CONCLUSION

Traditionally, increased hydrostatic pressure was considered to cause lung pathology by a passive increase of fluid filtration, while cellular mechanisms were poorly understood. In contrast, recent in vitro studies using cultured endothelial cells and our own experiments in the intact lung microvasculature have demonstrated a complex scenario of pressure- and stretch-induced active cellular responses, which are mediated through endothelial second-messenger signaling and seem to be relevant in the pathogenesis of pressure-induced lung disease. Specifically, hydrostatic stress evokes complex $[Ca^{2+}]_i$ responses in lung capillary endothelium (**Fig. 4**). Mean endothelial $[Ca^{2+}]_i$ increases because of Ca^{2+} influx through mechanosensitive membrane channels, whereas pacemaker-generated $[Ca^{2+}]_i$ oscillations are induced through Ca^{2+} release from intracellular stores, and propagated as an intercellular Ca^{2+} wave through gap junctional communication. Although the significance of this dual response remains unclear at present, the rise in mean $[Ca^{2+}]_i$ may provide the critical step that initiates vesicular secretion and induces a pro-inflammatory endothelial phenotype, for example by expression of P-selectin. $[Ca^{2+}]_i$ oscillations may activate effectors responsive to oscillation amplitude or frequency, such as mitochondrial dehydrogenases, calmodulin-dependent protein kinases, or transcription factors. Intercellular Ca^{2+} waves may coordinate these phenomena to achieve a homogeneous response to pressure stress in lung capillaries.

Additional Ca^{2+}-dependent and Ca^{2+}-independent endothelial responses to hydrostatic pressure and cell strain have been proposed in vitro and may be relevant in pressure-induced lung pathology. However, care should be taken in extrapolating these results to the intact lung, since endothelial responses in vitro may differ markedly from the in vivo situation. In addition, little is known yet on endothelial responses and adaptation mechanisms to chronic pressure stress, although chronic pulmonary capillary hypertension is clinically the more relevant condition. The introduction of cellular and molecular biology techniques to the *in situ* or in vivo situation provides new tools to study endothelial responses in an integrative approach, but we are just beginning to understand the complex cellular mechanisms and underlying second-messenger pathways in pressure-induced lung disease.

ACKNOWLEDGMENTS

This work was supported by the Deutsche Forschungsgemeinschaft (KU 1218/1-1) and a grant from the Medical Faculty of the University of Munich (FöFoLe No. 136). The author gratefully acknowledges the helpful suggestions and criticisms by Prof. Dr. A. R. Pries.

REFERENCES

1. Wagner, P. D., Gale, G. E., Moon, R. E., Torre-Bueno, J. R., Stolp, B. W., Saltzman, H. A. (1986) Pulmonary gas exchange in humans exercising at sea level and simulated altitude. *J. Appl. Physiol.* **61,** 260–270.
2. Maggiorini, M., Melot, C., Pierre, S., et al. (2001) High-altitude pulmonary edema is initially caused by an increase in capillary pressure. *Circulation* **103,** 2078–2083.
3. Pabst, R. and Tschernig, T. (2002) Perivascular capillaries in the lung: an important but neglected vascular bed in immune reactions? *J. Allergy Clin. Immunol.* **110,** 209–214.
4. Bärtsch, P. (1997) High altitude pulmonary edema. *Respiration* **64,** 435–443.
5. Audi, S. H., Dawson, C. A., Rickaby, D. A., and Linehan, J. H. (1991) Localization of the sites of pulmonary vasomotion by use of arterial and venous occlusion. *J. Appl. Physiol.* **70,** 2126–2136.
6. West, J. B. (2000) Pulmonary capillary stress failure. *J. Appl. Physiol.* **89,** 2483–2489.
7. Parker, J. C. and Ivey, C. L. (1997) Isoproterenol attenuates high vascular pressure-induced permeability increases in isolated rat lung. *J. Appl. Physiol.* **83,** 1962–1967.
8. Minnear, F. L., Barie, P. S., and Malik, A. B. (1983) Effects of transient pulmonary hypertension on pulmonary vascular permeability. *J. Appl. Physiol.* **55,** 983–989.
9. Bhattacharya, J., Nakahara, K., and Staub, N. C. (1980) Effect of pulmonary blood flow in the isolated perfused dog lung lobe. *J. Appl. Physiol.* **48,** 444–449.
10. Gotoh, N., Kambara, K., Jiang, X. W., et al. (2000) Apoptosis in microvascular endothelial cells of perfused rabbit lungs with acute hydrostatic edema. *J. Appl. Physiol.* **88,** 518–526.
11. Saldias, F. J., Azzam, Z. S., Ridge, K. M., et al. (2001) Alveolar fluid reabsorption is impaired by increased atrial pressures in rats. *Am. J. Physiol. Lung Cell Mol. Physiol.* **281,** L591–L597.
12. Kuebler, W. M., Parthasarathi, K., Wang, P. M., and Bhattacharya, J. (2000) A novel signaling mechanism between gas and blood compartments of the lung. *J. Clin. Invest.* **105,** 905–913.
13. Ying, X., Minamiya, Y., Fu, C., and Bhattacharya, J. (1996) Ca^{2+} waves in lung capillary endothelium. *Circ. Res.* **79,** 898–908.
14. Naruse, K. and Sokabe, M. (1993) Involvement of stretch-activated ion channels in Ca^{2+} mobilization to mechanical stretch in endothelial cells. *Am. J. Physiol.* **264,** C1037–C1044.
15. Kohler, R., Distler, A., and Hoyer, J. (1998) Pressure-activated cation channel in intact rat endocardial endothelium. *Cardiovasc. Res.* **38,** 433–440.
16. Kuebler, W. M., Ying, X., and Bhattacharya, J. (2002) Pressure-induced endothelial Ca^{2+} oscillations in lung capillaries. *Am. J. Physiol. Lung Cell Mol. Physiol.* **282,** L917–L923.
17. Rosales, O. R., Isales, C. M., Barrett, P. Q., Brophy, C., and Sumpio, B. E. (1997) Exposure of endothelial cells to cyclic strain induces elevations of cytosolic Ca^{2+} concentration through mobilization of intracellular and extracellular pools. *Biochem. J.* **326,** 385–392.
18. Monck, J. R. and Fernandez, J. M. (1996) The fusion pore and mechanisms of biological membrane fusion. *Curr. Opin. Cell Biol.* **8,** 524–533.
19. Betz, W. J. and Bewick, G. S. (1992) Optical analysis of synaptic vesicle recycling at the frog neuromuscular junction. *Science* **255,** 200–203.
20. Smith, C. B. and Betz, W. J. (1996) Simultaneous independent measurement of endocytosis and exocytosis. *Nature* **380,** 531–534.
21. Kuebler, W. M., Ying, X., Singh, B., Issekutz, A. C., and Bhattacharya, J. (1999) Pressure is pro-inflammatory in lung venular capillaries. *J. Clin. Invest.* **104,** 495–502.
22. Bless, N. M., Tojo, S. J., Kawarai, H., et al. (1998) Differing patterns of P-selectin expression in lung injury. *Am. J. Pathol.* **153,** 1113–1122.

23. Kuebler, W. M., Kuhnle, G. E. H., Groh, J., and Goetz, A. E. (1997) Contribution of selectins to sequestration of leukocytes in pulmonary microvessels by intravital microscopy in rabbits. *J. Physiol.* **501,** 375–386.
24. Mulligan, M. S., Polley, M. J., Bayer, R. J., Nunn, M. F., Paulson, J. C., and Ward, P. A. (1992) Neutrophil dependent lung injury. Requirement for P-selectin (GMP-140). *J. Clin. Invest.* **90,** 1600–1607.
25. Moore, T. M., Khimenko, P., Adkins, W. K., Miyasaka, M., and Taylor, A. E. (1995) Adhesion molecules contribute to ischemia and reperfusion-induced injury in the isolated rat lung. *J. Appl. Physiol.* **78,** 2245–2252.
26. Kuebler, W. M., Borges, J., Sckell, A., et al. (2000) Role of L-selectin in leukocyte sequestration in lung capillaries in a rabbit model of endotoxemia. *Am. J. Respir. Crit. Care Med.* **161,** 36–43.
27. Kuebler, W. M. and Goetz, A. E. (2002) The marginated pool. *Eur. Surg. Res.* **34,** 92–100.
28. Sakamaki, F., Kyotani, S., Nagaya, N., et al. (2000) Increased plasma P-selectin and decreased thrombomodulin in pulmonary arterial hypertension were improved by continuous prostacyclin therapy. *Circulation* **102,** 2720–2725.
29. Geppert, A., Zorn, G., Heinz, G., Huber, K., and Siostrzonek, P. (2001) Soluble selectins in the pulmonary and systemic circulation in acute cardiogenic and non-cardiogenic pulmonary failure. *Intensive Care Med.* **27,** 521–527.
30. Nakos, G., Pneumatikos, J., Tsangaris, I., Tellis, C., and Lekka, M. (1997) Proteins and phospholipids in BAL from patients with hydrostatic pulmonary edema. *Am. J. Respir. Crit. Care Med.* **155,** 945–951.
31. Kubo, K., Hanaoka, M., Hayano, T., et al. (1998) Inflammatory cytokines in BAL fluid and pulmonary hemodynamics in high-altitude pulmonary edema. *Respir. Physiol.* **111,** 301–310.
32. De Pasquale, C. G., Arnolda, L. F., Doyle, I. R., Grant, R. L., Aylward, P. E., and Bersten, A. D. (2003) Prolonged alveolocapillary barrier damage after acute cardiogenic pulmonary edema. *Crit. Care Med.* **31,** 1060–1067.
33. Wang, P. M., Fujita, E., and Bhattacharya, J. (2002) Vascular regulation of type II cell exocytosis. *Am. J. Physiol. Lung Cell Mol. Physiol.* **282,** L912–L916.
34. Kuebler, W. M., Uhlig, U., Goldmann, T., et al. (2003) Stretch activates nitric oxide production in pulmonary vascular endothelial cells in situ. *Am. J. Respir. Crit. Care Med.* **168,** 1391–1398.
35. Ichimura, H., Parthasarathi, K., Quadri, S., Issekutz, A. C., and Bhattacharya, J. (2003) Mechano-oxidative coupling by mitochondria induces proinflammatory responses in lung venular capillaries *J. Clin. Invest.* **111,** 691–699.
36. Dschietzig, T., Richter, C., Bartsch, C., et al. (2001) Flow-induced pressure differentially regulates endothelin-1, urotensin II, adrenomedullin, and relaxin in pulmonary vascular endothelium. *Biochem. Biophys. Res. Commun.* **289,** 245–251.
37. Fisslthaler, B., Popp, R., Michaelis, U. R., Kiss, L., Fleming, I., and Busse, R. (2001) Cyclic stretch enhances the expression and activity of coronary endothelium-derived hyperpolarizing factor synthase. *Hypertension* **38,** 1427–1432.
38. Okada, M., Matsumori, A., Ono, K., et al. (1998) Cyclic stretch upregulates production of interleukin-8 and monocyte chemotactic and activating factor/monocyte chemoattractant protein-1 in human endothelial cells. *Arterioscler. Thromb. Vasc. Biol.* **18,** 894–901.
39. Acevedo, A. D., Bowser, S. S., Gerritsen, M. E., and Bizios, R. (1993) Morphological and proliferative responses of endothelial cells to hydrostatic pressure: role of fibroblast growth factor. *J. Cell Physiol.* **157,** 603–614.
40. Iba, T., Shin, T., Sonoda, T., Rosales, O., and Sumpio, B. E. (1991) Stimulation of endothelial secretion of tissue-type plasminogen activator by repetitive stretch. *J. Surg. Res.* **50,** 457–460.
41. Sumpio, B. E., Widmann, M. D., Ricotta, J., Awolesi, M. A., and Watase, M. (1994) Increased ambient pressure stimulates proliferation and morphologic changes in cultured endothelial cells. *J. Cell Physiol.* **158,** 133–139.
42. Shin, H. Y., Gerritsen, M. E., and Bizios, R. (2002) Regulation of endothelial cell proliferation and apoptosis by cyclic pressure. *Ann. Biomed. Eng.* **30,** 297–304.
43. Du, W., Mills, I., and Sumpio, B. E. (1995) Cyclic strain causes heterogeneous induction of transcription factors, AP-1, CRE binding protein and NF-κB, in endothelial cells: species and vascular bed diversity. *J. Biomech.* **28,** 1485–1491.
44. Naruse, K., Sai, X., Yokoyama, N., and Sokabe, M. (1998) Uni-axial cyclic stretch induces c-src activation and translocation in human endothelial cells via SA channel activation. *FEBS Lett.* **441,** 111–115.
45. Hishikawa, K. and Luscher, T. F. (1997) Pulsatile stretch stimulates superoxide production in human aortic endothelial cells. *Circulation* **96,** 3610–3616.
46. Letsou, G. V., Rosales, O., Maitz, S., Vogt, A., and Sumpio, B. E. (1990) Stimulation of adenylate cyclase activity in cultured endothelial cells subjected to cyclic stretch. *J. Cardiovasc. Surg.* **31,** 634–639.

9

Regulation of Endothelial Barrier Function

Contributions of the Transcellular and Paracellular Pathways

Dolly Mehta, Richard D. Minshall, and Asrar B. Malik

SUMMARY

The vascular endothelium, consisting of a monolayer of endothelial cells and extracellular matrix, represents the major barrier to exchange of liquid and solutes across the vessel wall. Thus, minute changes in the endothelial monolayer with respect to its permeability to plasma proteins can have marked effects on the tissue fluid balance and can lead to edema. The *paracellular* and *transcellular* pathways control endothelial barrier function. Under physiological conditions, the endothelial barrier is described as being restrictive in that only small molecules (<3 nm) can move through the barrier via the paracellular route, whereas macromolecules are actively transported via the transcellular pathway. This restrictive barrier is required to establish the transendothelial oncotic pressure gradient that maintains tissue fluid homeostasis. Endothelial permeability to albumin, the main plasma protein, is the primary determinant of the oncotic pressure gradient and hence maintains the barrier function of the endothelium. The transcellular pathway, by transporting albumin through the endothelial cell, contributes to maintenance of the barrier function of the endothelium. This pathway is comprised of cargo-containing plasmalemmal vesicles, the caveolae. Recent data indicate that the formation, fission, and transport of caveolae in endothelial cells are dynamic processes that are regulated by coherent actions of the albumin-binding proteins caveolin-1 and dynamin. The activity of these proteins is positively regulated by *Src*-mediated phosphorylation. Pro-inflammatory mediators and growth factors, by binding endothelial cell-surface receptors, initiate a series of events that lead to the opening of intercellular junctions, thereby allowing passage of albumin across the endothelial monolayer by the paracellular route, disrupting the barrier function of the endothelium. Activation of the small-guanosine-5'-triphosphate (GTP)-binding protein RhoA has been shown to play a primary role in regulating paracellular permeability by modulating the integrity of the intercellular junctional protein complexes. This review focuses on the distinct contributions of caveolae-mediated transcellular and Rho-mediated paracellular pathways and their respective roles in regulating endothelial permeability.

1. INTRODUCTION

Studies of the biology of endothelial cells over the past three decades have led to the understanding that the endothelium is not a simple, inert barrier with fixed permeability, but rather a dynamic structure composed of metabolically active and functionally responsive cells. Regulation of tissue fluid balance is the most important function of endothelial cells. Endothelial cells act as an interface between the plasma and interstitial fluid because of their unique location in the vasculature. Thus, minute changes in the permeability of the endothelial monolayer to plasma proteins can have marked effects on the tissue fluid balance and can lead to edema. The transport of substances across the endothelium was initially proposed to be regulated by two types of endothelial pores, each with a

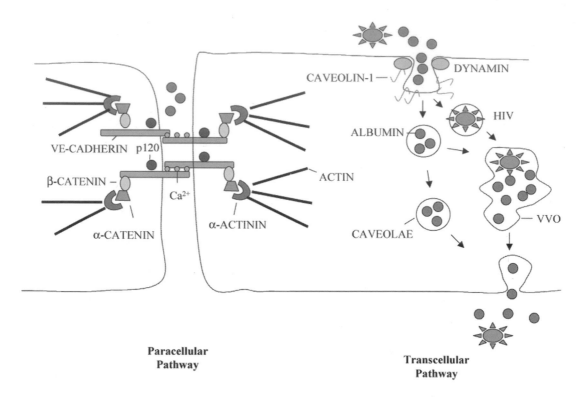

Fig. 1. Schematic of mechanisms regulating transport of albumin via transcellular and paracellular pathways. The transport of albumin through the transcellular pathway is mediated by caveolae. Caveolin-1 is the primary scaffold protein associated with the caveolae. Dynamin, a GTPase localized at the neck of caveolae, activates the release of caveolae from the endothelial cell surface. Released caveolae then shuttle across the cell and/or form VVOs (clusters of caveolae), which mediate transport of albumin across the endothelium. The transcellular pathway may also be involved in the transport of larger molecules, such as human immunodeficiency virus. The paracellular pathway describes transit of proteins through intercellular junctions, i.e., tight junctions and adherens junctions. This figure shows the typical arrangement of adherens junction proteins by which endothelial cells adhere and communicate with each other. VE-cadherin is the backbone of adherens junctions. While the extracellular domains maintain cell-cell contact through Ca^{2+}-dependent homotypic adhesion of VE-cadherin molecules, the intracellular domains provide junctional stability through their linkage with the actin cytoskeleton via catenins.

discrete radius. One pore was thought to allow passage of small solutes (approx 3 nm) and the other, larger molecules (approx 25 nm) *(1,2)*. However, the lack of convincing structural data demonstrating the existence of these pores has promoted an intensive re-evaluation of the pore theory.

With the use of electron microscopy and molecular biology techniques, a general consensus has been reached. It is now believed that solutes cross the endothelium not through pores but by one of two mechanisms that appear to act in concert to regulate vascular permeability *(3,4)*, and hence the barrier function of the endothelium (**Fig. 1**). The first mechanism, known as the *paracellular pathway*, reported initially by Majno and Palade, is one in which solutes pass from the luminal to the abluminal side of the endothelium through gaps formed by the opening of junctions between individual endothelial cells *(5,6)*. The second mechanism, the transcellular pathway *(7–10)*, is one in which the material to be transported is internalized at the luminal surface into specialized vesicles, transported across the cell, and subsequently released at the abluminal surface. The latter process is mediated by plasmalemmal structures known as *caveolae (7–10)*.

Under physiological conditions, the endothelial barrier is described as being restrictive, in that it is semipermeable to solutes based on solute size *(3,4)*. This restrictive barrier function is required to establish the transendothelial oncotic pressure gradient, which maintains tissue fluid homeostasis *(3,4)*. The permeability to albumin, the main plasma protein, is the primary determinant of the oncotic pressure gradient; therefore, understanding how albumin permeability is regulated is of paramount importance. In **Subheadings 2** and **3**, the distinct contributions of the transcellular and paracellular pathways in regulating endothelial permeability are discussed.

2. ROLE OF THE TRANSCELLULAR PATHWAY IN REGULATING ENDOTHELIAL PERMEABILITY

The endothelial cell expresses a number of distinct cell-surface receptors, defined as albumin-binding proteins (ABPs), which regulate albumin endocytosis and its transcellular transport, and hence the transendothelial oncotic pressure gradient. ABPs and the signaling machinery that activate transcellular albumin transport are described below.

2.1. Endothelial Caveolae

Caveolae are non-clathrin-coated, approx 75-nm, flask-shaped invaginations of the plasma membrane. They were first described morphologically nearly 50 yr ago by Palade *(11)*. Caveolae are major structures in endothelial cells, as they account for 95% of the cell-surface invaginations and approx 15% of endothelial cell volume *(9)*. Caveolae have a unique lipid composition: their main components are cholesterol and sphingolipids (sphingomyelin and glycosphingolipid). Because sphingolipids are precursors of the intracellular second messenger ceramide, caveolae serve an important function in the signaling pathway requiring lipid intermediates *(12)*. The other main component, cholesterol, is essential for maintaining the caveolae structure, as it creates the framework in which all other elements of the caveolae are inserted *(13)*. This is consistent with the finding that endocytosis of fluorescently tagged albumin is blocked by filipin *(14)* or methyl-β-cyclodextrin *(15)*, sterol-binding agents that disassemble cholesterol-rich caveolae *(16–18)*. The specific marker and major structural component of caveolae is caveolin-1, an integral membrane protein (20–22 kDa) having both amino- and carboxy-temini on the cytoplasmic face of the membrane. The caveolin gene family consists of caveolins 1, 2, and 3 *(19)*. Caveolins 1 and 2 are co-expressed in many cell types, such as endothelial cells, fibroblasts, smooth muscle cells, and adipocytes *(19,20)*. In contrast, the expression of caveolin-3 is muscle specific *(19,20)*. Caveolin proteins form homo- and hetero-oligomers that are stabilized by cholesterol *(21)*. Caveolin oligomers may also interact with glycosphingolipids *(22)*, and these protein–protein and protein–lipid interactions may act as the driving force for caveolae formation *(23)*. It is also possible that caveolin oligomers serve as docking sites for other important signaling molecules, such as receptors coupled to monomeric or heterotrimeric G proteins *(24)*. Since the 1950s, when caveolae were first discovered, they have been implicated in transcytosis of both large and small molecules across endothelial cells *(15,24,25)*.

2.2. Role of ABP gp60 in Regulating Endothelial Permeability

Studies have provided evidence that the 60-kDa glycoprotein gp60 (or albondin), found in the microvascular endothelial cell membrane, may regulate transendothelial permeability through its ability to bind native albumin *(14,15,25–34)*. The binding of albumin to cell-surface gp60 may be an important event, initiating endocytosis and the consequent release of caveolae from the membrane. Vesicles containing gp60-bound albumin as well as albumin in the fluid phase compartment are transported to the basolateral membrane, where the vesicle contents are released into the subendothelial space by exocytosis *(7,9,14,25,34,35)*.

The 60-kDa ABP was initially characterized by its unique affinity for the galactose-binding lectins *Limax flavus* agglutinin and *Ricinus communis* agglutinin, which in competition experiments inhib-

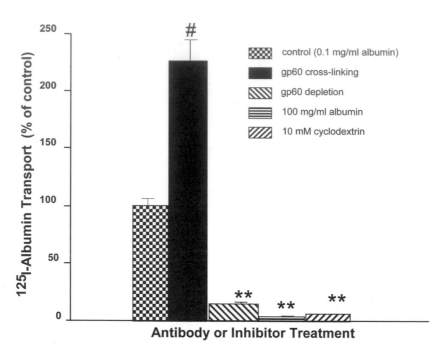

Fig. 2. 60-kDa albumin-binding protein (gp60)-dependent ^{125}I-albumin transport in bovine lung microvascular endothelial cells (BLMVEC). Endothelial monolayers were washed twice with HEPES-buffered DMEM at 4°C and incubated for 30 min with anti-gp60 antibody (10 μg/mL) at 4°C and with secondary antibody (goat antirabbit, 10 μg/mL) for 30 min to induce crosslinking. Cells were rewarmed to 37°C to activate uptake of ^{125}I-albumin and 1.5 μ*M* unlabeled albumin. Crosslinking of gp60 increased ^{125}I-albumin permeability 2.3-fold from a control value of 38 ± 15 nL/min/cm². To deplete cell-surface gp60, monolayers were washed twice with HEPES-buffered DMEM and incubated with anti-gp60 antibody (10 μg/mL) for 2 h at 37°C. Depletion of gp60 reduced ^{125}I-albumin transport 85%. ^{125}I-albumin flux was also blocked 95% when cells were co-incubated with 1.5 m*M* unlabeled albumin (100 mg/mL) or 10 m*M* cyclodextrin. Reproduced from ref. *102*, by copyright permission from The Rockefeller University Press.

ited albumin binding to rat fat-tissue microvessel endothelial gp60 *(26,36)*. Siflinger-Birnboim et al. showed that *Ricinus communis* agglutinin precipitated gp60 in bovine lung endothelial cell membranes, and, importantly, that it inhibited transendothelial albumin transport *(36)*.

With the availability of anti-gp60 antibodies, an important functional role for gp60 in inducing albumin-specific endothelial permeability was shown in cultured endothelial cells (**Fig. 2**) *(14,29,31)*. The specificity of the interaction of albumin with gp60 in caveolae was further demonstrated by measuring albumin uptake in rat lung endothelial cell monolayers using cholera toxin subunit B, a specific marker for caveolae, because it labels the caveolae-specific ganglioside GM1 *(37)*.

Albumin uptake in caveolae was found to be sensitive to the cholesterol-depleting agent methyl-β-cyclodextrin. It was shown that cyclodextrin blocked iodinated albumin uptake in a dose-dependent manner with a maximal inhibition occurring at 10 m*M* cyclodextrin. The inhibition appears to be due to cyclodextrin depletion of cell-surface caveolin-1 (**Figs. 2** and **3**) *(15)*. A similar role for gp60 in regulating the uptake of albumin in vivo in intact rat microcirculation was shown by Vogel et al. *(32,33)*. These investigators showed that gp60 activation is capable of inducing active transport of albumin across a continuous endothelial cell barrier in both skeletal muscle and pulmonary microvessels, but did so without increasing permeability to liquids (as measured by hydraulic conductivity) *(32,33)*. Thus, gp60 activation uncouples hydraulic conductivity (likely regulated by the diffusive paracellular pathway) from the transcellular pathway involving vesicular transport. All

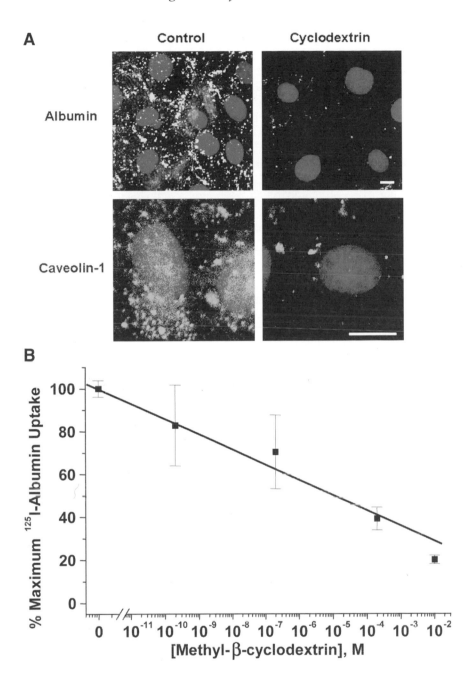

Fig. 3. Inhibitory effect of methyl-β-cyclodextrin on flux of ^{125}I-albumin. (**A**) Rat lung microvessel endothelial cells (RLMVEC) monolayers on glass coverslips were pretreated with vehicle or 2 mM methyl-β-cyclodextrin for 15 min, incubated with HBSS containing 50 μg/mL Alexa 488 albumin and 1.5 μM unlabeled albumin for 30 min, fixed, and stained with anti-caveolin-1 Ab (1 μg/mL) followed by goat-anti-mouse Alexa 568 and DAPI. Uptake of fluorescent albumin was blocked when cells were first treated with cyclodextrin. In addition, cyclodextrin significantly reduced cell-surface caveolin-1 immunostaining. (**B**) RLMVEC grown on transwell inserts were preincubated for 15 min with 0.2 nM–10 mM methyl-β-cyclodextrin or vehicle and then with ^{125}I-albumin in Hanks' balanced salt solution (HBSS) containing 1.5 μM free albumin for 15 min. A dose-dependent inhibition of ^{125}I-albumin flux from a control value of 7.7 ± 0.3 fmol/min/10^6 cells was observed. From John et al. *(15)*, with permission.

together, these studies indicate that gp60 activates membrane trafficking and regulates endothelial permeability to albumin by such a mechanism.

A recent report by our group described two binding affinities for albumin on the microvascular endothelial cell surface ($K_{D1} = 13.5$ nM and $K_{D2} = 1.6$ µM) that may reflect unclustered and clustered states of gp60 *(15)*. By comparing albumin's binding kinetics to its uptake and transport, this study suggested that the majority of albumin is transported through caveolae in the fluid phase rather than by receptor-mediated endocytosis, although receptor activation appears to be required for fluid-phase transport. Interestingly, despite the relatively high affinity of gp60 for albumin, the capacity of receptor-mediated albumin transport was submaximal in the presence of saturating levels of albumin, since further activation of gp60 by antibody crosslinking more than doubled the amount of albumin transported *(15)*. Thus, endothelial cells could use the transcellular pathway to increase albumin transport under pathological conditions associated with inflammation. Future studies are required to define the contribution of gp60-induced albumin transport in inflammatory states.

2.3. Caveolar Dynamics

Transcytosis via caveolae consists of two basic steps: budding (vesicle formation at the "donor" membrane) and fusion (vesicle fusion with the "acceptor" membrane) *(38)*. Endothelial caveolae are, indeed, like other carrier vesicles that undergo budding and fusion steps in a NEM-sensitive manner *(39)*. Caveolae are enriched for the molecular machinery required for vesicle formation, including v-SNAREs, VAMP-2, monomeric and heterotrimeric guanine nucleotide-binding proteins (GTPases), annexin II and VI, and NEM-sensitive fusion factor and its attachment protein SNAP, all of which contribute to the vesicular budding and fission processes *(39,40)*. Additionally, dynamin, a cytosolic GTPase, is found in endothelial caveolae. Dynamin mediates internalization and fission of caveolae *(41,42)*. Dynamin was found to be concentrated in the caveolar neck region, where, upon GTP hydrolysis, it mediates vesicular fission, releasing the caveolae from the plasma membrane into the cytosol. Additional components of endothelial caveolae include Rab 5, the ganglioside GM1, and the cholera toxin docking protein *(43,44)*. The functional roles of Rab 5 and gangliosides in caveolar trafficking are not known. The transport of caveolae following fission is facilitated by their association with actin cytoskeleton-associated proteins such as myosin, gelsolin, spectrin, and dystrophin *(45)*.

The dynamin-based mechanism mediating the release of caveolae from the plasma membrane is poorly understood. Phosphorylation events are likely important, since caveolar fission is increased by inhibiting phosphatases and decreased by inhibiting kinases *(46)*. Caveolin-1 is known to be phosphorylated *(47)* on tyrosine residue 14 by *Src* kinase *(48)*, suggesting a link between tyrosine kinase activity and release of caveolae. Studies show that the binding of albumin to gp60 induces tyrosine phosphorylation of both gp60 and caveolin-1 and facilitates their association *(14,31)*. This suggests that the activation of a gp60–caveolin-1 complex may induce the fission of the membrane-associated caveolae, resulting in albumin endocytosis *(14)*. The functional importance of this event is evident from the finding that the tyrosine kinase inhibitors herbimycin A and genistein, as well as the expression of a dominant-negative *Src*, prevented gp60-activated vesicle formation and albumin endocytosis *(14,31,37)* (**Fig. 4**). It is possible that *Src* may regulate dynamin function by regulating its phosphorylation, since in other cell types, dynamin is known to be a substrate for *Src* and has also been shown to promote actin cytoskeleton reorganization *(49,50,51)*, suggesting that *Src*-dynamin interactions may be an important component of the transcytosis signaling machinery.

The activation of a G protein-coupled pathway may also be involved in signaling albumin transcytosis *(14,19,52)*. This is evidenced by the findings that the inhibition of $G_{\alpha i}$ function with pertussis toxin inhibited ^{125}I-albumin uptake induced by gp60 antibody crosslinking in rat lung endothelial cells (**Fig. 5A**). Similarly, inhibition of $G_{\alpha i}$ function by expression of a $G_{\alpha i}$ minigene construct that competitively inhibits endogenous $G_{\alpha i}$-receptor interactions prevented the albumin-activated endocytosis of RH414 (a styryl piridinium dye that fluoresces once intercalated into the membrane

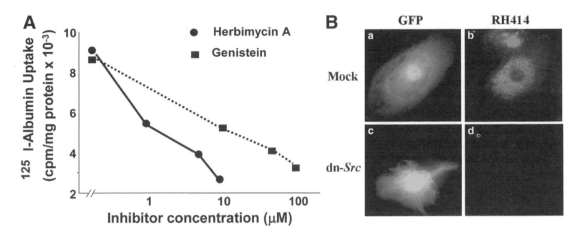

Fig. 4. Activation of *Src* kinase is required to induce ^{125}I-albumin uptake. (**A**) bovine pulmonary microvascular endothelial cells (BPMVEC) grown in six-well plates were incubated with the tyrosine kinase inhibitors for 30 min at 37°C, after which they were used for uptake of ^{125}I-albumin and 1.5 μM unlabeled albumin at 37°C. (**B**) BPMVEC were transfected with pcDNA3.1 alone (mock) or dn-*Src* cDNA, after which they were grown to confluence (48 h posttransfection). Whereas albumin induced the endocytosis of RH414, a styryl piridinium dye that fluoresces once intercalated in the membrane bilayer of the endocytic vesicle, it failed to induce the endocytosis of RH414 in cells expressing dn-*Src*, indicating that *Src* activation is required to induce albumin endocytosis. From Tiruppathi et al. *(31)* with permission, and reproduced from ref. *14*, by copyright permission from The Rockefeller University Press.

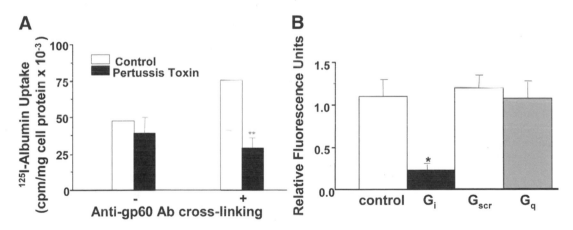

Fig. 5. Albumin endocytosis by crosslinking gp60 Ab occurs by a Gi-linked signaling pathway. (**A**) Endothelial monolayers were pretreated for 18 h with 100 ng/mL pertussis toxin, after which albumin uptake was induced by gp60 crosslinking. (**B**) Cells were transfected with a minigene construct that encodes the C-terminus of Gαi, a Gαq peptide, or a scrambled version of the Gαi minigene. After 48 h, these cells were activated with albumin and RH414 endocytosis was measured. Whereas the Gαi minigene blocked RH414 endocytosis, the Gαq minigene peptide or a scrambled version of the Gαi minigene had no effect. Reproduced from ref. *14*, by copyright permission from The Rockefeller University Press.

bilayer of the endocytic vesicle), whereas it was not affected by $G_{\alpha q}$ minigene expression in these cells (**Fig. 5B**). Attenuation of gp60-induced vesicle formation was also observed to be accompanied by overexpression of wild-type caveolin-1 by a mechanism involving the sequestration of endogenous $G_{\alpha i}$ by caveolin-1, thereby inhibiting its function *(14)*.

The pathway by which G_i signals the release of caveolae has not yet been elucidated. It is possible that *Src* may play an important role, because *Src* activation has been shown to occur downstream of G_i *(53,54)*. The finding that the expression of a catalytically inactive *Src* mutant prevented vesicle formation in endothelial cells *(14)* is consistent with this hypothesis. Interestingly, the catalytically inactive *Src* mutant also interfered with the binding of $G_{\alpha i}$ to caveolin-1 *(14)*. Thus, the release of caveolae may require *Src* to be in the active state. As the binding of this *Src* mutant to caveolin-1 displaced $G_{\alpha i}$ from caveolin-1, it is possible that *Src* and $G_{\alpha i}$ compete for a common binding site on the caveolin-1 scaffold domain *(19,55,56)*. This possibility is supported by the data showing that $G_{\alpha i}$ binds less caveolin-1 in cells transfected with the inactive *Src* mutant than with wild-type *Src*.

2.4. Role of Caveolin-1 in Regulating Endothelial Permeability

Caveolin-1 sequesters proteins such as endothelial nitric oxide synthase (eNOS), *Src*, and $G_{\alpha i}$, and is thought to maintain them in an inactive conformation *(19,56)*. These signaling molecules are thus concentrated in cholesterol-rich microdomains and stand ready to mediate a variety of cellular signaling functions. Caveolin-1 oligomerization and insertion into the cytoplasmic face of the plasma membrane not only serves as a scaffold for signaling molecules *(55)*, but may also facilitate membrane invagination and formation of the classic flask-shaped structure of the caveolae *(19,56)*. Further studies are needed to determine the precise role *Src*-induced phosphorylation of caveolin-1 plays in activating caveolae formation and thereby initiating transcytosis. The recent generation of caveolin-1 null mice is an important advance in this field *(57–59)*. These mice are viable but show a loss of endothelial caveolae; uncontrolled endothelial cell proliferation and lung fibrosis; a constitutively active eNOS, which accounts for an approximately fivefold increase in plasma NO levels *(59)*; and, importantly, defective endocytosis of albumin. These defects could be reversed by introduction of caveolin-1 cDNA *(57,58)*. However, despite the important role of caveolin-1 in regulating endothelial barrier function under normal conditions, caveolin-1 knockout mice are viable. This raises the possibility that a compensatory pathway regulating albumin transport is functional in these mice. One possibility is that the endothelial junctions open, allowing passage of albumin by the paracellular pathway *(59)*. Lisanti and colleagues showed that in caveolin-1 knockout mice, lung capillaries had defects in tight-junction morphology and abnormalities in capillary endothelial cell adhesion to the basement membrane *(59)*. These findings are significant, as they indicate that caveolin-1 may not only be involved in the caveolar transcytosis pathway, but may also play a regulatory role in the mechanisms that regulate permeability by the paracellular pathway. Future studies will clarify the role of caveolin-1 in the regulation of both the transcellular and paracellular pathways.

Figure 6 describes our model of albumin-stimulated endocytosis in endothelial cells. Caveolin-1 plays a central role in this model, as it serves as a scaffold for components of the caveolar release complex, G_i and *Src*, the signaling machinery responsible for gp60-induced endocytosis. *Src* kinases, which are activated by G_i upon stimulation of G protein-coupled receptors *(53)*, phosphorylated tyrosine residues on caveolin-1 *(14,31,48,55)*, as well as gp60 *(31)*. This model will need to be evaluated further to determine the precise relationship between gp60 and caveolin-1, as well as between gp60, G_i, and *Src*.

3. ROLE OF THE PARACELLULAR PATHWAY IN REGULATING ENDOTHELIAL PERMEABILITY

The endothelial cell is a target for many proinflammatory and thrombogenic mediators and growth factors. Proinflammatory mediators (thrombin, histamine, bradykinin, and substance P) and some growth factors (vascular endothelial growth factor [VEGF] and platelet-derived growth factor [PDGF]) disrupt interendothelial junctions, increasing endothelial permeability and allowing the passage of plasma proteins through intercellular gaps *(3,60)*. This pathway, known as the *paracellular pathway*, is enhanced in inflammatory diseases such as acute lung injury, acute respiratory distress

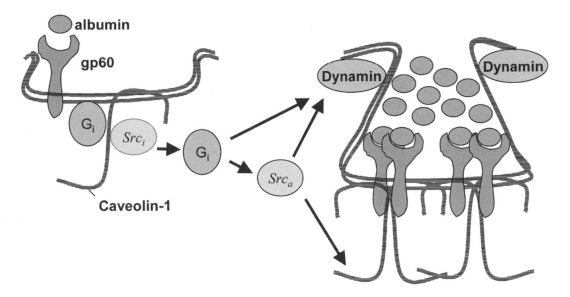

Fig. 6. Hypothesized mechanisms of gp60-activated vesicle formation. Albumin binding to endothelial cell-surface 60-kDa glycoprotein (gp60) induces clustering of gp60 and its physical interaction with caveolin-1. The heterotrimeric guanosine 5'-triphosphate (GTP)-binding protein, Gi, and *Src* tyrosine kinase, bind to the caveolin-1 scaffolding domain in their inactive conformations, and are activated upon albumin binding to gp60. Activated *Src* in turn is thought to phosphorylate caveolin-1, gp60, and dynamin to initiate plasmalemmal vesicle fission and transendothelial vesicular transport. Thus, the high-affinity albumin-binding protein, gp60, induces high-capacity receptor-bound and fluid-phase albumin transport via caveolae.

syndrome, and sepsis. Specific adhesion molecules, organized at cell-cell junctions, are responsible for endothelial integrity and thus contribute to the barrier function of the endothelium. There are two types of intercellular junctions—adherens junctions (AJ) and tight junctions (TJ) *(61–63)*. Studies have shown that disassembly of AJs is the principal mechanism of increased endothelial permeability via the paracellular pathway and of the resultant pulmonary edema *(64–67)*. The structural organization of the AJs and the signals that regulate their integrity are described later.

3.1. Adherens Junctions

Vascular endothelial specific type II cadherin (VE-cadherin) constitutes the backbone of the AJ (**Fig. 1**). The extracellular cadherin repeats are involved in mediating adhesion via specific Ca^{2+} binding sites *(61–63)*. Cadherins oligomerize in the same cell (*cis* oligomers) or with cadherins in adjacent cells (*trans* oligomers). The cytoplasmic domain contains two identified functional domains: the juxtamembrane domain (JMD), where p120 catenin binds, and the C-terminal domain (CTD), where β-catenin or plakoglobin (γ-catenin) bind in a mutually exclusive manner. β-catenin and plakoglobin associate with α-catenin, which in turn links VE-cadherin to the actin cytoskeleton. The homologous catenins p120, β-catenin, and plakoglobin belong to the *armadillo* like family (containing 40 amino acid motifs originally described in the *Drosophila* gene *armadillo*). Catenins bind to cadherins through domains containing these *armadillo* repeats. p120 is distinct in that it interacts only with the VE-cadherin JMD, where it has no interaction with either α-catenin or the actin cytoskeleton *(62,63)* but is involved in regulation of the adhesive interaction between cells. p120 also has other activities relevant to permeability, such as inhibition or activation of Rho *(68,69)* and Rac, through which it may regulate AJ function. However, the mechanisms by which p120 and β-catenin regulate AJ function in endothelial cells remains to be elucidated.

3.1.1. Role of RhoA in Regulating Adherens Junction Integrity

A critical factor controlling endothelial barrier integrity may be the modifications of VE-cadherin/catenin binding, which may shift AJ adhesive strength from strong to weak *(3,60,62,63)*. Pro-inflammatory mediators such as thrombin, histamine, bradykinin, and substance P act on their cognate endothelial surface receptors, activate second messengers, and induce increased endothelial permeability responses by reducing the adhesive strength of AJs *(3,60,62,63)*. Thrombin has been widely used to study endothelial cell signaling because it is a multi-functional mediator involved in both thrombosis and inflammation *(3,60,70)*. Thrombin binds to the protease activated receptor (PAR-1) in endothelial cells and cleaves and releases its N-terminus, generating a new PAR-1 N-terminus *(71–73)*. This new terminus functions as a tethered ligand, activating the heterotrimeric G proteins $G_{12/13}$, G_q, and G_i *(72)*. Both direct activation of $G_{12/13}$ and its cross-activation by G_q may activate the monomeric Rho family of GTPases *(74–77)*.

Recent studies have shown that thrombin induces the activation of RhoA in human endothelial cells in a PKCα-dependent manner (**Fig. 7**) *(75–79)*. Inhibition of RhoA by C3 transferase (a specific inhibitor of Rho) also blocks thrombin-induced decrease in transendothelial electrical resistance (reflecting increased paracellular endothelial permeability) (**Fig. 8**). Previous studies have shown that RhoA, by activating its downstream effector Rho kinase, stimulates actin-myosin-driven contractile forces, which may be transmitted to actin filaments linked to the endothelial adherens junction complex *(78–80)*. This series of events may cause the disruption of adherens junctions, inducing endothelial gap formation and increased paracellular permeability *(3,60)*.

The multiple functions of Rho are mediated by its tightly controlled GTPase cycle. Rho is regulated by a number of proteins, including: (1) guanine nucleotide exchange factors (GEFs), which stimulate GDP to GTP exchange; (2) GTPase-activating proteins (GAPs), which stimulate GTP-hydrolysis; and (3) guanine nucleotide dissociation inhibitors (GDIs), which bind and stabilize Rho-GDP *(74,81–83)*. The GDP-bound form of Rho complexed with GDI is not activated by RhoGEFs, suggesting that Rho activation critically depends upon upstream factors mediating the dissociation of GDI from Rho *(81)*. We have shown that thrombin induces the phosphorylation of GDI and that GDI phosphorylation occurs concurrently with the thrombin-induced activation of Rho *(76)*. Furthermore, the inhibition of protein kinase C (PKC)α abrogates not only thrombin-induced Rho activation, but also GDI phosphorylation and the increase in transendothelial electrical resistance (**Figs. 7–9**). These observations indicate that phosphorylation/dephosphorylation of GDI may play a role in the mechanism of PKCα-induced activation of Rho and endothelial barrier dysfunction.

Several studies show that an increase in cytosolic Ca^{2+} ($[Ca^{2+}]_i$) is a critical factor in activating the disassembly of adherens junctions *(67,84,85)*. PKCα may regulate these events by directly or indirectly regulating the phosphorylation/dephosphorylation state of AJ components *(67)*. Because PKCα regulates Rho activation *(76)*, it is possible that Rho may contribute to the regulation of AJ integrity by way of modulating the increase in $[Ca^{2+}]_i$.

Thrombin increases $[Ca^{2+}]_i$ through the G_q-coupled PLCβ pathway, which triggers Ca^{2+} mobilization from the endoplasmic reticulum (ER). This series of events is followed by Ca^{2+} entry into the cell through the plasmalemma by a process known as capacitative (or store operated) Ca^{2+} entry (CCE) *(86–91)*. The key feature of CCE is that it is activated by a signal generated by the emptying of ER Ca^{2+} stores *(86–91)*. Molecular cloning and functional expression studies have shown that products of the *Drosophila* transient receptor potential (TRP) family of proteins serve as Ca^{2+} channels in non-excitable cells, e.g., endothelial cells *(86–91)*. These channels are activated in response to stimulation of heterotrimeric G-protein-coupled receptors, such as PAR-1. TRP-1, -2, -4, and -5 channels are likely candidates for endogenous store-operated channels (SOCs) since they are activated by Ca^{2+} store depletion *(90)*. TRP channel-1 (TRPC-1) has been demonstrated to mediate Ca^{2+} entry upon store depletion in a variety of cell types, including endothelial cells *(90,92,93)*. However, the identity of the signal that links depletion of ER stores to the activation of Ca^{2+} entry through TRPC remains

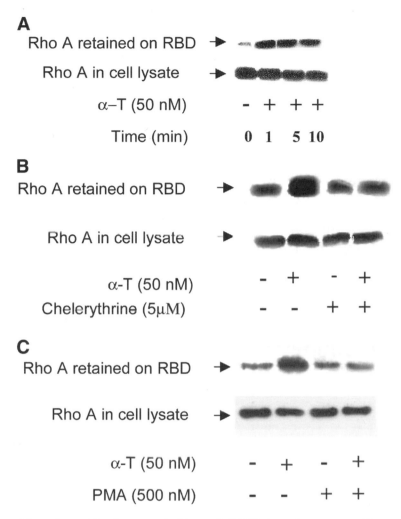

Fig. 7. Thrombin activates Rho in a protein kinase C (PKC)-dependent manner. Human umbilical vein endothelial cells (HUVEC), grown to confluence, were serum starved, then stimulated with thrombin. Rho activity was assayed by pull-down assay at the indicated times. **(A)** Thrombin stimulated Rho activity in a time-dependent manner, with the maximum response occurring at 1 min followed by a slow decline at 10 min. Top panel shows Rho activity as indicated by the amount of Rho bound to beads, whereas bottom panel shows amount of Rho in whole-cell lysates. **(B)** HUVEC were treated with chelerythrine (a broad-spectrum PKC inhibitor) for 30 min, or **(C)** were treated overnight with PMA to deplete conventional and novel PKC isozymes. Cells were lysed after 1 min of thrombin challenge to assay Rho activity. Overnight treatment of HUVEC with PMA prevented Rho activation in response to thrombin, indicating that phorbol-sensitive PKC isozymes induce the activation of Rho. Top panel shows Rho activity as indicated by the amount of Rho bound to beads, whereas bottom panel shows amount of Rho in whole-cell lysates. α-T, α-thrombin; PMA, phorbol 12-myristate 13-acetate. From ref. *76*, with permission.

unclear. Coupling between depleted ER stores with SOC channels has been proposed as the mechanism that activates SOC channels and increases Ca^{2+} influx *(86–91)*. Both chemical and/or conformational coupling has been indicated as a basis for activation of TRPC-1 upon store depletion *(86–91)*. In the chemical-coupling model, Ca^{2+} entry through TRPC may occur as a result of release of a chemical from ER that carries the message for activation of the cell-surface SOC channels; however, identity of these mediator(s) is not known *(94–96)*. In the conformational coupling model,

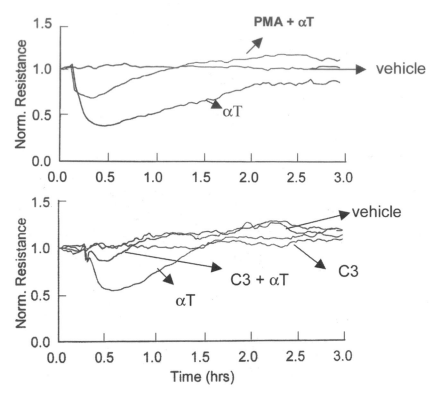

Fig. 8. Effects of inhibition of Rho or depletion of protein kinase C (PKC) on thrombin-induced endothelial cell retraction. Monolayers of Human umbilical vein endothelial cells (HUVEC) grown on gold electrodes were either pretreated overnight with 500 n*M* PMA to deplete phorbol ester-sensitive PKC isozymes (top), or pretreated for 16 h with 10 µg/mL C3 transferase (bottom). Serum-deprived cells were stimulated with 50 n*M* thrombin to measure the changes in transendothelial electrical resistance in real time. The inhibition of Rho or depletion of phorbol-sensitive isozyme markedly attenuated thrombin-induced endothelial cell retraction, indicating that PKC induces the permeability increase activated by thrombin via the Rho-mediated pathway. From ref. *76*, with permission.

store depletion causes inositol 1,4,5-trisphosphate (IP_3) R conformational change, enabling it to interact with TRPC, thereby resulting in channel opening *(86–91)*. If a change in IP_3R conformation is the sole requirement for its coupling to TRPC and its activation, Ca^{2+} entry through these channels should be essentially complete upon store depletion *(86)*. Furthermore, this model fails to explain Ca^{2+} entry by TRPC-1, as these channels have been shown to localize within intracellular membranes *(97)*. Thus, it is possible that this coupling may be induced by a protein that is known to shuttle between the cytosol and PM upon activation.

Small-GTP-binding proteins, such as Rho, have the ability to move from the cytosol to plasmalemma *(83)*. These proteins were initially implicated in inducing SOC activation *(98,99)*. Spatial reorganization of actin filaments in the cell (a Rho-regulated phenomenon) has been shown to regulate Ca^{2+} entry *(100,101)*. In a recent report, we showed that thrombin activated Rho in a time frame corresponding to store depletion-induced Ca^{2+} entry *(91)*. Thrombin stimulation of endothelial cells also induced translocation of Rho and subsequent co-localization of Rho with TRPC-1 and IP_3R at the plasmalemma *(91)*. The present results also demonstrated that appearance of IP_3R and TRPC-1 at the membrane required the activated form of Rho, since thrombin failed to induce PM translocation of these components in endothelial cells pretreated with C3. Inhibition of Rho function with either

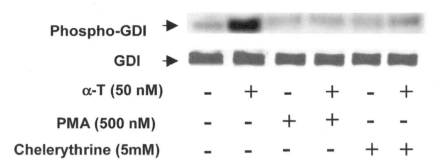

Phospho-GDI ➤						
GDI ➤						
α-T (50 nM)	−	+	−	+	−	+
PMA (500 nM)	−	−	+	+	−	−
Chelerythrine (5mM)	−	−	−	−	+	+

Fig. 9. Thrombin induces guanine nucleotide dissociation inhibitor (GDI) phosphorylation in a phorbol-ester-sensitive protein kinase C (PKC) isozyme-dependent manner. Human umbilical vein endothelial cells (HUVEC) were depleted of phorbol-sensitive PKC isozymes by overnight treatment with 500 nM PMA. Serum-starved cells were then labeled with [^{32}P]-orthophosphate for 4 h in phosphate-free medium. In parallel, labeled cells were treated with chelerythrine (a broad-spectrum PKC inhibitor) for 30 min. Cells were then stimulated with thrombin for 1 min, lysed, and Rho-GDI was immunoprecipitated. Immunoprecipitated proteins were electrophoresed, transferred to nitrocellulose membrane for analysis of phosphorylation (top) and Rho-GDI by Western blotting (bottom). Thrombin induced the phosphorylation of GDI within 1 min, which was not observed in the absence of phorbol-sensitive PKC-isozyme activation. α''-T, ''α-thrombin; PMA, phorbol 12-myristate 13-acetate; P-GDI, phosphorylated GDI. From ref. *76*, with permission.

dn-Rho or C3 transferase significantly reduced Ca^{2+} entry as well as SOC current in single-cell recordings (**Fig. 10**). This was the result of Rho activation of TRPC-1, since overexpression of TRPC-1 in endothelial cells produced a sustained C3 transferase-sensitive increase in [Ca^{2+}]$_i$ in response to thrombin exposure. All together, our results demonstrate an important role of Rho in inducing interaction of the key proteins required for activation of SOC-induced Ca^{2+} entry. Thus, Ca^{2+} entry by this mechanism is important in increasing endothelial permeability, as inhibition of Rho attenuated thrombin-induced increase in endothelial permeability (**Fig. 10**). The present results are consistent with the Rho-activated coupling model, in which Rho, by signaling trafficking of IP$_3$R and TRPC-1 to PM, promotes the interaction of these components of the complex (**Fig. 11**). Membrane insertion of this complex thereby triggers Ca^{2+} entry through TRPC-1 after Ca^{2+} store depletion. Rho-induced actin polymerization also participates in this process by maintaining stable interaction of IP$_3$R and TRPC-1 channels at the PM. Thus, Rho, by regulating [Ca^{2+}]$_i$, may provide an additional regulatory mechanism by which thrombin induces disruption of adherens junctions and increases endothelial permeability due to the paracellular pathway.

4. FUTURE PERSPECTIVES

Studies over the past several years have greatly advanced our understanding of the transcellular and paracellular pathways that regulate endothelial barrier function. Recent studies suggest that these two pathways function in a compensatory way, such that albumin transit across the endothelium is tightly regulated. However, additional research is needed to more fully understand the mechanisms that maintain these pathways in proper balance regulating endothelial permeability.

ACKNOWLEDGMENTS

This work was supported by NIH grants HL45638 and HL71794. We thank Dr. Laura Kelly Price for excellent editorial assistance.

REFERENCES

1. Pappenheimer, J. R., Renkin, E. M., Borrero, L. M. (1951) Filtration, diffusion and molecular sieving through peripheral capillary membranes; a contribution to the pore theory of capillary permeability. *Am. J. Physiol.* **167,** 13–46.

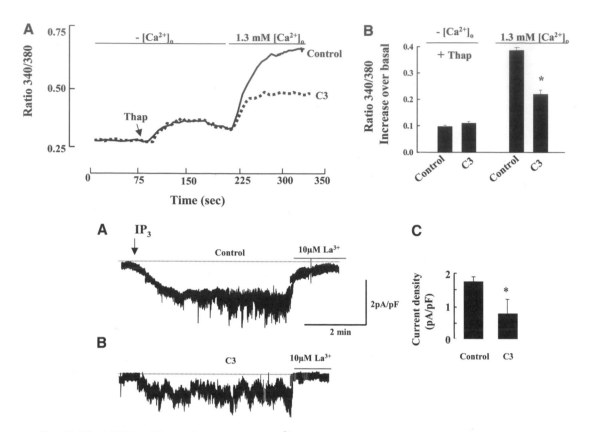

Fig. 10. Rho inhibitor C3 transferase prevents Ca^{2+} entry (top). Human pulmonary arterial endothelial cells transfected without or with 3 μg/mL C3 transferase were loaded with fura2-AM and stimulated with thapsigargin (thap) in the absence of extracellular Ca^{2+} to deplete ER Ca^{2+}. This was followed by re-addition of 1.3 mM $[Ca^{2+}]_o$ to determine Ca^{2+} entry. (A) Trace showing the average of real time data from 25 control or C3-treated cells from a single experiment. (B) Mean ± S.E. of the release of Ca^{2+} from stores, and Ca^{2+} entry from multiple experiments calculated as the maximum increase over basal value in each condition ($n = 3$) (bottom). After establishment of whole-cell patch in human microvascular endothelial cells pretreated without (A or C) or with C3 (B or C), the store-operated channel (SOC) current developed at the holding potential (–50 mV) because of store depletion induced by 30 μM inositol 1,4,5-trisphosphate (F-IP_3) diffusing from the pipet solution. (A–B) Representative trace showing IP_3-induced store-operated channel (SOC) current from control or C3-treated cell. (C) Mean ± S.E. of current density from control or C3-treated cells ($n = 7$ for each condition). *, values different from untreated cells ($p < 0.05$). From ref. *91*, with permission.

2. Renkin, E. M., Watson, P. D., Sloop, C. H., Joyner, W. M., and Curry, F. E. (1977) Transport pathways for fluid and large molecules in microvascular endothelium of the dog's paw. *Microvasc. Res.* **14,** 205–214.
3. Lum, H. and Malik, A. B. (1994) Regulation of vascular endothelial barrier function. *Am. J. Physiol.* **267,** L223–L241.
4. Michel, C. C. and Curry, F. E. (1999) Microvascular permeability. *Physiol. Rev.* **79,** 703–761.
5. Majno, G., Palade, G. E., and Schoefl, G. I. (1961) Studies on inflammation. II. The site of action of histamine and serotonin along the vascular tree: a topographic study. *J. Biophys. Biochem. Cytol.* **11,** 607–626.
6. Majno, G. and Palade, G. E. (1961) Studies on inflammation. 1. The effect of histamine and serotonin on vascular permeability: an electron microscopic study. *J. Biophys. Biochem. Cytol.* **11,** 571–605.
7. Milici, A. J., Watrous, N. E., Stukenbrok, H., and Palade, G. E. (1987) Transcytosis of albumin in capillary endothelium. *J. Cell Biol.* **105,** 2603–2612.
8. Palade, G. F., Simionescu, M., and Simionescu, N. (1981) Differentiated microdomains on the luminal surface of the capillary endothelium. Biorheology **18,** 563–568.
9. Predescu, D. and Palade, G. E. (1993) Plasmalemmal vesicles represent the large pore system of continuous microvascular endothelium. *Am. J. Physiol.* **265,** H725–H733.
10. Schnitzer, J. E., Liu, J., and Oh, P. (1995) Endothelial caveolae have the molecular transport machinery for vesicle budding, docking, and fusion including VAMP, NSF, SNAP, annexins, and GTPases. *J. Biol. Chem.* **270,** 14,399–14,404.

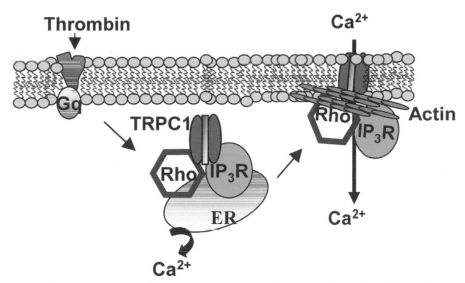

Fig. 11. Model of Rho-activated Ca^{2+} entry. Upon activation, Rho associates with IP_3R and transient receptor potential channel 1 (TRPC-1), and the complex is translocated to the plasma membrane. Rho couples IP_3R to TRPC-1 in an actin filament polymerization-dependent manner, thereby linking Ca^{2+} store emptying to Ca^{2+} entry. From ref. *91*, with permission.

11. Palade, G. E. (1953) Fine structure of blood capillaries. *J. Appl. Physiol.* **24,** 1424–1436.
12. Liu, P. and Anderson, R. G. (1995) Compartmentalized production of ceramide at the cell surface. *J. Biol. Chem.* **270,** 27,179–27,185.
13. Smart, E. J., Graf, G. A., McNiven, M. A., et al. (1999) Caveolins, liquid-ordered domains, and signal transduction. *Mol. Cell. Biol.* **19,** 7289–7304.
14. Minshall, R. D., Tiruppathi, C., Vogel, S. M., et al. (2000) Endothelial cell-surface gp60 activates vesicle formation and trafficking via G(i)-coupled Src kinase signaling pathway. *J. Cell Biol.* **150,** 1057–1070.
15. John, T. A., Vogel, S. M., Tiruppathi, C., Malik, A. B., and Minshall, R. D. (2003) Quantitative analysis of albumin uptake and transport in the rat microvessel endothelial monolayer. *Am. J. Physiol. Lung Cell Mol. Physiol.* **284,** L187–L196.
16. Rothberg, K. G., Ying, Y. S., Kamen, B. A., and Anderson, R. G. (1990) Cholesterol controls the clustering of the glycophospholipid-anchored membrane receptor for 5-methyltetrahydrofolate. *J. Cell Biol.* **111,** 2931–2938.
17. Rothberg, K. G., Heuser, J. E., Donzell, W. C., Ying, Y. S., Glenney, J. R., and Anderson, R. G. (1992) Caveolin, a protein component of caveolae membrane coats. *Cell* **68,** 673–682.
18. Schnitzer, J. E., Oh, P., Pinney, E., and Allard, J. (1994) Filipin-sensitive caveolae-mediated transport in endothelium: reduced transcytosis, scavenger endocytosis, and capillary permeability of select macromolecules. *J. Cell Biol.* **127,** 1217–1232.
19. Okamoto, T., Schlegel, A., Scherer, P. E., and Lisanti, M. P. (1998) Caveolins, a family of scaffolding proteins for organizing "preassembled signaling complexes" at the plasma membrane. *J. Biol. Chem.* **273,** 5419–5422.
20. Scherer, P. E., Lewis, R. Y., Volonte, D., et al. (1997) Cell-type and tissue-specific expression of caveolin-2. Caveolins 1 and 2 co-localize and form a stable hetero-oligomeric complex in vivo. *J. Biol. Chem.* **272,** 29,337–29,346.
21. Monier, S., Parton, R. G., Vogel, F., Behlke, J., Henske, A., Kurzchalia, T. V. (1995) VIP21-caveolin, a membrane protein constituent of the caveolar coat, oligomerizes in vivo and in vitro. *Mol. Biol. Cell* **6,** 911–927.
22. Fra, A. M., Masserini, M., Palestini, P., Sonnino, S., and Simons, K. (1995) A photo-reactive derivative of ganglioside GM1 specifically cross-links VIP21-caveolin on the cell surface. *FEBS Lett.* **375,** 11–14.
23. Sargiacomo, M., Scherer, P. E., Tang, Z., et al. (1995) Oligomeric structure of caveolin: implications for caveolae membrane organization. *Proc. Natl. Acad. Sci. USA* **92,** 9407–9411.
24. Simionescu, M., Gafencu, A., and Antohe, F. (2002) Transcytosis of plasma macromolecules in endothelial cells: a cell biological survey. *Microsc. Res. Tech.* **57,** 269–288.
25. Minshall, R. D., Tiruppathi, C., Vogel, S. M., and Malik, A. B. (2002) Vesicle formation and trafficking in endothelial cells and regulation of endothelial barrier function. *Histochem. Cell. Biol.* **117,** 105–112.
26. Schnitzer, J. E., Carley, W. W., and Palade, G. E. (1988) Albumin interacts specifically with a 60-kDa microvascular endothelial glycoprotein. *Proc. Natl. Acad. Sci. USA* **85,** 6773–6777.
27. Schnitzer, J. E., Ulmer, J. B., and Palade, G. E. (1990) A major endothelial plasmalemmal sialoglycoprotein, gp60, is immunologically related to glycophorin. *Proc. Natl. Acad. Sci. USA* **87,** 6843–6847.
28. Schnitzer, J. E. (1992) gp60 is an albumin-binding glycoprotein expressed by continuous endothelium involved in albumin transcytosis. *Am. J. Physiol.* **262,** H246–H254.

29. Schnitzer, J. E. and Oh, P. (1994) Albondin-mediated capillary permeability to albumin. Differential role of receptors in endothelial transcytosis and endocytosis of native and modified albumins. *J. Biol. Chem.* **269,** 6072–6082.
30. Tiruppathi, C., Finnegan, A., and Malik, A. B. (1996) Isolation and characterization of a cell surface albumin-binding protein from vascular endothelial cells. *Proc. Natl. Acad. Sci. USA* **93,** 250–254.
31. Tiruppathi, C., Song, W., Bergenfeldt, M., Sass, P., and Malik, A. B. (1997) Gp60 activation mediates albumin transcytosis in endothelial cells by tyrosine kinase-dependent pathway. *J. Biol. Chem.* **272,** 25,968–25,975.
32. Vogel, S. M., Easington, C. R., Minshall, R. D., et al. (2001) Evidence of transcellular permeability pathway in microvessels. *Microvasc. Res.* **61,** 87–101.
33. Vogel, S. M., Minshall, R. D., Pilipovic, M., Tiruppathi, C., and Malik, A. B. (2001) Albumin uptake and transcytosis in endothelial cells in vivo induced by albumin-binding protein. *Am. J. Physiol. Lung Cell Mol. Physiol.* **281,** L1512–L1522.
34. Ghitescu, L., Fixman, A., Simionescu, M., and Simionescu, N. (1986) Specific binding sites for albumin restricted to plasmalemmal vesicles of continuous capillary endothelium: receptor-mediated transcytosis. *J. Cell Biol.* **102,** 1304–1311.
35. Predescu, S. A., Predescu, D. N., and Palade, G. E. (1997) Plasmalemmal vesicles function as transcytotic carriers for small proteins in the continuous endothelium. *Am. J. Physiol.* **272,** H937–H949.
36. Siflinger-Birnboim, A., Schnitzer, J., Lum, H., et al. (1991) Lectin binding to gp60 decreases specific albumin binding and transport in pulmonary artery endothelial monolayers. *J. Cell. Physiol.* **149,** 575–584.
37. Niles, W. D. and Malik, A. B. (1999) Endocytosis and exocytosis events regulate vesicle traffic in endothelial cells. *J. Membr. Biol.* **167,** 85–101.
38. Rothman, J. E. (2002) Lasker Basic Medical Research Award. The machinery and principles of vesicle transport in the cell. *Nat. Med.* **8,** 1059–1062.
39. Schnitzer, J. E., Allard, J., and Oh, P. (1995) NEM inhibits transcytosis, endocytosis, and capillary permeability: implication of caveolae fusion in endothelia. *Am. J. Physiol.* **268,** H48–H55.
40. Predescu, D., Horvat, R., Predescu, S., and Palade, G. E. (1994) Transcytosis in the continuous endothelium of the myocardial microvasculature is inhibited by N-ethylmaleimide. *Proc. Natl. Acad. Sci. USA* **91,** 3014–3018.
41. Schnitzer, J. E., Oh, P., and McIntosh, D. P. (1996) Role of GTP hydrolysis in fission of caveolae directly from plasma membranes. *Science* **274,** 239–242.
42. Oh, P., McIntosh, D. P., and Schnitzer, J. E. (1998) Dynamin at the neck of caveolae mediates their budding to form transport vesicles by GTP-driven fission from the plasma membrane of endothelium. *J. Cell Biol.* **141,** 101–114.
43. Parton, R. G. (1994) Ultrastructural localization of gangliosides; GM1 is concentrated in caveolae. *J. Histochem. Cytochem.* **42,** 155–166.
44. Predescu, S. A., Predescu, D. N., Palade, G. E. (2001) Endothelial transcytotic machinery involves supramolecular protein-lipid complexes. *Mol. Biol. Cell* **12,** 1019–1033.
45. Lisanti, M. P., Scherer, P. E., Vidugiriene, J., et al. (1994) Characterization of caveolin-rich membrane domains isolated from an endothelial-rich source: implications for human disease. *J. Cell Biol.* **126,** 111–126.
46. Parton, R. G., Joggerst, B., and Simons, K. (1994) Regulated internalization of caveolae. *J. Cell Biol.* **127,** 1199–215.
47. Glenney, J. R., Jr. (1989) Tyrosine phosphorylation of a 22-kDa protein is correlated with transformation by Rous sarcoma virus. *J. Biol. Chem.* **264,** 20,163–20,166.
48. Li, S., Seitz, R., Lisanti MP. (1996) Phosphorylation of caveolin by src tyrosine kinases. The alpha-isoform of caveolin is selectively phosphorylated by v-Src in vivo. *J. Biol. Chem.* **271,** 3863–8.
49. Ahn, S., Maudsley, S., Luttrell, L. M., Lefkowitz, R. J., and Daaka, Y. (1999) Src-mediated tyrosine phosphorylation of dynamin is required for beta2-adrenergic receptor internalization and mitogen-activated protein kinase signaling. *J. Biol. Chem.* **274,** 1185–1188.
50. Ahn, S., Kim, J., Lucaveche, C. L., et al. (2002) Src-dependent tyrosine phosphorylation regulates dynamin self-assembly and ligand-induced endocytosis of the epidermal growth factor receptor. *J. Biol. Chem.* **277,** 26,642–26,651.
51. Orth, J. D., Krueger, E. W., Cao, H., and McNiven, M. A. (2002) The large GTPase dynamin regulates actin comet formation and movement in living cells. *Proc. Natl. Acad. Sci. USA* **99,** 167–172.
52. Murthy, K. S. and Makhlouf, G. M. (2000) Heterologous desensitization mediated by G protein-specific binding to caveolin. *J. Biol. Chem.* **275,** 30,211–30,219.
53. Igishi, T. and Gutkind, J. S. (1998) Tyrosine kinases of the Src family participate in signaling to MAP kinase from both Gq and Gi-coupled receptors. *Biochem. Biophys. Res. Commun.* **244,** 5–10.
54. Ellis, C. A., Malik, A. B., Gilchrist, A., et al. (1999) Thrombin induces proteinase-activated receptor-1 gene expression in endothelial cells via activation of Gi-linked Ras/mitogen-activated protein kinase pathway. *J. Biol. Chem.* **274,** 13,718–13,727.
55. Li, S., Couet, J., and Lisanti, M. P. (1996) Src tyrosine kinases, Galpha subunits, and H-Ras share a common membrane-anchored scaffolding protein, caveolin. Caveolin binding negatively regulates the auto-activation of Src tyrosine kinases. *J. Biol. Chem.* **271,** 29,182–29,190.
56. Anderson, R. G. (1998) The caveolae membrane system. *Annu. Rev. Biochem.* **67,** 199–225.
57. Drab, M., Verkade, P., Elger, M., et al. (2001) Loss of caveolae, vascular dysfunction, and pulmonary defects in caveolin-1 gene-disrupted mice. *Science* **293,** 2449–2452.
58. Razani, B., Engelman, J. A., Wang, X. B., et al. (2001) Caveolin-1 null mice are viable but show evidence of hyperproliferative and vascular abnormalities. *J. Biol. Chem.* **276,** 38,121–38,138.
59. Schubert, W., Frank, P. G., Woodman, S. E., et al. (2002) Microvascular hyperpermeability in caveolin-1 (-/-) knockout mice. Treatment with a specific nitric-oxide synthase inhibitor, L-name, restores normal microvascular permeability in Cav-1 null mice. *J. Biol. Chem.* **277,** 40,091–40,098.

60. Dudek, S. M. and Garcia, J. G. (2001) Cytoskeletal regulation of pulmonary vascular permeability. *J. Appl. Physiol.* **91,** 1487–1500.
61. Bazzoni, G., Dejana, E., and Lampugnani, M. G. (1999) Endothelial adhesion molecules in the development of the vascular tree: the garden of forking paths. *Curr. Opin. Cell Biol.* **11,** 573–581.
62. Dejana, E. (1997) Endothelial adherens junctions: implications in the control of vascular permeability and angiogenesis. *J. Clin. Invest.* **100,** S7–S10.
63. Dejana, E., Spagnuolo, R., and Bazzoni, G. (2001) Interendothelial junctions and their role in the control of angiogenesis, vascular permeability and leukocyte transmigration. *Thromb. Haemost.* **86,** 308–315.
64. Rabiet, M. J., Plantier, J. L., Rival, Y., Genoux, Y., Lampugnani, M. G., and Dejana, E. (1996) Thrombin-induced increase in endothelial permeability is associated with changes in cell-to-cell junction organization. *Arterioscler. Thromb. Vasc. Biol.* **16,** 488–496.
65. Corada, M., Mariotti, M., Thurston, G., et al. (1999) Vascular endothelial-cadherin is an important determinant of microvascular integrity in vivo. *Proc. Natl. Acad. Sci. USA* **96,** 9815–9820.
66. Hordijk, P. L., Anthony, E., Mul, F. P., Rientsma, R., Oomen, L. C., and Roos, D. (1999) Vascular-endothelial-cadherin modulates endothelial monolayer permeability. *J. Cell Sci.* **112,** 1915–1923.
67. Sandoval, R., Malik, A., Minshall, R., Kouklis, P., Ellis, C., and Tiruppathi, C. (2001) Ca(2+) signalling and PKCalpha activate increased endothelial permeability by disassembly of VE-cadherin junctions. *J. Physiol.* **533,** 433–445.
68. Anastasiadis, P. Z., Moon, S. Y., Thoreson, M. A., et al. (2000) Inhibition of RhoA by p120 catenin. *Nat. Cell Biol.* **2,** 637–644.
69. Noren, N. K., Liu, B. P., Burridge, K., and Kreft, B. (2000) p120 catenin regulates the actin cytoskeleton via Rho family GTPases. *J. Cell Biol.* **150,** 567–580.
70. Garcia, J. G., Verin, A. D., and Schaphorst, K. L. (1996) Regulation of thrombin-mediated endothelial cell contraction and permeability. *Semin. Thromb. Hemost.* **22,** 309–315.
71. Coughlin, S. R., Scarborough, R. M., Vu, T. K., and Hung, D. T. (1992) Thrombin receptor structure and function. *Cold Spring Harb. Symp. Quant. Biol.* **57,** 149–154.
72. Coughlin, S. R. (2000) Thrombin signalling and protease-activated receptors. *Nature* **407,** 258–264.
73. Vu, T. K., Hung, D. T., Wheaton, V. I., and Coughlin, S. R. (1991) Molecular cloning of a functional thrombin receptor reveals a novel proteolytic mechanism of receptor activation. *Cell* **64,** 1057–1068.
74. Kozasa, T., Jiang, X., Hart, M. J., et al. (1998) p115 RhoGEF, a GTPase activating protein for Galpha12 and Galpha13. *Science* **280,** 2109–2111.
75. Holinstat, M., Mehta, D., Kozasa, T., Minshall, R. D., and Malik, A. B. (2003) Protein kinase Calpha-induced p115RhoGEF phosphorylation signals endothelial cytoskeletal rearrangement. *J. Biol. Chem.* **278,** 28,793–28,798.
76. Mehta, D., Rahman, A., and Malik, A. B. (2001) Protein kinase C-alpha signals rho-guanine nucleotide dissociation inhibitor phosphorylation and rho activation and regulates the endothelial cell barrier function. *J. Biol. Chem.* **276,** 22,614–22,620.
77. Sah, V. P., Seasholtz, T. M., Sagi, S. A., and Brown, J. H. (2000) The role of Rho in G protein-coupled receptor signal transduction. *Annu. Rev. Pharmacol. Toxicol.* **40,** 459–489.
78. van Nieuw Amerongen, G. P., Draijer, R., Vermeer, M. A., and van Hinsbergh, V. W. (1998) Transient and prolonged increase in endothelial permeability induced by histamine and thrombin: role of protein kinases, calcium, and RhoA. *Circ. Res.* **83,** 1115–1123.
79. van Nieuw Amerongen, G. P., van Delft, S., Vermeer, M. A., Collard, J. G., and van Hinsbergh, V. W. (2000) Activation of RhoA by thrombin in endothelial hyperpermeability: role of Rho kinase and protein tyrosine kinases. *Circ. Res.* **87,** 335–340.
80. Essler, M., Amano, M., Kruse, H. J., Kaibuchi, K., Weber, P. C., and Aepfelbacher, M. (1998) Thrombin inactivates myosin light chain phosphatase via Rho and its target Rho kinase in human endothelial cells. *J. Biol. Chem.* **273,** 21,867–21,874.
81. Olofsson, B. (1999) Rho guanine dissociation inhibitors: pivotal molecules in cellular signalling. *Cell. Signal.* **11,** 545–554.
82. Sasaki, T. and Takai, Y. (1998) The Rho small G protein family-Rho GDI system as a temporal and spatial determinant for cytoskeletal control. *Biochem. Biophys. Res. Commun.* **245,** 641–645.
83. Ridley, A. J. (2001) Rho family proteins: coordinating cell responses. *Trends Cell Biol.* **11,** 471–477.
84. Sandoval, R., Malik, A. B., Naqvi, T., Mehta, D., and Tiruppathi, C. (2001) Requirement for Ca2+ signaling in the mechanism of thrombin-induced increase in endothelial permeability. *Am. J. Physiol. Lung Cell Mol. Physiol.* **280,** L239–L247.
85. Gao, X., Kouklis, P., Xu, N., et al. (2000) Reversibility of increased microvessel permeability in response to VE-cadherin disassembly. *Am. J. Physiol. Lung Cell Mol. Physiol.* **279,** L1218–L1225.
86. Venkatachalam, K., van Rossum, D. B., Patterson, R. L., Ma, H. T., and Gill, D. L. (2002) The cellular and molecular basis of store-operated calcium entry. *Nat. Cell Biol.* **4,** E263–E272.
87. Berridge, M. J. (1995) Capacitative calcium entry. Biochem. J. **312,** 1–11.
88. Putney, J. W., Jr. (1999) TRP, inositol 1,4,5-trisphosphate receptors, and capacitative calcium entry. *Proc. Natl. Acad. Sci. USA* **96,** 14,669–14,671.
89. Putney, J. W., Jr., Broad, L. M., Braun, F. J., Lievremont, J. P., and Bird, G. S. (2001) Mechanisms of capacitative calcium entry. *J. Cell Sci.* **114,** 2223–2229.
90. Nilius, B. and Droogmans, G. (2001) Ion channels and their functional role in vascular endothelium. *Physiol. Rev.* **81,** 1415–1459.

91. Mehta, D., Ahmmed, G. U., Paria, B. C., et al. (2003) RhoA interaction with inositol 1,4,5-trisphosphate receptor and transient receptor potential channel-1 regulates Ca2+ entry. Role in signaling increased endothelial permeability. *J. Biol. Chem.* **278,** 33,492–33,500.

92. Moore, T. M., Brough, G. H., Babal, P., Kelly, J. J., Li, M., and Stevens, T. (1998) Store-operated calcium entry promotes shape change in pulmonary endothelial cells expressing Trp1. *Am. J. Physiol.* **275,** L574–L582.

93. Brough, G. H., Wu, S., Cioffi, D., et al. (2001) Contribution of endogenously expressed Trp1 to a Ca2+-selective, store-operated Ca2+ entry pathway. *FASEB J.* **15,** 1727–1738.

94. Parekh, A. B., Terlau, H., and Stuhmer, W. (1993) Depletion of InsP3 stores activates a Ca2+ and K+ current by means of a phosphatase and a diffusible messenger. *Nature* **364,** 814–818.

95. Randriamampita, C. and Tsien, R. Y. (1993) Emptying of intracellular Ca2+ stores releases a novel small messenger that stimulates Ca2+ influx. *Nature* **364,** 809–814.

96. Su, Z., Csutora, P., Hunton, D., Shoemaker, R. L., Marchase, R. B., and Blalock, J. E. (2001) A store-operated nonselective cation channel in lymphocytes is activated directly by Ca(2+) influx factor and diacylglycerol. *Am. J. Physiol. Cell Physiol.* **280,** C1284–C1292.

97. Hofmann, T., Schaefer, M., Schultz, G., and Gudermann, T. (2002) Subunit composition of mammalian transient receptor potential channels in living cells. *Proc. Natl. Acad. Sci. USA* **99,** 7461–7466.

98. Bird, G. S. and Putney, J. W., Jr. (1993) Inhibition of thapsigargin-induced calcium entry by microinjected guanine nucleotide analogues. Evidence for the involvement of a small G- protein in capacitative calcium entry. *J. Biol. Chem.* **268,** 21,486–21,488.

99. Fasolato., C., Hoth, M., and Penner, R. (1993) A GTP-dependent step in the activation mechanism of capacitative calcium influx. *J. Biol. Chem.* **268,** 20,737–20,740.

100. Rosado, J. A. and Sage, S. O. (2000) A role for the actin cytoskeleton in the initiation and maintenance of store-mediated calcium entry in human platelets. *Trends Cardiovasc. Med.* **10,** 327–332.

101. Rosado, J. A. and Sage, S. O. (2000) Regulation of plasma membrane Ca2+-ATPase by small GTPases and phosphoinositides in human platelets. *J. Biol. Chem.* **275,** 19,529–19,535.

102. Minshall, R. D., Tiruppathi, C., Vogel, S. M., et al. (2000) Endothelial cell-surface gp60 activates vesicle formation and trafficking via G i -coupled Src kinase signaling pathway. *J. Cell Biol.* **150,** 1057–1070.

10

Sphingolipid Signaling

Implications for Vascular Biology

Margaret M. Harnett

SUMMARY

Sphingolipids comprise a family (>300) of lipids that are characterized by their sphingoid backbone but differ in their headgroup constituents. Complex headgroups involving β-glucose or galactose linkages (cerebrosides), sialic acid (gangliosides), or sulphated-galactosyl linkages (sulphatides) are known as glycosphingolipids and have long been recognized as playing roles in maintaining the structural integrity of membranes and mediating cell-cell recognition and interactions. In contrast, the addition of phosphorylcholine to ceramide by sphingomyelin synthase generates the prototypic phosphosphingolipid, sphingomyelin. These phosphosphingolipids are present in much lower concentrations, and recent interest has focused on the role of three sphingomyelin-derived second messengers—ceramide, sphingosine, and sphingosine-1-phosphate (S1P)—in regulating cell fate (death/survival) decisions. Moreover, there is increasing evidence that sphingolipids can also signal by modulating receptor function by regulating the formation of lipid rafts, specialized membrane signaling domains that are enriched in cholesterol and sphingolipids. This review will discuss the signaling roles of the sphingolipid-derived second messengers and the implications for vascular biology.

Key Words: Sphingolipids; signal transduction; ceramide; sphingosine-1-phosphate; Edg receptors; calcium.

1. INTRODUCTION

Until the late 1970s, lipids were considered to play simply a structural role in the generation and maintenance of cell-membrane permeability barriers due to their amphipathic nature and ability to form bilayers. However, at this time it was discovered that the "second messenger" molecule required for the receptor-mediated mobilization of intracellular stores of calcium was inositol 1,4,5-trisphosphate (IP_3), a product of the phospholipase C-mediated hydrolysis of a minor phospholipid species phosphatidylinositol 4,5-bisphosphate (PIP_2) *(1)*. Moreover, the alternative product of PIP_2 hydrolysis, diacylglycerol (DAG), was found to be the physiological activator of a family of key downstream signaling serine/threonine protein kinases known generically as protein kinase C (PKC), which had previously been identified as the target of the tumor promoter phorbol myristate acetate (PMA). The importance of these lipid-derived second messengers was underlined by the finding that receptor-mediated responses such as exocytosis or proliferation of many cell types could be mimicked by pharmacological activation of PKC by PMA and calcium mobilization by calcium ionophores *(2)*. Moreover, PIP_2 was also found to be the substrate for the lipid kinase phosphoinositide

From: *Cell Signaling in Vascular Inflammation*
Edited by: J. Bhattacharya © Humana Press Inc., Totowa, NJ

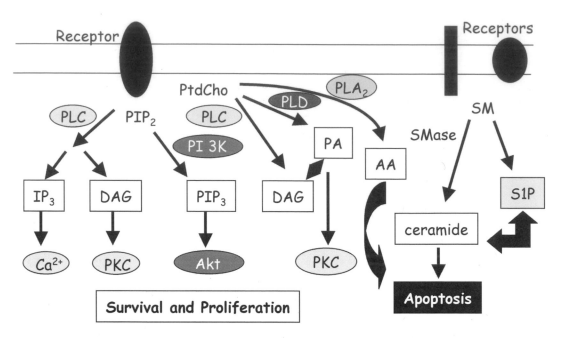

Fig. 1. Receptor-coupled lipid signal transduction. G protein-coupled receptors or growth-factor receptor tyrosine kinases couple to one or more phospholipid and sphingolipid signaling pathways to transduce signals leading to apoptosis, survival, differentiation, or proliferation. These signals may crosstalk: for example, in many cell types tumor necrosis factor receptor (TNF-R) coupling to SMase-mediated generation of ceramide is dependent on prior induction of AA via cPLA$_2$. Likewise, in monocytes, FcγRI coupling to sphingosine kinase and S1P generation is dependent on upstream coupling to PI 3K and PtdCho-PLD. Abbreviations: AA, arachidonic acid; Akt, the proto-oncogene ser/thr kinase, Akt; DAG, diacylglycerol; IP$_3$, inositol 1,4,5-trisphosphate; PA, phosphatiditic acid; PI 3K, phosphoinositide 3-kinase; PIP$_2$, phosphatidylinositol 4,5-bisphosphate; PIP$_3$, phosphatidylinositol 3,4,5-trisphosphate; PKC, protein kinase C; PLA$_2$, phospholipase A$_2$; PLC, phospholipase C; PLD, phospholipase D; PtdCho, phosphatidylcholine; S1P, sphingosine-1-phosphate; SM, sphingomyelin; SMase, sphingomyelinase.

3-kinase (PI 3K), which generates the lipid second messenger PI (3,4,5)P$_3$, a key player in many cellular responses, including the movement of organelle membranes, shape alteration through rearrangement of cytoskeletal actin, rescue from apoptosis, transformation, and chemotaxis (3). These findings triggered an explosive burst of research into the role of lipids and their products as key players in receptor-mediated signal transduction (1–4).

The fact that PIP$_2$ was a minor phospholipid species found in the inner leaflet of the plasma membrane fitted with the then current dogma that second-messenger signals had to be transient signals. However, it became apparent that for many prolonged responses such as proliferation, sustained and substantial generation of DAG and/or PKC activation was required, suggesting that such DAG was generated from alternative sources (Fig. 1). This proposal led to the finding that hydrolysis of the major phospholipid phosphatidylcholine (PtdCho; <40% plasma membrane lipid) provided a range of lipid second messengers. Indeed, PtdCho can be hydrolyzed by (1) PLC, to generate phosphocholine (PC) and DAG; (2) phospholipase D (PLD), to generate choline and phosphatiditic acid (PA); and (3) phospholipase A$_2$, to produce arachidonic acid (AA) and lysophosphatidylcholine (5,6). It is now widely established that DAG, PA (these are interconvertible), and AA all can have second-messenger function (7,8), and there is increasing evidence that PC can also function in this manner (9).

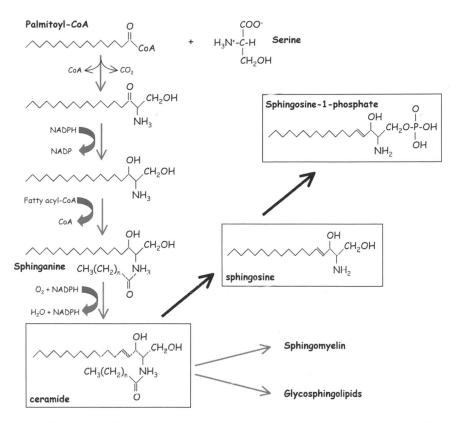

Fig. 2. Sphingolipid metabolic pathways. Serine palmitoyltransferase condenses palmitoyl-CoA plus serine to generate 3-oxosphinganine, which is then converted to sphinganine by oxosphinganine reductase. Sphinganine is then converted to dihydroceramide by dihydroceramide synthase, the target of the inhibitor fumonisin B. Dihydroceramide is then converted to ceramide by dihydroceramide desaturase (*de novo* ceramide generation). Ceramide can then be incorporated into phosphosphingolipids such as sphingomyelin by sphingomelin synthase or alternatively, into glycosphingolipids by enzymes such as glucosylceramide synthase. During prosurvival signaling ceramide may be metabolized to sphingosine by ceramidase and subsequently to sphingosine-1-phosphate by sphingosine kinase. Sphingosine-1-phosphate can then be degraded by sphingosine-1-phosphate lyase or reconverted to sphingosine by sphingosine-1-phosphatase. Ceramide can also be generated by sphingomyelinase-mediated hydrolysis of sphingomyelin.

The finding that PtdCho is generally found in the outer leaflet of the plasma membrane also demonstrated that bioactive lipids need not be located in the inner leaflet of the plasma membrane, and suggested that all membrane lipids could potentially act as sources of lipid second messengers. Indeed, a wealth of data in the last 10–15 yr has implicated key signaling roles for another major class of lipids, the sphingolipids. Sphingolipids, which are found in all eukaryotes and can be broadly subdivided into glycophingolipids and phosphosphingolipids, comprise a family (>300) of lipids that are characterized by their sphingoid backbone but differ in their headgroup constituents (**Fig. 2**). Complex headgroups involving β-glucose or galactose linkages (cerebrosides), sialic acid (gangliosides), or sulphated-galactosyl linkages (sulphatides) are known as glycosphingolipids and have long been recognized as playing roles in maintaining the structural integrity of membranes and mediating cell–cell recognition and interactions. In contrast, the addition of phosphorylcholine to ceramide by sphingomyelin synthase generates the prototypic phosphosphingolipid sphingomyelin. These phosphosphingolipids are present in much lower concentrations, and recent interest has focused on the role of three sphingomyelin-derived second messengers—ceramide, sphingosine, and sphingosine-1-phosphate (S1P)—in regulating cell fate (death/survival) decisions *(10–16)*. Moreover, there is increasing evidence that sphingolipids can also signal by modulating receptor function by regulating the formation of lipid rafts, specialized membrane signaling domains that are enriched in cholesterol and sphingolipids *(17–20)*. This review will discuss the signaling roles of the sphingolipid-derived second messengers and the implications for vascular biology.

2. CERAMIDE AND APOPTOSIS

Ceramide, which can be generated either by hydrolysis of the sphingolipid sphingomyelin (SM) by a family of acid and neutral sphingomyelinases (SMase) or by *de novo* synthesis, has been proposed to be a coordinator of stress responses *(10,12,18,21,22)*. Indeed, stress signals such as cytokines (e.g., tumor necrosis factor [TNF]), heat, ultraviolet (UV) irradiation, hypoxia, and chemotherapeutic agents (e.g., doxorubicin, etoposide) all induce SMase and/or *de novo* generation of ceramide, and this induction of ceramide correlates with apoptosis. Indeed, it is well established that such apoptosis can be mimicked by pharmacological application of the short ceramides C2-ceramide or C6-ceramide.

Ceramide-mediated apoptosis appears to act by disrupting mitochondrial integrity, leading to the activation of caspases and consequent cellular disassembly. Thus, the role of SMase activation and ceramide generation in the outer leaflet of the plasma membrane in transducing apoptosis is not clear, and indeed the generation of acid SMase knockout mice have further questioned the likelihood of an essential role of this pool of ceramide in transducing apoptotic signals. In contrast, the recent complete delineation of the pathways of sphingolipid metabolism in yeast indicated that the enzymes involved in *de novo* synthesis of ceramide are localized to the endoplasmic reticulum, golgi, and mitochondrial membranes. Together with the finding that inhibitors of this pathway induce apoptosis in vitro, the localization of these enzymes has suggested a key role for receptor-driven *de novo* synthesis of ceramide in the transduction of apoptosis *(21,22)*. This proposal has been supported by the finding that inhibition of enzymes such as dihydroceramide synthase (by the fungal agent fumonisin B, **Fig. 2**) in vivo results in disorders associated with disruption of apoptosis, such as various cancers, pulmonary edema, kidney toxicity, and neural tube disorders *(15,18,21,22)*. Care should be taken when interpreting the effects of fumonisin B, however, as blockage of dihydroceramide synthase could lead to generation of the anti-apoptotic/promitogenic homolog of S1P, sphinganine-1-phosphate. Nevertheless, mutations in the first enzyme of the pathway, serine palmitoyl transferase (SPTLC1), similarly cause hereditary type-1 sensory neuropathy, the most common hereditary disorder of peripheral sensory neurons *(21,22)*.

Although the precise mechanisms underlying ceramide-induced apoptosis are unclear, disruption of mitochondrial potential, regulated by pro- and anti-apoptotic members of the Bcl-2 family, results in the release of cytochrome C to the cytoplasm and activation of effector caspases or other executioner proteases, such as cathepsins. Loss of mitochondrial integrity results in cell-cycle arrest, and activation of caspases/cathepsins leads to endonuclease activation and cellular disassembly, hallmarks of apoptosis (**Fig. 3**). Growth factor-derived signals can rescue/prevent such mitochondrial targeted apoptosis by coupling to the PI 3K-dependent generation of PIP_3 and consequent activation of the proto-oncogene serine/threonine kinase Akt (or protein kinase B; PKB). Akt acts, in least in part, to phosphorylate and deactivate pro-apoptotic Bcl-2 family members, such as Bad, and thus protects mitochondrial integrity. Ceramide impacts on these signals in a number of ways *(10,12,18,21,22)*: firstly, ceramide signaling generally acts to oppose mitogenic PLD, PKC, and Ras signaling. In addition, ceramide can induce the activation of the stress kinases p38 and Jnk MAPK, which have been implicated in the transduction of apoptosis *(23)*. Moreover, ceramide can induce the activation of the serine/threonine protein phosphatases PP1 and PP2A, which can act to switch off survival signals by, for example, dephosphorylating and inactivating Akt, dephosphorylating and activating Bad, and/or regulating induction and activation of Bcl-2/Bcl-$_X$ and caspase 9 *(10,12,24)*. Similarly, dephosphorylation of the retinoblastoma protein that regulates the transcription of genes required for mitogenesis (Rb) results in cell-cycle arrest at the G1-S-phase transition point. Finally, it

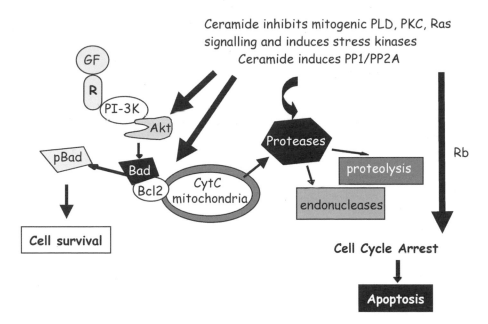

Fig. 3. Mechanisms of ceramide induction of apoptosis. Disruption of mitochondrial potential, regulated by pro- (Bad) and anti-apoptotic (Bcl-2) members of the Bcl-2 family, leads to the release of cytochrome C to the cytoplasm and activation of effector caspases or other executioner proteases, such as cathepsins, and results in apoptosis. Growth factor-derived signals can rescue/prevent such mitochondrial-targeted apoptosis by coupling to the activation of Akt. Akt phosphorylates and deactivates Bad and thus protects mitochondrial integrity. Ceramide opposes mitogenic signaling and induces the activation of the stress kinases p38 and Jnk MAPK and the serine/threonine protein phosphatases PP1 and PP2A. PP1 and PP2A switch off survival/proliferation signals by dephosphorylating and inactivating Akt, Bad, and Rb. Finally, it appears that ceramide can also bind directly to, and activate, executioner proteases such as cathepsin D.

appears that ceramide can also bind directly to and activate executioner proteases such as cathepsin D *(10,12).*

3. THE CERAMIDE-SPHINGOSINE-1-PHOSPHATE RHEOSTAT

The identification of S1P as an anti-apoptotic/promitogenic lipid second messenger led to the proposal that the receptor-driven interconversion of ceramide and S1P provided a dynamic switch mechanism, "the ceramide-sphingosine-1-phosphate rheostat," for regulating commitment to and rescue from apoptosis (**Fig. 4**). As S1P is derived from ceramide via sphingosine by the consecutive actions of ceramidase and sphingosine kinase, and the actions of ceramide and S1P are mutually antagonistic, the balance of signal dictates the functional outcome *(13–16,25)*. Indeed, this rheostat provides a dynamic and amplifying system of regulation. Thus, while ceramide acts to downregulate mitogenic signals such as PKC and Erk, and induces apoptotic signals such as stress kinases and caspases, conversion to S1P both relieves such negative signaling and actively promotes positive signaling by downregulating apoptotic signals and inducing mitogenic signals such as PKC and Erk *(13–16)*.

The importance of S1P in mitogenic signaling has been indicated not only by studies involving the addition of exogenous S1P or sphingosine kinase (SPHK) inhibitors, but also by recent genetic studies overexpressing wild-type or dominant-negative constructs of the recently cloned SPHK *(14,25)* or S1P phosphatases (S1PPases) *(26)*. Two forms of human SPHK have recently been cloned— SPHK1 and SPHK2, which although cytosolic appear to be able to associate and be active in membrane preparations *(14,25,27)*. Overexpression of SPHK1 in NIH3T3 fibroblasts was found to be

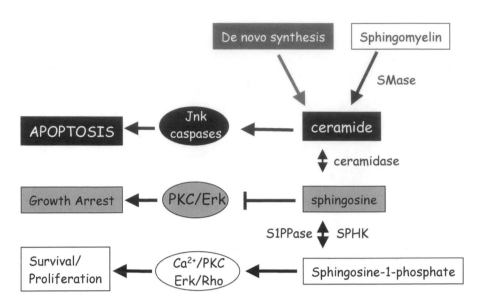

Fig. 4. The ceramide-sphingosine-1-phosphate rheostat. Ceramide, sphingosine, and sphingosine-1-phosphate are in dynamic equilibrium, with the functional outcome of apoptosis, growth arrest, or proliferation dependent on the balance of receptor-driven levels of these sphingolipid second messengers and the mitogenic vs apoptotic signals they elicit.

protective against apoptosis, and these protective effects appeared to be mediated by the inhibition of Jnk and caspase 2, 3, and 7 activity *(14,15,25)*. Moreover, such overexpression of SPHK1 enhances growth and proliferation of NIH3T3 cells and tumor formation when such cells are transplanted in NOD or SCID mice *(28,29)*. Consistent with this, sphingosine kinase inhibitors such as dimethylsphingosine or dominant-negative constructs of SPHK can inhibit the effects of SPHK and block Ras-mediated transformation *(14,25,28,29)*. Furthermore, a family of membrane-bound S1P phosphatases (S1PPases) have recently been identified and cloned. Thus, S1PPase and SPHK act in concert to keep sphingosine and S1P in dynamic equilibrium (**Fig. 4**). Loss of S1PPase in yeast results in elevation of S1P and protection from stress, whereas transfection of mammalian cells with S1PPase results in the elevation of ceramide and the induction of apoptosis. Similarly, S1P can also be metabolized by S1P lyase, an endoplasmic reticulum-located enzyme whose deletion in yeast mutants results in growth arrest *(14,26)*. Interestingly, platelets, which have high levels of SPHK, do not express S1P lyase, and this is thought to be the basis of the ability of platelets to act as stores of high concentrations of S1P. Because S1P can mediate many of the essential endothelial responses required for neovascularization, this has implicated platelet release of S1P as a key regulator in the process of angiogenesis during clotting and wound healing *(30,31)*.

4. SPHINGOSINE-1-PHOSPHATE: AN INTRACELLULAR AND EXTRACELLULAR SIGNALING MOLECULE

S1P is a particularly interesting second messenger as there is increasing evidence that it can signal both intracellularly and extracellularly *(13,14,32–35)*. Following growth factor stimulation of receptors such as PDGFR, SPHK is translocated to the membranes, resulting in generation of S1P. Such S1P can be released from the cells, and although it is not clear how this release is mediated, it has recently been shown that the cystic fibrosis transmembrane regulator (CFTR), a member of the ABC family of translocators, can regulate uptake of S1P *(20,36)*. Following release from the cells, S1P can act either in an autocrine or paracrine manner, on a family of G protein coupled receptors (GPCRs)

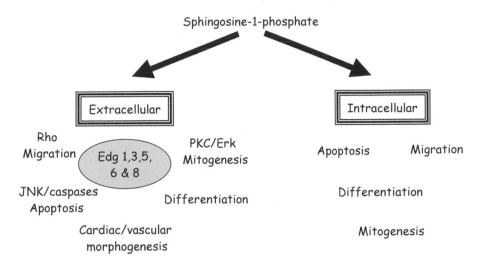

Fig. 5. Mechanism of action of sphingosine-1-phosphate. Sphingosine-1-phosphate may be released from cells to act in an autocrine or paracrine fashion via Edg receptors to induce a variety of functional outcomes. Alternatively, sphingosine-1-phosphate can act as an intracellular second messenger.

that are specific for S1P (**Fig. 5**). These receptors are members of the endothelial differentiation gene (Edg) receptors, and to date S1P has been shown to be a natural ligand for the Edg-1, -3, -5, -6 and -8 receptors, which have been renamed S1PRs—namely $S1P_1$, $S1P_3$, $S1P_2$, $S1P_4$, and $S1P_5$ respectively *(13,14,32–35)*. S1PRs appear to be ubiquitously expressed, and while $S1P_1$ and $S1P_5$ mainly couple to Gi, it appears that $S1P_2$ can couple to all classes of G proteins; $S1P_3$ couples to Gi, Gq, and $G_{12/13}$; and $S1P_4$ couples to Gi and G_{12}. Thus, the differential functional outcomes of S1P-signaling are likely to depend on the specific profile of S1PR and G protein expression in particular cell types. Nevertheless, S1PR signaling has been reported to induce migration via Rho GTPase signaling, which is widely established to be important for cytoskeletal rearrangement and motility, and proliferation and differentiation via PKC and ErkMAPK. Rather surprisingly, $S1P_5$, which appears to be restricted to the neural system, mediates anti-proliferative, apoptotic signaling and couples to inhibition of Erk by activation of a tyrosine phosphatase and induction of Jnk MAPK and caspase activation *(13,14,32–35)*.

The finding that the Edg-1/$S1P_1$ knockout mouse was embryonically lethal as a result of the failure of vascular smooth-muscle cells to migrate around arteries and capillaries and reinforce them, has focused considerable attention on the role of S1P and Edg receptors in directing vascular maturation and pathophysiological lesions such as atherogenesis *(14,15,30–34,37–41)*. Moreover, the PDGF-BB and PDGFR-β knockout mice exhibited similar phenotypes to the Edg-1 null mice and revealed that crosstalk between the PDGF-R and the $S1P_1$-GPCR plays a vital role in mediating angiogenesis *(14,37)*. Interestingly, the S1PRs appear to undergo several novel forms of crosstalk with growth factor receptors, and this is likely to provide additional levels of specificity of functional responses. For example, it has recently been shown that the PDGFR and $S1P_1$ form tethered receptor complexes in order to promote the integrative, synergistic signaling required for endothelial migration essential in vascular maturation. By contrast, the insulin-like growth factor-1 receptor (IGF-1R) activates $S1P_1$ in an SPHK-independent manner by inducing the AKT-dependent phosphorylation of $S1P_1$ at Thr-236, resulting in the coupling of the receptor to Rac GTPase activation and chemotaxis *(13,14,32–35)*.

Although this is still controversial, there is increasing evidence that S1P can also signal to regulate calcium mobilization, exocytosis, survival, differentiation, and proliferation by acting as an intracellular second messenger *(13,14,32–35)*. For example, while many of the effects of S1P cannot be mimicked by addition of exogenous S1P, microinjection of S1P or caged S1P has been shown to mobilize calcium and promote survival and proliferation. Similarly, while the S1P analog sphinganine-1-phosphate can bind to and activate all S1PRs, it does not mimic the pro-survival effects of S1P. Moreover, yeast do not express GPCRs, yet S1P promotes their cell survival *(13,14,32–35)*.

Consistent with this, we have recently shown that the high-affinity IgG receptor on monocytes, FcγRI, is coupled to a novel S1P-dependent pathway that is responsible for mobilizing calcium in an IP_3-independent manner. Moreover, FcγRI plays a central role in the clearance of immune complexes, and this SPHK-dependent pathway is essential for trafficking internalized immune complexes for degradation *(42–44)*. This novel pathway involves the tyrosine kinase-dependent activation of PI 3K (p85- and G protein-regulated isoforms) and PtdCho-PLD in the absence of any measurable activation of PIP_2-PLC. The immediate product of PLD is PA, and this has been shown to directly activate SPHK in vitro, indicating that PLD activation is upstream of the SPHK activity responsible for generating S1P and resultant calcium transients. Moreover, antisense knockdown experiments demonstrated a specific role for PLD1 and not PLD2 in coupling this receptor to SPHK activation and calcium transients *(42–44)*. It has recently been shown *(45)* that this pathway is also responsible for the FcεR-mediated, S1P-dependent release of calcium and exocytosis from mast cells *(46)*. Although S1P has been frequently proposed to play a role in mobilizing calcium from intracellular stores *(47)*, the ability of S1P to directly mobilize calcium has proved controversial due to the ability of the Edg receptors to mobilize calcium through conventional IP_3-dependent pathways *(13,14,47)*. Nevertheless, there are increasing data suggesting that S1P can access the same intracellular calcium pools as IP_3 but in an IP_3-insensitive (i.e., insensitive to the IP_3 antagonist heparin) manner *(47)*. The recent cloning of the SCaMPER (sphingolipid calcium release-mediating protein of endoplasmic reticulum) receptor provides additional evidence that sphingoid derivatives are able to engage intracellular receptors and effect calcium release from stores independently of IP_3 generation *(48)*. This putative calcium channel comprises 181 amino acids with two potential transmembrane spanning domains, and therefore constitutes a completely different structure from either the IP_3 or ryanodine receptors. Moreover, such responses to sphingolipids are not blocked by La^{3+}, ryanodine, or heparin, indicating that SCaMPER does not simply act as an accessory molecule for either the IP_3 or ryanodine receptors. However, it remains to be determined whether SCaMPER represents the receptor-coupled S1P-sensitive calcium channel in vivo *(47)*. It should also be borne in mind that alternative mechanisms may contribute to S1P-mediated calcium mobilization. For example, sphingosine has been shown to inhibit the receptor-coupled store-operated calcium release–activated calcium channel (I_{CRAC}), and thus, in addition to mobilizing calcium directly, generation of S1P from sphingosine should also alleviate the inhibition of I_{CRAC} and result in elevated intracellular calcium *(14,49)*.

5. SPHINGOLIPIDS AND LIPID RAFTS

Much interest has focused recently on the role of sphingolipid-enriched membrane microdomains, called *lipid rafts*, in promoting receptor-driven intracellular signaling, particularly of immune cells *(17–20)*. These lipid rafts act to recruit or sequester receptors and signaling molecules such that foci of signaling are organized around activated receptor complexes. These domains are enriched in certain proteins, such as GPI-anchored proteins and signaling molecules, e.g., Src kinases (via acylation) and Ras (via farnesylation), while others, e.g., negative regulatory receptors, are excluded *(17–20)*. In certain cell types, such as endothelial cells and smooth-muscle cells, lipid-raft domains are associated with caveolae, which are also enriched with signaling elements such as Erk MAPKs, GPCRs, and growth-factor receptors *(18)*.

Indeed, Src kinases appear to exhibit optimal activity only in lipid rafts, and are inhibited in nonraft domains, providing additional layers of regulation to prevent aberrant receptor activation. Thus, in naïve T-cells, the T-cell antigen receptors (TCR) are excluded from lipid rafts, but enter following ligation due to increased affinity of the ligated receptors for these microdomains. Entry into rafts allows Src kinase-mediated phosphorylation of immunoreceptor tyrosine-based activation motifs

(ITAMs) localized in the cytoplasmic domains of these receptors, resulting in recruitment of signaling molecules via phosphotyrosine–SH2 domain interactions. Naïve T-cells have few and small plasma membrane rafts, but mitogenic signaling targets rafts normally sequestered intracellularly in vesicles to the surface to promote rapid and sustained signaling. Such rafts coalesce to form polarized centers of signaling at the point of antigen recognition. Activated or memory T-cells, have more and larger lipid rafts, allowing rapid and amplified responses *(19)*. Furthermore, recruitment or exclusion of receptors from lipid rafts can dictate the differential functional responses of receptors during immune cell development. Thus, while in mature B-cells, signaling through the B-cell antigen receptor (BCR) occurs in lipid rafts and leads to activation, in immature B-cells, the BCR is excluded from rafts, and signaling leads to apoptosis *(50)*.

Interestingly, recent studies investigating the role of lipid rafts in transducing Fas-mediated apoptosis may finally have identified the role for the stress signal-mediated activation of SMase and resultant ceramide generation in the plasma membrane. Indeed, SM hydrolysis and ceramide generation in the outer leaflet of the plasma membrane appears to be required for the clustering of Fas receptors (CD95) required for apoptotic signaling. Disruption of lipid-raft formation by cholesterol depletion prevented such ceramide generation and Fas aggregation, suggesting important roles for plasma membrane localized sphingolipid metabolism and lipid rafts in receptor signaling *(51,52)*.

6. IMPLICATIONS FOR VASCULAR BIOLOGY

The finding that the Edg-1/S1P$_1$ knockout mouse was embryonically lethal due to failure of vascular smooth-muscle cells to migrate around arteries and capillaries and reinforce them, has focused considerable attention on the role of S1P in directing vascular maturation *(14,15,30–34,37–41)*. Indeed, S1P mediates many important endothelial cell responses associated with angiogenesis, including detachment of endothelial cells, chemotactic migration, survival, proliferation, adhesion, recruitment of smooth-muscle cells, and maturation into capillary-like structures in vivo *(14,15,30–34,37–41)*. The source of this S1P in vivo is controversial, but it is likely that it is released from platelets, which, due to their high SPHK activity and lack of S1P lyase, accumulate and store high concentrations of S1P until stimulation during clotting and wound healing. Although dysfunctional regulation is apparent in certain disease states, such as atherogenesis, it would appear that aberrant angiogenesis is normally prevented by the dynamic interactions of sphingolipid metabolic enzymes in regulating serum levels of S1P. Indeed, the challenge now is to dissect the precise roles of the ceramide S1P rheostat in directing differentiation, migration adhesion, proliferation, and death of all vascular cell types in order to define the signaling mechanisms underlying normal physiology that can be targeted for therapeutic manipulation during pathophysiology and disease.

ACKNOWLEDGMENTS

Grant support from the Medical Research Council, the Biotechnology and Biological Sciences Research Council, the Wellcome Trust, the Scottish Hospital Endowment Research Trust, and the McFeat Bequest at the University of Glasgow.

REFERENCES

1. Michell, R. H., Kirk, C. J., Jones, L. M., Downes, C. P., Creba, and J. A. (1981) The stimulation of inositol lipid metabolism that accompanies calcium mobilization in stimulated cells: defined characteristics and unanswered questions. *Philos. Trans. R. Soc. Lond. B Biol. Sci.* **296,** 123–138.
2. Berridge, M. J. (1987) Inositol trisphosphate and diacylglycerol: two interacting second messengers. *Annu. Rev. Biochem.* **56,** 159–163.
3. Toker, A. and Cantley, L. C. (1997) Signalling through the lipid products of phosphoinositide-3-OH kinase. *Nature* **387,** 673–676.
4. Berridge, M. J. (1993) Inositol trisphosphate and calcium signalling. *Nature* **361,** 315–325.
5. Wakelam, M. J. O., Pettitt, T. R., Kaur, P., et al. (1993) Phosphatidylcholine hydrolysis: a multiple messenger generating system. *Adv. Second Messenger Phosphoprotein Res.* **28,** 73.
6. Wakelam, M. J. (1997) Introduction: Signal activated phospholipases. *Semin. Cell Dev. Biol.* **8,** 285.

7. Wakelam, M. J. (1998) Diacylglycerol—when is it an intracellular messenger? *Biochim. Biophys. Acta* **1436,** 117–126.
8. Piomelli, D. (1993) Arachidonic acid in cell signaling. *Curr. Opin. Cell Biol.* **5,** 274–280.
9. Jimenez, B., del Peso, L., Montaner, S., Esteve, P., and Lacal, J. C. (1995) Generation of phosphorylcholine as an essential event in the activation of Raf-1 and MAP-Kinases in growth factors-induced mitogenic stimulation. *J. Cell. Biochem.* **57,** 141–149.
10. Hannun, Y. A. and Luberto, C. (2000) Ceramide in the eukaryotic stress response. *Trends Cell. Biol.* **10,** 73–80.
11. Hannun YA, Luberto C, Argraves KM. (2001) Enzymes of sphingolipid metabolism: from modular to integrative signaling. *Biochemistry* **40,** 4893–903.
12. Hannun, Y. A. and Obeid, L. M. (2002) The Ceramide-centric universe of lipid-mediated cell regulation: stress encounters of the lipid kind. *J. Biol. Chem.* **277,** 25,847–25,850.
13. Spiegel, S. and Milstien, S. (2000) Sphingosine-1-phosphate: signaling inside and out. *FEBS Lett.* **476,** 55–57.
14. Spiegel, S. and Milstien, S. (2002) Sphingosine 1-phosphate, a key cell signaling molecule. *J. Biol. Chem.* **277,** 25,851–25,854.
15. Pyne, S. and Pyne, N. (2000) Sphingosine 1-phosphate signalling in mammalian cells. *Biochem. J.* **349,** 385–402.
16. Pyne, S. (2002) Cellular signaling by sphingosine and sphingosine 1-phosphate. Their opposing roles in apoptosis. *Subcell. Biochem.* **36,** 245–268.
17. Dykstra, M., Cherukuri, A., and Pierce, S. K. (2001) Rafts and synapses in the spatial organization of immune cell signaling receptors. *J. Leukoc. Biol.* **70,** 699–707.
18. Ohanian, J. and Ohanian, V. (2001)Sphingolipids in mammalian cell signalling. *Cell Mol. Life Sci.* **58,** 2053–2068.
19. Viola, A. (2001) The amplification of TCR signaling by dynamic membrane microdomains. *Trends Immunol.* **22,** 322–327.
20. van Meer, G. and Lisman, Q. (2002) Sphingolipid transport: rafts and translocators. *J. Biol. Chem.* **277,** 25,855–25,858.
21. Merrill, A. H., Jr. (2002) De novo sphingolipid biosynthesis: a necessary, but dangerous, pathway. *J. Biol. Chem.* **277,** 25,843–28,846.
22. Linn, S. C., Kim, H. S., Keane, E. M., Andras, L. M., Wang, E., and Merrill, A. H., Jr. (2001) Regulation of de novo sphingolipid biosynthesis and the toxic consequences of its disruption. *Biochem. Soc. Trans.* **29,** 831–835.
23. Pelech, S. L. Kinase (1996) Connections on the cellular internet. *Curr. Biol.* **6,** 551–554.
24. Chalfant, C. E., Rathman, K., Pinkerman, R. L., et al. (2002) De novo ceramide regulates the alternative splicing of caspase 9 and Bcl-x in A549 lung adenocarcinoma cells. Dependence on protein phosphatase-1. *J. Biol. Chem.* **277,** 12,587–12,595.
25. Olivera, A. and Spiegel, S. (2001) Sphingosine kinase: a mediator of vital cellular functions. *Prostaglandins Other Lipid Mediat.* **64,** 123–134.
26. Mandala, S. M. (2001) Sphingosine-1-phosphate phosphatases. *Prostaglandins Other Lipid Mediat.* **64,** 143–156.
27. Liu, H., Chakravarty, D., Maceyka, M., Milstien, S., and Spiegel, S. (2002) Sphingosine kinases: a novel family of lipid kinases. *Prog. Nucleic Acid Res. Mol. Biol.* **71,** 493–511.
28. Xia, P., Gamble, J. R., Wang, L., et al. (2000) An oncogenic role of sphingosine kinase. *Curr. Biol.* **10,** 1527–1530.
29. Xia, P., Wang, L., Moretti, P. A., et al. (2002) Sphingosine kinase interacts with TRAF2 and dissects tumor necrosis factor-alpha signaling. *J. Biol. Chem.* **277,** 7996–8003.
30. Yatomi, Y., Ozaki, Y., Ohmori, T., and Igarashi, Y. (2001) Sphingosine 1-phosphate: synthesis and release. *Prostaglandins Other Lipid Mediat.* **64,** 107–122.
31. English, D., Garcia, J. G., and Brindley, D. N. (2001) Platelet-released phospholipids link haemostasis and angiogenesis. *Cardiovasc. Res.* **49,** 588–599.
32. Spiegel, S. (2000) Sphingosine 1-phosphate: a ligand for the EDG-1 family of G-protein-coupled receptors. *Ann. NY Acad. Sci.* **905,** 54–60.
33. Spiegel, S. and Milstien, S. (2000) Functions of a new family of sphingosine-1-phosphate receptors. *Biochim. Biophys. Acta* **1484,** 107–116.
34. Pyne, S. and Pyne, N. (2000) Sphingosine 1-phosphate signalling via the endothelial differentiation gene family of G-protein-coupled receptors. *Pharmacol. Ther.* **88,** 115–131.
35. Hla, T., Lee, M. J., Ancellin, N., et al. (2000) Sphingosine-1-phosphate signaling via the EDG-1 family of G-protein-coupled receptors. *Ann. NY Acad. Sci.* **905,** 16–24.
36. Boujaoude, L. C., Bradshaw-Wilder, C., Mao, C., et al. (2001) Cystic fibrosis transmembrane regulator regulates uptake of sphingoid base phosphates and lysophosphatidic acid: modulation of cellular activity of sphingosine 1-phosphate. *J. Biol. Chem.* **276,** 35,258–35,264.
37. Spiegel, S., English, D., and Milstien, S. (2002) Sphingosine 1-phosphate signaling: providing cells with a sense of direction. *Trends Cell. Biol.* **12,** 236–242.
38. English, D., Brindley, D. N., Spiegel, S., and Garcia, J. G. (2002) Lipid mediators of angiogenesis and the signalling pathways they initiate. *Biochim. Biophys. Acta* **1582,** 228–239.
39. Racke, K., Hammermann, R., and Juergens, U. R. (2000) Potential role of EDG receptors and lysophospholipids as their endogenous ligands in the respiratory tract. *Pulm. Pharmacol. Ther.* **13,** 99–114.
40. Auge, N., Negre-Salvayre, A., Salvayre, R., and Levade, T. (2000) Sphingomyelin metabolites in vascular cell signaling and atherogenesis. *Prog. Lipid Res.* **39,** 207–229.
41. Levade, T., Auge, N., Veldman, R. J., Cuvillier, O., Negre-Salvayre, A., and Salvayre, R. (2001) Sphingolipid mediators in cardiovascular cell biology and pathology. *Circ. Res.* **89,** 957–968.
42. Melendez, A., Floto, R. A., Cameron, A. J., Gillooly, D., Harnett, M. M., Allen, J. M. (1998) A molecular switch changes the signalling pathway used by the FcγRI antibody receptor to mobilise calcium. *Curr. Biol.* **8,** 210–221.

43. Melendez, A., Floto, R. A., Gillooly, D., Harnett, M. M., and Allen, J. M. (1998) FcγRI-coupling to phospholipase D initiates sphingosine kinase mediated calcium mobilisation and vesicular trafficking. *J. Biol. Chem.* **273,** 9393–9407.

44. Melendez, A. J., Bruetschy, L., Floto, R. A., Harnett, M. M., and Allen, J. M. (2001) Functional coupling of FcgammaRI to nicotinamide adenine dinucleotide phosphate (reduced form) oxidative burst and immune complex trafficking requires the activation of phospholipase D1. *Blood* **98,** 3421–3428.

45. Melendez, A. J. and Khaw, A. K. (2002) Dichotomy of Ca^{2+} signals triggered by different phospholipid pathways in antigen stimulation of human mast cells. *J. Biol. Chem.* **277,** 17,255–17,262.

46. Choi, O. H., Kim, J. H., and Kinet, J. P. (1996) Calcium mobilization via sphingosine kinase in signalling by the Fc epsilon RI antigen receptor. *Nature* **380,** 634–636.

47. Young, K. W. and Nahorski, S. R. (2001) Intracellular sphingosine 1-phosphate production: a novel pathway for Ca^{2+} release. *Semin. Cell Dev. Biol.* **12,** 19–25.

48. Mao, C., Kim, S. H., Almenoff, J. S., Rudner, X. L., Kearney, D. M., and Kindman, L. A. (1996) Molecular cloning and characterization of SCaMPER, a sphingolipid Ca2+ release-mediating protein from endoplasmic reticulum. *Proc. Natl. Acad. Sci. USA* **93,** 1993–1996.

49. Mathes, C., Fleig, A., and Penner, R. (1998) Calcium release-activated calcium current (ICRAC) is a direct target for sphingosine. *J. Biol. Chem.* **273,** 25,020–25,030.

50. Pierce, S. K. (2002) Lipid rafts and B-cell activation. *Nat. Rev. Immunol.* **2,** 96–105.

51. Grassme, H., Jekle, A., and Riehle, A., et al. (2001) CD95 signaling via ceramide-rich membrane rafts. *J. Biol. Chem.* **276,** 20,589–20,596.

52. Cremesti, A., Paris, F., and Grassme, H., et al. (2001) Ceramide enables fas to cap and kill. *J. Biol. Chem.* **276,** 23,954–23,961.

11

Regulation of Cytokine Signaling

Bao Q. Vuong, Lisa McKeag, Julie A. Losman, Jianze Li, Alex Banks, Scott Fay, Peter Chen, and Paul Rothman

SUMMARY

Cytokines are important modulators of the immune response that underlies the inflammatory process in atopic forms of asthma. Interleukin (IL)-4 and IL-13 are important cytokines for the regulation of these asthmatic immune responses. However, the cellular mechanisms that regulate IL-4 and IL-13 signaling remain unknown. Recently, a new family of proteins, termed *suppressors of cytokine signaling* (SOCS), has been identified. We have previously shown that SOCS-1 is a potent inhibitor of JAK-STAT signaling activated by IL-4. SOCS-1 expression is regulated both at the RNA and protein stability level. To identify proteins that bind and potentially regulate SOCS-1, we used the yeast two-hybrid system. We have identified the serine-threonine kinase Pim-2 as a binding partner for SOCS-1. Our preliminary studies demonstrate that SOCS-1 can interact with all three Pim kinases in mammalian cells. Co-expression of SOCS-1 with Pim kinases leads to the expression of novel SOCS-1 isoforms to require serine-threonine kinase activity. Pim kinases can directly phosphorylate SOCS-1. In addition, co-expression of SOCS-1 with Pim-2 increases the levels of SOCS-1 protein. Finally, expression of Pim-2 increases the inhibition of IL-4 signaling by SOCS-1. These data lead to a model by which the expression of Pim kinases alters SOCS-1 function through a phosphorylation event that stabilizes the SOCS-1 protein. This chapter proposes experiments to test this model and determine the role Pim kinases play in regulating IL-4 signaling in vivo. In addition, we propose to study the role of Pim kinases in a murine model of asthma.

Key Words: PIM kinases; SOCS (suppressor of cytokine signaling); interleukin-4 (IL-4); interferon-γ (IFN-γ); cytokine signaling; allergy.

1. INTRODUCTION

The immune response responsible for the inflammation found in allergic states is extremely complex and involves a variety of inflammatory cells, including B and T lymphocytes, mast cells, eosinophils, macrophages, and dendritic cells. For example, in response to challenge with allergen, cells in the lung initiate a cascade of events characterized by the production of TH2 cytokines and the recruitment of inflammatory cells including eosinophils into the lung (reviewed in ref. *1*). The resulting inflammation results in bronchial hyper-responsiveness and the clinical manifestations of asthma. Current research in this field has been directed at understanding this inflammatory process to identify essential molecules responsible for this immune response. These molecules would be targets for the development of therapeutic interventions. Recent work has demonstrated that a variety of molecules participate in the inflammatory immune response. Although the importance of many of these molecules in atopic immune responses remains unclear, interleukin (IL)-4, IL-13, and molecules regulating the signal transduction of these cytokines have been demonstrated to be essential for the development of atopic immune responses (reviewed in ref. *2*).

From: *Cell Signaling in Vascular Inflammation*
Edited by: J. Bhattacharya © Humana Press Inc., Totowa, NJ

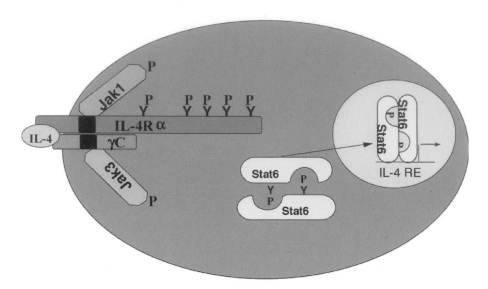

Fig. 1. Model for interleukin (IL)-4 signal transduction. The binding of IL-4 to its heterodimeric receptor results in the activation of two Jak kinases. These kinases phosphorylate conserved tyrosines present on the cytoplasmic tail of the IL-4Rα chain. The signaling molecule Stat6 docks on these residues via its SH-2 domain. Stat6 is itself tyrosine-phosphorylated by the Jak kinases, allowing Stat6 to form homodimers via reciprocal SH2-phosphotyrosyl interactions. Stat6 homodimers are found in the nucleus, where they bind IL-4 response elements present within promoters of genes that are induced by IL-4.

The pathways by which cytokines exert their biological effects have been a major focus of research over the past several years. Much of this work has defined the mechanisms by which binding of cytokines to their cognate receptors activates downstream signaling pathways. For type I and II cytokines, one of these pathways is the JAK-STAT signaling pathway. Our laboratory has been focused on defining the signaling pathway of IL-4, a cytokine involved in the activation, proliferation, and differentiation of a variety of hematopoietic cells, including B-cells, T-cells, and mast cells (3). When IL-4 is provided to a cell, it initiates signaling by oligomerizing the heterodimeric IL-4 receptor (**Fig. 1**), which in hematopoietic cells is composed of the ligand-specific IL-4 receptor α chain (IL-4Rα) and the common gamma chain (γ_c) (reviewed in ref. 4). This oligomerization initiates signaling by activating two nonreceptor tyrosine kinases (JAK1 and JAK3), which are constitutively associated with the cytokine receptor chains (JAK1 with IL-4Rα and JAK3 with γ_c). The activated JAK kinases phosphorylate specific tyrosines (Tyr-497, 575, 603, 631, and 713) on the cytoplasmic domain of IL-4Rα, which act as docking sites for signaling molecules that contain either PTB or SH2 domains. One molecule that binds to the phosphorylated IL-4Rα is a member of the STAT (signal transducer and activator of transcription) family of transcription factors, STAT6. Binding of STAT6 to the phosphorylated IL-4Rα induces the phosphorylation of STAT6 on Tyr-641 by the receptor-associated JAK kinases. Phosphorylated STAT6 dimerizes, translocates into the nucleus, and activates transcription of genes involved in B-cell differentiation, including the germline Iε gene and the low-affinity FcεII receptor CD23. The observations that cell lines deficient in JAK1 are unable to phosphorylate STAT6 (5) and that B-cells from STAT6-deficient mice are deficient in class switching to IgE (6–8) underscore the essential role of JAK1 and STAT6 in IL-4 function.

Although the effect of most cytokines is limited in both magnitude and duration, the mechanisms responsible for this limitation have not been well studied. The activity of cytokines is partly regulated by their production. In addition, we and others have demonstrated that the developmentally regulated expression of cytokine receptors is an important mechanism utilized by the immune system to limit

- **Expression of Cell Surface Receptor**
- **Regulated Activation of Receptor**
  - **SHP-1, SHP-2, CD45**
- **Regulation of Signaling Molecules**
  - **Cytoplasm**
    - **PIAS, SOCS**
  - **Nucleus**
    - **TC-PTP**

Fig. 2. Mechanisms to regulate cytokine signaling. Both the duration and amplitude of cytokine signaling are regulated at multiple steps in the process.

the biological effects of cytokines (9,10). Recent research has been focused on the intracellular mechanisms used to limit cytokine signaling (**Fig. 2**). Several mechanisms regulating cytokine signaling in the cell have been identified. Tyrosine phosphatases regulate the phosphorylation of various components in the signaling pathway. For example, the recruitment of SHP-1 to cytokine receptors (e.g., erythropoietin) is believed to regulate the duration and/or magnitude of cytokine signaling (11–14). Recent data have also demonstrated that STATs are dephosphorylated by nuclear phosphatases (15) and targeted for degradation by the proteosome (16). In addition, PIAS (protein inhibitor of activated STAT) proteins can limit the ability of STATs to bind DNA (17).

More recently, suppressors of cytokine signaling (SOCS) proteins have been identified as potent inhibitors of cytokine signaling (**Fig. 3**). The first family member, cytokine-induced SH2-containing protein (CIS) is induced by erythropoietin (EPO) and IL-3, and associates with tyrosine-phosphorylated EPO or IL-3 receptors (18). CIS is thought to regulate cytokine signaling by acting as an adapter protein that recruits a negative regulator, or by blocking the phosphotyrosines of the activated receptor that normally bind to STATs. Although transgenic mice overexpressing CIS have severe defects in T-cell development (19), the importance of CIS in vivo is undefined. The second SOCS family member, SOCS-1 (a.k.a. JAB and SSI-1), was cloned by three different groups (20–22). The same gene was cloned as an inhibitor of IL-6 signaling, a JAK-binding protein, and a protein with an SH2 domain similar to STAT's. Other members of the SOCS family, SOCS-2 through SOCS-7, were identified in an analysis of DNA databases (23). All of the SOCS family members have a conserved carboxyl terminal motif, termed the *SOCS box*, a central SH2 domain, and a divergent N-terminus.

A number of cytokines that signal through JAKs, including IL-4, have been shown to induce expression of SOCS mRNA in bone marrow (20). Therefore, we examined the effect of SOCS-1, SOCS-2, and SOCS-3 expression on IL-4 signaling (24). We found that expression of SOCS-1, but not SOCS-2, inhibited IL-4-induced phosphorylation of JAK1 and STAT6 and activation of STAT6 DNA-binding and transcriptional activity in stable cell lines. Furthermore, transient overexpression of SOCS-3 was capable of inhibiting IL-4-induced gene transcription, although stable expression of SOCS-3 had no detectable effect on IL-4 signaling. Analysis of cells from socs1$^{-/-}$ mice confirmed the importance of SOCS-1 in the regulation of STAT6 activation by IL-4 (25).

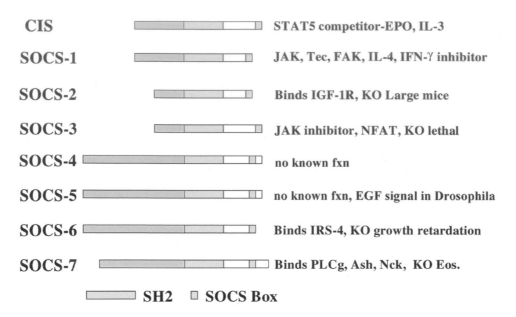

CIS   STAT5 competitor-EPO, IL-3

SOCS-1   JAK, Tec, FAK, IL-4, IFN-γ inhibitor

SOCS-2   Binds IGF-1R, KO Large mice

SOCS-3   JAK inhibitor, NFAT, KO lethal

SOCS-4   no known fxn

SOCS-5   no known fxn, EGF signal in Drosophila

SOCS-6   Binds IRS-4, KO growth retardation

SOCS-7   Binds PLCg, Ash, Nck, KO Eos.

SH2   ▫ SOCS Box

Fig. 3. Domain structure of the suppressors of cytokine signaling (SOCS) family of proteins. SOCS family of proteins contain a conserved SOCS box motif at the carboxyl-terminal, a central SH2 domain, and amino-terminal domains that are not conserved between the eight family members.

SOCS protein levels are regulated by several different mechanisms. The transcription of SOCS genes is induced by cytokines and other mitogens. In bone-marrow cells, CIS, SOCS-1, SOCS-2, and SOCS-3 mRNA is expressed at low levels and upregulated by many cytokines *(20)*. Recent data suggest that translation of SOCS-1 mRNA is regulated by its 5' untranslated region *(26,27)*. In addition, the half-life of the SOCS proteins is tightly controlled. SOCS proteins are unstable, and proteosome inhibitors decrease their turnover *(28)*. Some data suggest that the conserved C-terminal SOCS box may regulate the turnover of SOCS proteins *(28)*; however, the role of the SOCS box in regulating the levels of SOCS proteins remains controversial *(29–31)*. Interestingly, the SOCS box shares homology to the F box, which is present in proteins such as VHL and Cdc4 *(32)*. Both the F box and the SOCS box have been shown to interact with the elongin BC complex to regulate the degradation of proteins by the ubiquitin proteosome pathway *(32)* (**Fig. 4**).

Structure-function analysis of SOCS-1 has suggested that its SH2 domain, SOCS box, and amino terminus are important for its function or protein stability *(31,33,34)*, suggesting that SOCS-1 might interact with other proteins to regulate its activity. To identify proteins that regulate the function of SOCS-1, we used a yeast two-hybrid screen to isolate SOCS-1-interacting proteins. One of the clones isolated in the screen encoded the kinase domain of PIM2. Additional experiments using yeast two-hybrids and GST fusion proteins confirmed that the PIM2/SOCS-1 interaction was specific and that domains in the amino terminus of SOCS-1 were required for this interaction.

PIM2 is a member of the PIM family of serine-threonine kinases. The first PIM family member to be identified was *PIM1*, which was isolated as a common proviral insertion site in Moloney murine leukemia virus-induced T-cell lymphomas in mice *(35)*. Subsequently, PIM1 was shown to be involved in the generation of B-cell lymphomas *(36,37)* as well as erythroleukemias *(38)*. By sequence similarity with *PIM1*, van der Lugt and colleagues cloned *PIM2*, which also encodes a serine/threonine kinase *(39)*. Transgenic overexpression of either *PIM1* or *PIM2* predisposes mice to T-cell lymphomas *(40,41)*. Moreover, both *PIM1* and *PIM2* exhibit potent synergy with other oncogenes such as c-*myc* and bcl-2 in lymphomagenesis *(37,41)*. Consistent with their roles in lymphomagenesis,

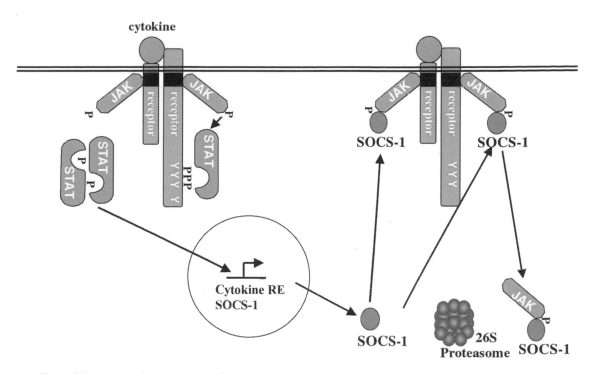

Fig. 4. Mechanisms for regulation of Jak/STAT signaling by suppressor of cytokine signaling (SOCS)-1. SOCS-1 functions in an autofeedback loop to affect Jak/STAT signaling. Activation of Jak-STAT signaling by cytokines induces STAT activation, which leads to induction of SOCS-1. SOCS-1 can inhibit Jak kinases function both by acting as a pseudosubstrate and by targeting activated Jak kinases for proteasomal degradation.

both *PIM1* and *PIM2* are found to be expressed at high levels in activated lymphocytes *(41)*. In addition, PIM1 and PIM2 mRNA and protein are induced and stabilized by a variety of cytokines *(42–45)*. Surprisingly, mice deficient for *PIM1* or *PIM2* show no obvious phenotypic alterations in their hematopoietic system *(46)*, suggesting some functional redundancy between *PIM1*, *PIM2*, and other genes. Recently, *PIM3* was cloned from an EST database search (B. Vuong and P. Rothman, unpublished data). The amino acid homology of the PIM2 and PIM3 proteins to PIM1 is 53% and 65%, respectively *(39)* (B. Vuong and P. Rothman, unpublished data). However, despite intensive studies, the precise in vivo role of the PIM kinases and the identity of their cellular substrates remains unclear.

To confirm the interaction of PIM2 and SOCS-1 in mammalian cells, cDNAs expressing full-length PIM2 and SOCS-1 were transfected into 293T-cells. Co-immunoprecipitation experiments demonstrated that these proteins interact when overexpressed in mammalian cells. Similarly, PIM1 and PIM3 interact with SOCS-1 when overexpressed in mammalian cells. Recently, we demonstrated co-immunoprecipitation of SOCS-1 and PIM1 in murine thymocytes, which were cultured with PMA/ionomycin for 4 h to induce PIM1 protein levels. Immunoprecipitation of endogenous SOCS-1 demonstrated that PIM1 co-immunoprecipitates with SOCS-1, suggesting that SOCS-1 can interact with PIM1 in lymphocytes. Two forms of PIM1 are expressed in mice and are encoded by different translation initiation sites in the PIM1 mRNA *(47)*. Interestingly, SOCS-1 preferentially interacts with the smaller 34-kD isoform of PIM1, which has been shown to have a shorter half-life than the 44-kD isoform.

In 293T-cells, co-expression of SOCS-1 with the PIM kinases induced the appearance of another isoform of SOCS-1, which migrated at a slower mobility on Western blots. Similar experiments performed with other SOCS proteins did not result in new species. Because SOCS-1 and PIM2 can interact, we sought to determine whether SOCS-1 might be a substrate for the PIM kinases. Overexpression of SOCS-1 with a PIM2 mutant that lacks kinase activity (K61M) does not induce the formation of the slower-migrating SOCS-1 isoforms. In addition, the presence of the slower-migrating SOCS-1 species was sensitive to the kinase inhibitor H7. Novel SOCS-1 species were also observed when either PIM1 or PIM3 was co-expressed with SOCS-1. These results suggest that overexpression of the PIM kinases with SOCS-1 induces a posttranslational modification of SOCS-1.

To determine whether PIM2 can directly phosphorylate SOCS-1, we generated recombinant GST-SOCS-1 and GST-PIM2 proteins. Subsequently, an in vitro kinase assay was performed with the recombinant SOCS-1 and PIM2 proteins in the presence of $\gamma[^{32}P]$-ATP. SDS-PAGE analysis of the in vitro kinase assay demonstrated that PIM2 can directly phosphorylate SOCS-1 in vitro. In addition, experiments with deletion mutants of SOCS-1 showed that the N-terminal domain of SOCS-1 is required for the PIM2-induced phosphorylation. Similar results were obtained with PIM1 and PIM3. Interestingly, the Pim-induced slower-mobility isoforms of SOCS-1 are lost when whole-cell extracts containing these isoforms are treated with lambda phosphatase in vitro. These data thus demonstrate that SOCS-1 is a direct substrate for the PIM kinases in vivo.

Because overexpression of the PIM kinases with SOCS-1 induces a posttranslational modification of SOCS-1, we sought to determine whether the PIM-induced modification of SOCS-1 altered the function of SOCS-1. Recent data suggest that the protein stability of SOCS-1 may be regulated posttranslationally *(29–31)*. Interestingly, co-expression of SOCS-1 with PIM2 in 293T-cells dramatically increases the protein levels of SOCS-1. The levels of SOCS-1 are similarly increased if SOCS-1-expressing cells are grown in the presence of the proteasomal inhibitor LLnL *(28,48)*. In cells expressing only SOCS-1, the levels of SOCS-1 protein decrease rapidly in the presence of a protein synthesis inhibitor such as cycloheximide. However, in cells expressing both SOCS-1 and PIM2, the levels of SOCS-1 protein decrease more slowly. Interestingly, the slower-migrating, PIM-dependent form of SOCS-1 degrades more slowly than the faster-migrating, PIM-independent form of SOCS-1. Pulse chase analysis with $[^{35}S]$-methionine in cells expressing SOCS-1 in the presence or absence of PIM2 confirmed that PIM2 could alter the protein stability of SOCS-1. Thus, these data demonstrate that expression of PIM2 increases the stability of the SOCS-1 protein.

Our studies in cell lines demonstrated that the PIM kinases bind and phosphorylate SOCS-1. To complement these results genetically, thymocytes from $PIM1^{-/-}PIM2^{-/-}$ or wild-type mice were isolated and stimulated with PMA/ionomcyin for 4 h to induce PIM kinase and/or SOCS-1 expression *(49)*. Protein extracts from these cells were immunoprecipitated with SOCS-1 antisera, and the levels of SOCS-1 protein were examined. Consistent with our previous observations using cell lines, SOCS-1 protein levels were 5–10 times higher in activated thymocytes from wild-type mice as compared to levels in $PIM1^{-/-}PIM2^{-/-}$ mice. Interestingly, PMA/ionomcyin stimulates SOCS-1 protein levels but does not alter the levels of SOCS-1 mRNA in wild-type thymocytes. To determine whether SOCS-1 protein levels are similarly altered in mice overexpressing PIM1, thymocytes from Em-*PIM1* transgenic (TG) or wild-type mice were isolated and stimulated with PMA/ionomcyin for 1 h to induce PIM1 and SOCS-1 expression *(40)*. A shorter time point for stimulation was chosen to ensure that the levels of PIM1 in wild-type and transgenic mice were different. Consistent with previously mentioned observations, SOCS-1 protein levels in thymocytes from PIM1 TG mice were higher than in wild-type controls.

To determine whether the PIM-mediated increase in SOCS-1 protein levels altered cytokine signaling, we examined the effects of SOCS-1 and PIM expression on IL-4 and interferon (IFN)-γ-mediated transcription. 293T-cells were transfected with a luciferase reporter construct under the control of a multimerized-STAT6 or -STAT1 promoter in the presence or absence of SOCS-1 and/or PIM2. Comparison of luciferase activity following stimulation with IL-4 or IFN-γ demonstrated that SOCS-1 could inhibit IL-4 and IFN-γ-induced transcription mediated by STAT6 and STAT1, respectively. Strikingly, co-expression of wild-type PIM2 with SOCS-1 increased the inhibition of STAT6

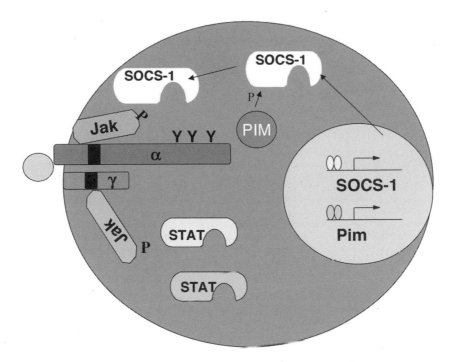

Fig. 5. PIM kinases modulate suppressor of cytokine signaling (SOCS)-1 regulation of Jak/STAT signaling. The levels of PIM kinases are induced in response to different cytokines. PIM kinases can phosphorylate SOCS-1. This phosphorylation can both alter SOCS-1 levels and SOCS-1 function, thereyby alteing SOCS-1's ability to regulate Jak kinases.

or STAT1 transcriptional activity; however, co-expression of a kinase-inactive PIM2 did not enhance the ability of SOCS-1 to regulate STAT6 or STAT1 transcriptional activity. These data are consistent with previously published data using cells from SOCS-1-deficient mice, which demonstrate prolonged STAT6 and STAT1 tyrosine phosphorylation downstream of IL-4 and IFN-γ signaling, respectively *(50,51)*. Together with the results presented above, these data suggest that PIM2 increases the protein levels of SOCS-1 to enhance the ability of SOCS-1 to inhibit JAK-STAT signaling activated by IL-4 and IFN-γ. As mentioned earlier, transient transfections in 293T-cells demonstrated that overexpression of the PIM kinases increases the ability of SOCS-1 to inhibit IL-4 signaling. To examine the role of the PIM kinases in regulating SOCS-1 function in vivo, thymocytes were isolated from wild-type and PIM1/PIM2-deficient mice and stimulated with IL-4. Interestingly, tyrosine phosphorylation of STAT6 downstream of IL-4 is prolonged in PIM1/PIM2-deficient cells as compared to wild-type cells. These data demonstrate that the PIM kinases act to regulate IL-4 signaling.

The data described herein suggest an intriguing model for the regulation of JAK-STAT signaling (**Fig. 5**). Cytokine stimulation up-regulates the expression of both SOCS-1 and the PIM kinases. Expression of the PIM kinases enhances the ability of SOCS-1 to negatively regulate JAK-STAT signaling by phosphorylating and stabilizing the protein levels of SOCS-1. The regulation of SOCS-1 protein stability by the PIM kinases may define tissue-specific cytokine responsiveness. SOCS-1 mRNA is found in many tissues *(20)*, whereas PIM2 is predominantly expressed in the hematopoietic system *(39)* and PIM1 and PIM3 are more ubiquitously expressed *(41)* (B. Vuong and P. Rothman, unpublished data). In addition, the cytokine-mediated regulation of PIM and SOCS-1 expression may play a role in the crosstalk between cytokines. IFN-γ signaling induces PIM and SOCS-1 protein expression *(20,43)*. Further, IFN-γ signaling inhibits IL-4 signaling, possibly through SOCS-1 *(52)*. Thus, expression of the PIM kinases and the subsequent stabilization of SOCS-1 may be important for the inhibition of IL-4 signaling by IFN-γ. The identification of SOCS-1 and the PIM kinases as critical regulators of IL-4 and IFN-γ signaling may allow for the development of novel anti-inflammatory agents that reduce the severity and/or development of atopic immune responses.

ACKNOWLEDGMENTS

This work was supported by grants from the Arthritis Foundation and NIH P01 AI50514 to P. R.

REFERENCES

1. Holt, P. G., et al. (1999) The role of allergy in the development of asthma. *Nature* **402 (6760 Suppl.)**, B12–B17.
2. Corry, D. B. and Kheradmand, F. (1999) Induction and regulation of the IgE response. *Nature* **402 (6760 Suppl.)**, B18–B23.
3. Nelms, K., et al. (1999) The IL-4 receptor: signaling mechanisms and biologic functions. *Annu. Rev. Immunol.* **17**, 701–738.
4. Jiang, H., Harris, M. B., and Rothman, P. (2000) IL-4/IL-13 signaling beyond JAK/STAT. *J. Allergy Clin. Immunol.* **105 (6 Pt. 1)**, 1063–1070.
5. Reichel, M., et al. (1997) The IL-4 receptor alpha-chain cytoplasmic domain is sufficient for activation of JAK-1 and STAT6 and the induction of IL-4-specific gene expression. *J. Immunol.* **158 (12)**, 5860–5867.
6. Shimoda, K., et al. (1996) Lack of IL-4-induced Th2 response and IgE class switching in mice with disrupted Stat6 gene. *Nature* **380 (6575)**, 630–633.
7. Kaplan, M. H., et al. (1996) Stat6 is required for mediating responses to IL-4 and for development of Th2 cells. *Immunity* **4 (3)**, 313–319.
8. Takeda, K., et al. (1996) Essential role of Stat6 in IL-4 signalling. *Nature* **380 (6575)**, 627–630.
9. Pernis, A., et al. (1995) Lack of interferon gamma receptor beta chain and the prevention of interferon gamma signaling in TH1 cells. *Science* **269 (5221)**, 245–247.
10. Bach, E. A., et al. (1995) Ligand-induced autoregulation of IFN-gamma receptor beta chain expression in T helper cell subsets. *Science* **270 (5239)**, 1215–1218.
11. David, M., et al. (1993) A nuclear tyrosine phosphatase downregulates interferon-induced gene expression. *Mol. Cell Biol.* **13 (12)**, 7515–7521.
12. Neel, B. G. (1997) Role of phosphatases in lymphocyte activation. *Curr. Opin. Immunol.* **9 (3)**, 405–420.
13. Neel, B. G. and Tonks, N.K. (1997) Protein tyrosine phosphatases in signal transduction. *Curr. Opin. Cell Biol.* **9 (2)**, 193–204.
14. Haque, S. J., et al. (1998) Protein-tyrosine phosphatase Shp-1 is a negative regulator of IL-4- and IL-13-dependent signal transduction. *J. Biol. Chem.* **273 (51)**, 33,893–33,896.
15. Venema, R. C., et al. (1998) Angiotensin II-induced tyrosine phosphorylation of signal transducers and activators of transcription 1 is regulated by Janus-activated kinase 2 and Fyn kinases and mitogen-activated protein kinase phosphatase 1. *J. Biol. Chem.* **273 (46)**, 30,795–30,800.
16. Kim, T. K. and Maniatis, T. (1996) Regulation of interferon-gamma-activated STAT1 by the ubiquitin-proteasome pathway. *Science* **273 (5282)**, 1717–1719.
17. Liu, B., et al. (1998) Inhibition of Stat1-mediated gene activation by PIAS1. *Proc. Natl. Acad. Sci. USA* **95 (18)**, 10,626–10,631.
18. Yoshimura, A., et al. (1995) A novel cytokine-inducible gene CIS encodes an SH2-containing protein that binds to tyrosine-phosphorylated interleukin 3 and erythropoietin receptors. *EMBO J.* **14 (12)**, 2816–2826.
19. Matsumoto, A., et al. (1999) Suppression of STAT5 functions in liver, mammary glands, and T cells in cytokine-inducible SH2-containing protein 1 transgenic mice. *Mol. Cell Biol.* **19 (9)**, 6396–6407.
20. Starr, R., et al. (1997) A family of cytokine-inducible inhibitors of signalling. *Nature* **387 (6636)**, 917–921.
21. Naka, T., et al. (1997) Structure and function of a new STAT-induced STAT inhibitor. *Nature* **387 (6636)**, 924–929.
22. Endo, T. A., et al. (1997) A new protein containing an SH2 domain that inhibits JAK kinases. *Nature* **387 (6636)**, 921–924.
23. Hilton, D. J., et al. (1998) Twenty proteins containing a C-terminal SOCS box form five structural classes. *Proc Natl Acad Sci USA* **95 (1)**, 114–119.
24. Losman, J. A., et al. (1999) Cutting edge: SOCS-1 is a potent inhibitor of IL-4 signal transduction. *J. Immunol.* **162 (7)**, 3770–3774.
25. Naka, T., et al. (1998) Accelerated apoptosis of lymphocytes by augmented induction of Bax in SSI-1 (STAT-induced STAT inhibitor-1) deficient mice. *Proc. Natl. Acad. Sci. USA* **95 (26)**, 15,577–15,582.
26. Gregorieff, A., et al. (2000) Regulation of SOCS-1 expression by translational repression. *J. Biol. Chem.* **275 (28)**, 21,596–21,604.
27. Schluter, G., Boinska, D., and Nieman-Seyde, S. C. (2000) Evidence for translational repression of the SOCS-1 major open reading frame by an upstream open reading frame. *Biochem. Biophys. Res. Commun.* **268 (2)**, 255–261.
28. Zhang, J.-G., et al. (1999) The conserved SOCS box motif in suppressors of cytokine signaling binds to elongins B and C and may couple bound proteins to proteasomal degradation. *Proc. Natl. Acad. Sci. USA* **96**, 2071–2076.
29. Hanada, T., et al. (2001) A mutant form of JAB/SOCS1 augments the cytokine-induced JAK/STAT pathway by accelerating degradation of wild-type JAB/CIS family proteins through the SOCS-box. *J. Biol. Chem.* **276 (44)**, 40,746–40,754.

30. Kamura, T., et al. (1998) The Elongin BC complex interacts with the conserved SOCS-box motif present in members of the SOCS, ras, WD-40 repeat, and ankyrin repeat families. *Genes Dev.* **12**, 3872–3881.
31. Narazaki, M., et al. (1998) Three distinct domains of SSI-1/SOCS-1/JAB protein are required for its suppression of interleukin 6 signaling. *Proc. Natl. Acad. Sci. USA* **95 (22)**, 13,130–13,134.
32. Tyers, M. and Rottapel, R. (1999) VHL: A very hip ligase. *Proc. Natl. Acad. Sci.* **96 (22)**, 12,230–12,232.
33. Nicholson, S. E., et al. (1999) Mutational analyses of the SOCS proteins suggest a dual domain requirement but distinct mechanisms for inhibition of LIF and IL-6 signal transduction. *EMBO J.* **18 (2)**, 375–385.
34. Yasukawa, H., et al. (1999) The JAK-binding protein JAB inhibits Janus tyrosine kinase activity through binding in the activation loop. *EMBO J.* **18 (5)**, 1309–1320.
35. Cuypers, H. T., et al. (1984) Murine leukemia virus-induced T-cell lymphomagenesis: integration of proviruses in a distinct chromosomal region. *Cell* **37 (1)**, 141–150.
36. Mucenski, M. L., et al. (1987) Common sites of viral integration in lymphomas arising in AKXD recombinant inbred mouse strains. *Oncogene Res.* **2 (1)**, 33–48.
37. Verbeek, S., et al. (1991) Mice bearing the E mu-myc and E mu-pim-1 transgenes develop pre-B-cell leukemia prenatally. *Mol. Cell Biol.* **11 (2)**, 1176–1179.
38. Dreyfus, F., et al. (1990) Rearrangements of the Pim-1, c-myc, and p53 genes in Friend helper virus-induced mouse erythroleukemias. *Leukemia* **4 (8)**, 590–594.
39. van der Lugt, N. M., et al. (1995) Proviral tagging in E mu-myc transgenic mice lacking the Pim-1 proto-oncogene leads to compensatory activation of Pim-2. *EMBO J.* **14 (11)**, 2536–2544.
40. van Lohuizen, M., et al. (1989) Predisposition to lymphomagenesis in pim-1 transgenic mice: cooperation with c-myc and N-myc in murine leukemia virus-induced tumors. *Cell* **56 (4)**, 673–682.
41. Allen, J. D., et al. (1997) Pim-2 transgene induces lymphoid tumors, exhibiting potent synergy with c-myc. *Oncogene* **15 (10)**, 1133–1141.
42. Dautry, F., et al. (1988) Regulation of pim and myb mRNA accumulation by interleukin 2 and interleukin 3 in murine hematopoietic cell lines. *J. Biol. Chem.* **263 (33)**, 17,615–17,620.
43. Yip-Schneider, M. T., Horie, M., and Broxmeyer, H. E. (1995) Transcriptional induction of pim-1 protein kinase gene expression by interferon gamma and posttranscriptional effects on costimulation with steel factor. *Blood* **85 (12)**, 3494–3502.
44. Domen, J., et al. (1993) Impaired interleukin-3 response in Pim-1-deficient bone marrow-derived mast cells. *Blood* **82 (5)**, 1445–1452.
45. Lilly, M., et al. (1992) Sustained expression of the pim 1 kinase is specifically induced in myeloid cells by cytokines whose receptors are structurally related. *Oncogene* **7 (4)**, 727–732.
46. Laird, P. W., et al. (1993) In vivo analysis of Pim-1 deficiency. *Nucleic Acids Res.* **21 (20)**, 4750–4755.
47. Saris, C. J., Domen, J., and Berns, A. (1991) The pim-1 oncogene encodes two related protein-serine/threonine kinases by alternative initiation at AUG and CUG. *EMBO J.* **10 (3)**, 655–664.
48. Chen, X. P., et al. (2002) Pim serine/threonine kinases regulate the stability of SOCS-1 protein. *Proc. Natl. Acad. Sci. USA* **99 (4)**, 2175–2180.
49. Wingett, D., et al. (1996) pim-1 proto-oncogene expression in anti-CD3-mediated T cell activation is associated with protein kinase C activation and is independent of Raf-1. *J. Immunol.* **156 (2)**, 549–557.
50. Starr, R., et al. (1998) Liver degeneration and lymphoid deficiencies in mice lacking suppressor of cytokine signaling-1. *Proc. Natl. Acad. Sci. USA* **95 (24)**, 14,395–14,399.
51. Morita, Y., et al. (2000) Signals transducers and activators of transcription (STAT)-induced STAT inhibitor-1 (SSI-1)/ suppressor of cytokine signaling-1 (SOCS-1) suppresses tumor necrosis factor alpha-induced cell death in fibroblasts. *Proc. Natl. Acad. Sci. USA* **97 (10)**, 5405–5410.
52. Dickensheets, H. L. and Donnelly, R. P. (1999) Inhibition of IL-4-inducible gene expression in human monocytes by type I and type II interferons. *J. Leukoc. Biol.* **65 (3)**, 307–312.

12

Cell Signaling by Vasoactive Agents

Barry L. Fanburg, Regina M. Day, Amy R. Simon, Sheu-Ling Lee, and Yuichiro J. Suzuki

SUMMARY

The vasoactive agents serotonin, endothelin-1, and angiotensin-2 have all been shown to produce proliferation of smooth muscle cells and thereby act as cellular mitogens. Although these vasoactive substances differ substantially in structure, their effects on cell signaling pathways are very similar. In general, following cellular ligation of the agents, reactive oxygen species (ROS) are generated through stimulation of NAD(P)H oxidase, and MAP kinases are subsequently activated. This leads to activation of multiple transcription factors, including AP-1, Egr-1, and GATA. Cell-cycling proteins are expressed to initiate the cell-growth response. Similar cellular responses by these vasoactive substances may be important in the production and release of cytokines, such as interleukin-6, which participate in vascular inflammation. The inflammatory responses of vasoactive substances are in need of further study.

Key Words: Cell signaling; serotonin; endothelin-1; angiotensin II; NAD(P)H oxidases; reactive oxygen species; MAP kinases; GATA; transcription factors; cytokines.

1. INTRODUCTION

It has been recognized since the early work of Owens and colleagues (1) that vasoactive substances may accelerate vascular smooth muscle cell (SMC) growth. More recent studies have indicated that vasoactive agents also regulate inflammatory responses (2). Three particular vasoactive substances—i.e., serotonin (5-HT), angiotensin II (Ang II), and endothelin-1 (ET-1) (see **Table 1**)—have been studied extensively for their actions, and their signaling intermediates have been defined.

Both 5-HT and ET-1 are potent vasoconstrictors, and an increase in their functions has been associated with pulmonary hypertension. The fawn-hooded rat with a genetic disorder in storage of 5-HT by platelets and elevated serum levels of 5-HT develops pulmonary hypertension spontaneously (3). Eddahibi et al. have demonstrated that treatment with 5-HT potentiates development of pulmonary hypertension in chronically hypoxic rats (4), and serotonin transporter (SERT) knockout mice show a comparatively muted response of the pulmonary vasculature to exposure to hypoxia (5). Furthermore, there is an enhanced expression of SERT in pulmonary artery SMCs of patients with pulmonary hypertension (6). Similarly, ET-1 expression is increased in the lungs of patients with pulmonary hypertension (7).

While 5-HT and ET-1 have been most closely associated with pulmonary hypertension (7,8), Ang II has been related to systemic hypertension, congestive heart failure, and pulmonary fibrosis (9,10). Ang II is upregulated in patients with systemic hypertension. Ang II receptor antagonists as well as inhibitors of angiotensin-converting enzyme (ACE, a protease that activates Ang II from its inactive precursor Ang I) are known to reduce hypertension. A growing literature implicates the activity of

From: *Cell Signaling in Vascular Inflammation*
Edited by: J. Bhattacharya © Humana Press Inc., Totowa, NJ

Table 1
Activation of Transcription Factors by Vasoactive Agents (*see* text for references)

5-HT	Ang II	ET-1
AP-1	AP-1	AP-1
GATA-4	CREB	GATA-4
Egr-1	GATA-4	NF-κB
STAT	Egr-1	
	NF-kB	
	STAT	

Ang II and ACE in fibrotic diseases, and recent studies with animal models show that inhibitors of these proteins block cardiovascular remodeling after ischemia/reperfusion *(11)*.

2. VASOACTIVE AGENTS AND THEIR RECEPTORS

Although they have all been classified as vasoactive agents, 5-HT, Ang II, and ET-1 bear little resemblance to each other. Ang II and ET-1 are peptides of 8 and 21 amino acids, respectively. Ang II affects cellular growth in SMCs through the Ang II type 1 and type 2 receptors (AT1R and AT2R, respectively), while ET-1 signals through the endothelin A and endothelin B (ETA and ETB) receptors. Although there are no sequence similarities between these factors, their receptors are all seven-membrane-spanning proteins in the G protein-coupled receptor (GPCR) family. Both Ang II and ET-1 appear to have pro- and anti-apoptotic effects on cells; the type of biological outcome of Ang II and ET-1 treatment appears to depend on a variety of factors, including the cell type observed, the receptor subtypes expressed, and the concentration of the factor. Apoptosis-inducing concentrations were roughly 10- to 100-fold higher than doses required for cell growth *(12)*. Studies have indicated that the ETA receptor and AT1R are most frequently associated with SMC proliferation in response to their respective factors *(12)*.

Unlike Ang II and ET-1, 5-HT (5-hydroxytryptamine) is a modified amino acid, not a peptide. Also unlike the ET-1 and Ang II receptors, 5-HT produces its mitogenic effect on pulmonary artery SMCs through an energy-dependent transport process via the serotonin transporter (SERT), a member of a sodium- and energy-dependent family of transporters *(13–15)*. In addition to the 5-HT transporter, at least 14 subtypes of the 5-HT receptor (also in the GPCR family) have been identified; many of these as well as SERT have been cloned *(16–19)*. While some studies have shown proliferation in other cell types downstream of 5-HT receptors *(20)*, studies in our laboratory have shown that cellular internalization of 5-HT via SERT is required for the mitogenic action to occur in SMCs. **Figure 1** shows a proliferative response of bovine pulmonary artery smooth muscle cells (BPSMC) to 5-HT at concentrations as low as 1 μ*M*. The stimulation is most marked in the presence of iproniazide, a monoamine oxidase inhibitor, which blocks intracellular degradation of 5-HT. 5-hydroxyindoleacetic acid, the end-product of 5-HT degradation, failed to stimulate smooth muscle cell proliferation. In contrast to Ang II and ET-1, 5-HT has not been found to induce apoptosis in any cell types examined to date.

3. FORMATION OF ROS IN RESPONSE TO VASOACTIVE SUBSTANCES, ROLE IN MITOGENESIS

Oxidants are well known to produce injury to the lung. It became recognized in the mid- to late-1980s that oxidants may also enhance cellular proliferation when induced through cell signaling processes. Much of our knowledge about this was initially derived from the oncologic literature *(21,22)* and was later transmitted to studies of nontransformed cells, including those of the lung and vasculature *(2)*.

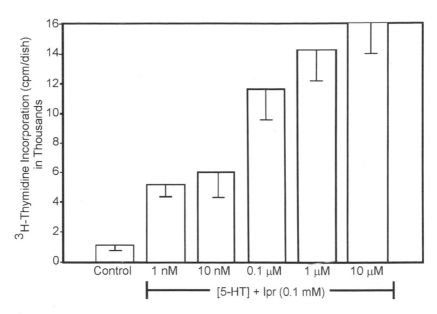

Fig. 1. 5-HT stimulates proliferation of smooth muscle cells (SMCs). Bovine pulmonary artery SMCs were incubated with 5-HT plus iproniazid (Ipr) for 24 h. DNA synthesis was determined by monitoring [^{3}H]thymidine incorporation. Values represent means ± SD. (*n* = 4). The figure was reproduced from Lee et al. *(13)*, with permission.

During the last several years, it has become apparent that the binding of many polypeptides to cell-membrane tyrosine kinases and GPCRs initiates reactive oxygen species (ROS)-generating reactions such as the activation of NAD(P)H oxidase *(24)*. Generation of ROS occurs similarly to that of the phagocyte, where ROS formation is initiated by bacterial engulfment. In fact, many of the same components of NAD(P)H oxidase present in phagocytic cells have also been identified in vascular cells and participate in ROS generation *(25,26)*.

Both ET-1 and Ang II produce intracellular ROS, which are believed to act as second messengers for signal transduction by their respective receptors. ET-1 has been shown to stimulate pulmonary artery smooth muscle cell proliferation through induction of ROS *(27)*. The increased relative dihydroethidium fluorescence, which was the measurement of ROS produced by ET-1, was reduced to control level by PD 156707, an inhibitor of MEK in the mitogen-activated protein kinase (MAPK) pathway, suggesting that MAPK activation was upstream to ROS production. Ang II also produces H_2O_2 formation in smooth muscle cells, and Ang II-induced cellular proliferation is dependent upon ROS generation *(28)*. Extensive studies in the Ang II/ROS system have helped in the identification of proteins such as p22phox, the gp91phox analogs nox1 and nox4, and the small G proteins Rho and/or Rac 1, which are critical components of the O_2^--generating system in SMCs *(29–32)*.

Studies in our laboratory have demonstrated that the mitogenic effect of 5-HT on pulmonary artery SMCs also requires activation of an NAD(P)H oxidase that produces O_2^- (**Fig. 2**) *(33)*. The SMC growth response appears to be dependent upon the dismutation of O_2^- to H_2O_2, which may be the actual ROS responsible for cellular growth *(34)*. Activation of the NAD(P)H oxidase requires active uptake of 5-HT by the cell since, like mitogenesis, it is blocked by the 5-HT transporter inhibitor imipramine. 5-HT-induced SMC growth is also blocked by diphenyliodonium (DPI) and quinacrine, inhibitors of NAD(P)H oxidase (**Fig. 3**), and a variety of antioxidants (**Fig. 4**), but not by allupurinol, an inhibitor of xanthine oxidase *(33)*. α-Hydroxyfarnesylphosphonic acid, which inhibits activation of p21ras, also blocks both cellular proliferation and ROS-linked chemiluminescence downstream of 5-HT (**Fig. 5**) *(33)*. Because of the role of Rac implied by ROS production in response to growth

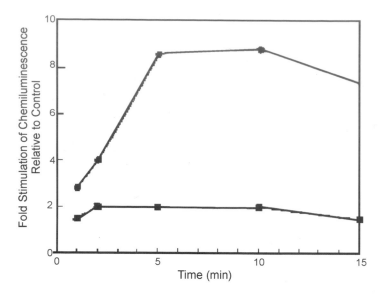

Fig. 2. Effect of 5-HT transporter inhibitor imipramine (IMP) on O_2^- generation. Bovine pulmonary artery smooth muscle cells (SMCs) were incubated with 1 μM 5-HT plus 0.1 mM iproniazid without (closed circles) or with 0.1 mM imipramine (closed squares). O_2^- generation was measured by a lucigenin-enhanced chemiluminescence assay. The figure was reproduced from Lee et al. *(33)*, with permission.

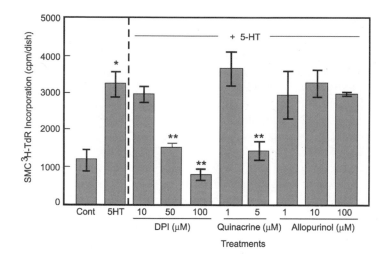

Fig. 3. Effects of NAD(P)H oxidase inhibitors on 5-HT-induced proliferation of SMCs. Bovine pulmonary artery smooth muscle cells (SMCs) were pretreated with diphenyliodonium (DPI), quinacrine (NAD[P]H oxidase inhibitors), or allopurinol (xanthine oxidase inhibitor), then incubated with 1 μM 5-HT for 24 h. DNA synthesis was determined by monitoring [^{3}H]thymidine incorporation. Values represent means ± SD. (*n* = 4). (*) denotes the value that is significantly different from control at $p < 0.05$. (**) denotes values significantly different from 5-HT alone at $p < 0.05$. The figure was reproduced from Lee et al. *(33)*, with permission.

factors in fibroblasts *(35)*, we examined Rac's role in 5-HT-mediated cell signaling. Overexpression of dominant-negative Rac 1 (N17Rac1) inhibited 5-HT-mediated activation of a c-*fos*-luciferase reporter gene expression (unpublished data). These results support a concept that 5-HT-mediated ROS production also utilizes a Rac-dependent mechanism. Interestingly, NAD(P)H oxidase is not activated by 5-HT in endothelial cells from the same vessels, where there is no growth response (data not shown).

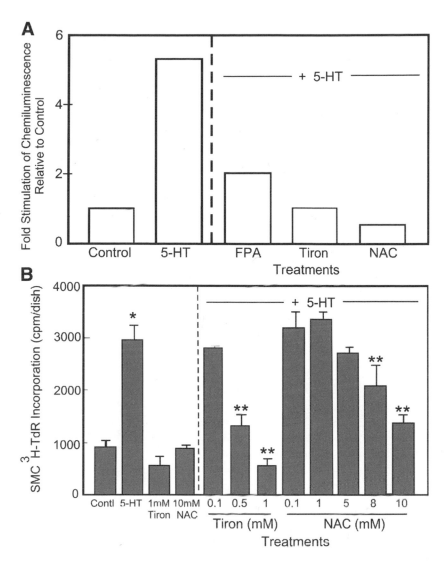

Fig. 4. Effects of antioxidants on 5-HT-induced O_2^- generation and proliferation of smooth muscle cells (SMCs). Bovine pulmonary artery SMCs were pretreated with α-hydroxyfarnesylphosphonic acid (FPA, 0.1 mM), tiron (10 mM), or N-acetylcysteine (NAC, 10 mM), then incubated with 1 μM 5-HT. (A) O_2^- generation was measured by a lucigenin-enhanced chemiluminescence assay. **(B)** DNA synthesis was determined by monitoring [^{3}H]thymidine incorporation. Values represent means ± SD. ($n = 4$). (*) denotes the value that is significantly different from control at $p < 0.05$. (**) denotes values significantly different from 5-HT alone at $p < 0.05$. The figure was reproduced from Lee et al. *(33),* with permission.

4. ACTIVATION OF MAPK

The MAP kinases provide an intermediate signal transduction pathway in response to stimuli that lead to cellular growth *(36,37)*. Receptor tyrosine kinases or G protein-coupled receptors may use Ras to activate this pathway, or activation may be Ras-independent. Both exogenous and endogenous ROS have been reported to activate MAP kinases via phosphorylation of tyrosine or threonine residues *(37–40)*. Similarly, phosphorylation may occur by inhibition of phosphatases.

As stated above, activation of MAPK by ET-1 appears to occur upstream of ROS production, as inhibitors of MAPK blocked ROS. However, activation of MAPK by Ang II can occur upstream and

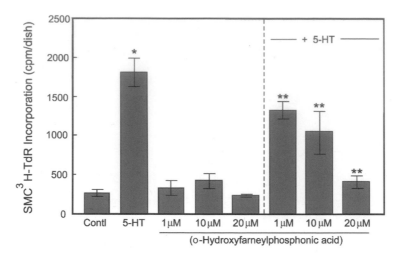

Fig. 5. Effect of the p21[ras] inhibitor on 5-HT-induced proliferation of smooth muscle cells (SMCs). Bovine pulmonary artery SMCs were pre-treated with α-hydroxyfarnesylphosphonic acid, then incubated with 1 μ*M* 5-HT for 24 h. DNA synthesis was determined by monitoring [³H]thymidine incorporation. Values represent means ± SD. (*n* = 4). (*) denotes the value that is significantly different from control at $p < 0.05$. (**) denotes values significantly different from 5-HT alone at $p < 0.05$. The figure was reproduced from Lee et al. *(33)*, with permission.

downstream of ROS. Ang II activates both the p42/p44 and p38 MAPK pathways in SMCs. Transfection of cells with catalase blocked phosphorylation of MAPKs produced by Ang II in the studies of Ushio-Fukai et al. *(29)*, and it was concluded that the p42/p44 and p38 MAPK pathways for this signaling were not in series, but rather occurred in parallel. Viedt et al. further showed that transfection of SMCs with p22phox antisense blocked p38 MAPK activation, indicating the requirement of NAD(P)H oxidase *(41)*. These findings are supported by recent studies of MAPK, which show that these kinases are activated in large complexes in coordination with scaffolding proteins, and the scaffolds for the p42/p44 and p38 MAPKs are distinct, independent modules *(42)*. However, no mechanism has yet been proposed for the differences in ROS-dependent or -independent activation of these complexes.

p42/p44 MAPKs are activated by 5-HT, and this activation is dependent upon the generation of ROS (**Fig. 6**) *(43)*. The MAPK inhibitor, PD98059, blocks MAPK activation, but fails to block ROS generation, indicating that ROS generation, in this case, is upstream of MAPK in the signaling cascade. As anticipated, activation of MAPK by 5-HT is blocked by a variety of anti-oxidants, including tiron, *N*-acetylcysteine, and *Ginkgo biloba* extract, and the NAD(P)H oxidase inhibitor DPI, which also blocks cellular proliferation induced by 5-HT *(43)*. Unlike Ang II, which activates both p42/p44 and p38 MAPKs *(28)*, 5-HT failed to activate p38 MAPK despite the ability of the p38 MAPK inhibitors SB202190 and SB203580 to block (³H)- thymidine incorporation by SMC treated with 5-HT *(34)*. We attributed this inhibition of cellular proliferation to the demonstrated ability of SB202190 and SB203580 to function as an O_2^--quenching antioxidant (**Fig. 7**). The specific oxidase involved in 5-HT-regulated pathways has not yet been identified.

5. TRANSCRIPTION FACTOR ACTIVATION AND GENE REGULATION BY VASOACTIVE AGENTS

There have been a number of previous studies on transcription factor activation by vasoactive peptides (**Table 1**). Many of the factors that have been found to be activated by the vasoactive peptides are associated with growth, e.g., activator protein-1 (AP-1), early growth response-1 (Egr-1),

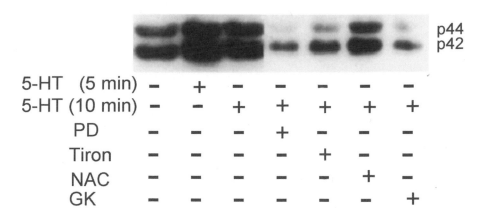

Fig. 6. Effects of MEK inhibitor and antioxidants on 5-HT-induced activation of p42/p44 MAPK. Bovine pulmonary artery smooth muscle cells (SMCs) were pretreated with PD98059 (PD, 10 μM), tiron (2 mM), N-acetylcysteine (NAC, 10 mM), or *Ginkgo biloba* (GK, 200 μg/mL), then incubated with 5-HT. Phosphorylation of p42/p44 MAPK was determined by Western blot analysis using the phospho-specific antibody. The figure was reproduced from Lee et al. *(43)*, with permission.

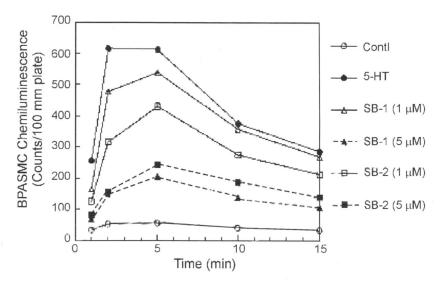

Fig. 7. Effect of SB-203580 (SB-1) and SB-202190 (SB-2) on O_2^- generation. Bovine pulmonary artery smooth muscle cells (SMCs) incubated with 1 μM 5-HT with varied concentrations of SB-1 and SB-2. O_2^- generation was measured by a lucigenin-enhanced chemiluminescence assay. The figure was reproduced from Lee et al. *(34)*, with permission.

and cyclic AMP-response element-binding protein (CREB) *(44,45)*. Nuclear factor-κB (NF-κB) is often considered for its role in anti-apoptotic gene activation, an activity often associated with but not required for growth. Some of these transcription factors are also associated with inflammation. The GATA family of transcription factors includes six genes with a highly conserved zinc finger DNA domain that interacts with DNA regulatory elements containing a consensus (A/T)GATA(A/G) sequence. Recently, our laboratory has uncovered a mitogenic function for GATA-4 in pulmonary vascular SMCs *(46)*.

The factors AP-1, Egr-1, GATA, and CREB are known to be activated downstream of MAPKs *(45)*. Signal transducers and activators of transcription (STATs) have been shown to be activated exclusively downstream of the Janus kinases (Jaks) or the related kinase Tyk2 *(44,45)*. Interestingly, the Jaks, which are often considered to be activated independently of MAPKs, have also recently been shown to be activated downstream of intracellular ROS *(47)*. NF-κB is most notably activated primarily in response to ROS, whether added exogenously or generated intracellularly by the NAD(P)H oxidase *(44,45,48)*. Activation of NF-κB is largely dependent upon degradation of its inhibitory subunit, IκB.

The most intensive investigation of transcription factor activation has been done for Ang II signaling. Cell growth in response to Ang II has been largely attributed to the activation of the AP-1, GATA-4, and Egr-1 factor activities (downstream of MAPK) *(44,49–51)*. Other factors have been shown to be activated as a part of Ang II-induced inflammation. Activation of CREB, NF-κB, STAT 1a, 2, 3, and 5, and, in some cell types, AP-1, are associated with the early activation of inflammatory effects and cytokine regulation after tissue damage *(52)*. The mechanisms of Ang II-induced transcription factor activation have been found to be largely downstream of ROS generation, with one intervening kinase as described above *(29,44,50)*.

Compared with the extensive literature available for Ang II activation of transcription factors, comparatively little is known about ET-1-induced transcription factor activation. The factors identified for ET-1 include AP-1, GATA-4, and NF-κB; the first two of these have been shown to play roles in ET-1-induced cell growth *(53,54)*. In SMCs, AP-1 was induced downstream of MAPK, but in a ROS-dependent manner, through the induction of Jun-amino-terminal kinase (JNK) activation *(53)*, although NF-κB has been shown to regulate the cytokine interleukin-6 *(55)*.

Our laboratory has been increasingly interested in the activation of transcription factors involved in SMC proliferation. A number of studies have shown that the 5-HT receptors can activate gene transcription through a variety of transcription factors *(56–58)*. Several of these activities are associated with the stimulation of cytokines or proteins associated with fibrosis. We studied the influence of 5-HT on GATA factors in pulmonary artery smooth muscle cells. 5-HT upregulated GATA DNA-binding activity fivefold, and supershift experiments showed this to be attributed at least in part to GATA-4 *(46)*. Pretreatment of cells with inhibitors of SERT, ROS, and MEK blocked the GATA-4 activation by 5-HT, and the dominant-negative mutant of GATA-4 blocked cell growth produced by 5-HT.

We also recently found that 5-HT induces sustained activation of the Egr-1 transcription factor (unpublished data). A number of studies have correlated Egr-1 activity with cell growth *(59,60)*, and the factor is activated through phosphorylation sites in a serine/threonine-rich region *(61)*. As stated above, Egr-1 nuclear translocation and DNA-binding activity are believed to be controlled largely through the activity of upstream MAP kinases, suggesting that this may be the mechanism by which 5-HT regulates this factor *(45,61,62)*.

Because 5-HT is mitogenic in vascular smooth muscle, candidate downstream target genes are those genes involved in cellular proliferation. Much is already known about how external stimuli, such as growth factors and cytokines, result in cell-cycle progression through the G1 phase of the cycle. This involves the activation of immediate early genes such as c-*myc*, with the subsequent activation of cyclin D1, which results in its association with and activation of cyclin-dependent kinases (CDK) and the inactivation of Rb *(63)*. We have verified that α- and β-actin *(64)* and the early response genes c-*fos* (unpublished data) and c-*myc (64)* are all upregulated by 5-HT in smooth muscle cells. In addition, we have determined that the cell-cycle regulator cyclin D is upregulated by 5-HT in vascular SMCs (unpublished data). This regulation of cyclin D1 by 5-HT is consistent with what others have reported in mouse fibroblasts that contain 5-HT 2B receptors *(65)*.

6. VASOACTIVE AGENTS AND INFLAMMATORY RESPONSES

Recently, the roles of vascular SMCs and vasoactive agents in the regulation of inflammatory events have been recognized. Mechanisms of these agents in mediating pro-inflammatory events

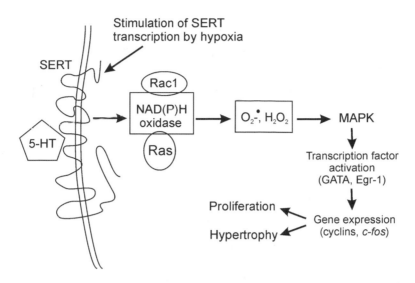

Fig. 8. Proposed pathway for 5-HT stimulation of smooth muscle cell growth.

may involve the activation of various transcription factors as described above. Gene transcription of pro-inflammatory cytokine interleukin-6 is regulated by STAT, CREB, and NF-κB transcription factors. 5-HT *(66)*, Ang II *(67,68)*, and ET-1 *(55)* all induce gene transcription of interleukin-6, perhaps through the activation of these transcription factors. Interleukin-6 is well-known to be an upstream regulator of a number of inflammatory cytokines. Further, these transcription factors also directly regulate other pro-inflammatory cytokines, such as interleukin-1 and tumor necrosis factor.

7. DISCUSSION

Research in our laboratory has focused on the mechanism of 5-HT-induced proliferation and hypertrophy of pulmonary artery SMCs. Despite the well known presence of a variety of subtypes of 5-HT receptors on cellular membranes, our studies demonstrate that active transport of 5-HT in SMCs is coupled to intracellular processes that activate the development of hyperplasia and hypertrophy. This fits well with the known pathology that occurs in pulmonary hypertension. The schema of signaling events that occur in this process is illustrated in **Fig. 8.** Cellular internalization of 5-HT activates GTPase-activating protein and initiates a probable combination of Rac 1 and other components of NAD(P)H oxidase, whose activation then produces O_2^-. Dismutation of O_2^- forms H_2O_2, which activates p42/p44 MAPKs. The specific physicochemical process by which this occurs is unknown, but presumably involves either its oxidation or the oxidation of a related phosphatase, thereby inactivating the phosphatase.

Subsequently, transcription factors are activated. We have found activation of GATA-4 and Egr-1 in pulmonary artery SMCs. Cyclin genes contain elements in promoter regions for both of these transcription factors. Similarly, early-response genes, including c-*fos*, and cellular structural genes, such as α- and β-actins, are stimulated. These signals initiate cell-cycle progression and result in hyperplasia and hypertrophy of SMCs. It appears from the literature that other vasoactive agents, such as ET-1 and Ang II, utilize similar pathways to 5-HT in their initiation of smooth-muscle hyperplasia and hypertrophy. Whether or not any other signaling pathways can produce a similar effect has not been determined. Furthermore, very little information is presently available about signaling pathways that lead vasoactive agents to produce an inflammatory response.

ACKNOWLEDGMENTS

This work was supported by NIH grant HL32723.

REFERENCES

1. Geisterfer, A. A., Peach, M. J., and Owens, G. K. (1988) Angiotension II induces hypertrophy, not hyperplasia, of cultured rat aortic smooth muscle cells. *Circ. Res.* **62,** 749–756.
2. Kranzhofer, R., Schmidt, J., Pfeiffer, C. A., Hagl, S., Libb,y P., and Kubler, W. (1999) Angiotensin induces inflammatory activation of human vascular smooth muscle cells. *Arterioscler. Thromb. Vasc. Biol.* **19,** 1623–1629.
3. Sato, K., Webb, S., Tucker, A., et al. (1992) Factors influencing the idiopathic development of pulmonary hypertension in the fawn hooded rat. *Am. Rev. Respir. Dis.* **145,** 793–797.
4. Eddahibi, S., Raffestin, B., Pham, I., et al. (1997) Treatment with 5-HT potentiates development of pulmonary hypertension in chronically hypoxic rats. *Am. J. Physiol.* **272,** H1173–H1181.
5. Eddahibi, S., Hanoun, N., Lanfumey, L., et al. (2000) Attenuated hypoxic pulmonary hypertension in mice lacking the 5-hydroxytryptamine transporter gene. *J. Clin. Invest.* **105,** 1555–1562.
6. Eddahibi, S., Humbert, M., Fadel, E., et al. (2001) Serotonin transporter overexpression is responsible for pulmonary artery smooth muscle hyperplasia in primary pulmonary hypertension. *J. Clin. Invest.* **108,** 1141–1150.
7. Giaid, A., Yanagisawa, M., Langleben, D., et al. (1993) Expression of endothelin-1 in the lungs of patients with pulmonary hypertension. *N. Engl. J. Med.* **328,** 1732–1739.
8. Herve, P., Drouet, L., Dosquet, C., et al. (1990) Primary pulmonary hypertension in a patient with a familial platelet storage pool disease: role of serotonin. *Am. J. Med.* **89,** 117–120.
9. Schunkert, H., Dzau, V. J., Tang, S. S., et al. (1990) Increased rat cardiac angiotensin converting enzyme activity and mRNA expression in pressure overload left ventricular hypertrophy. Effects on coronary resistance, contractility, and relaxation. *J. Clin. Invest.* **86,** 1913–1920.
10. McEwan, P. E., Gray, G. A., Sherry, L., et al. (1998) Differential effects of angiotensin II on cardiac cell proliferation and intramyocardial perivascular fibrosis in vivo. *Circulation* **98,** 2765–2773.
11. Sun, Y., Zhang, J. Q., Zhang, J., et al. (1998) Angiotensin II, transforming growth factor-β1 and repair in the infarcted heart. *J. Mol. Cell. Cardiol.* **30,** 1559–1569.
12. Filippatos, G. S., Gangopadhyay, N., Lalude, O., et al. (2001) Regulation of apoptosis by vasoactive peptides. *Am. J. Physiol.* **281,** L749–L761.
13. Lee, S. L., Wang, W. W., Moore, B. J., et al. (1991) Dual effect of serotonin on growth of bovine pulmonary artery smooth muscle cells in culture. *Circ. Res.* **68,** 1362–1368.
14. Fanburg, B. L. and Lee, S. L. (1997) A new role for an old molecule: serotonin as a mitogen. *Am. J. Physiol.* **272,** L795–L806.
15. Fanburg, B. L. and Lee, S. L. (2000) A role for the serotonin transporter in hypoxia-induced pulmonary hypertension. *J. Clin. Invest.* **105,** 1521–1523.
16. Fargin, A., Raymond, J. R., Lohse, M. J., et al. (1988) The geonomic clone G-21, which resembles a β-adrenergic receptor sequence encodes the 5-HT1A receptor. *Nature* **335,** 358–360.
17. Julius, D., Huang, K. N., Livelli, T. J., et al. (1990) The 5HT2 receptor defines a family of structurally distinct but functionally conserved serotonin receptors. *Proc. Natl. Acad. Sci. USA* **87,** 928–932.
18. Blakely, R. D., Berson, H. E., Fremeau, R. T. Jr., et al. (1991) Cloning and expression of a functional serotonin transporter from rat brain. *Nature* **354,** 66–70.
19. Ramamoorthy, S., Bauman, A. L., Moore, K. R., et al. (1993) Antidepressant- and cocaine-sensitive human serotonin transporter: molecular cloning, expression and chromosomal localization. *Proc. Natl. Acad. Sci. USA* **90,** 2542–2546.
20. Hinton, J. M., Hill, P., Jeremy, J., et al. (2000) Signalling pathways activated by 5-HT$_{1B}$/5-HT$_{1D}$ receptors in native smooth muscle and primary cultures of rabbit renal artery smooth muscle cells. *J. Vasc. Res.* **37,** 457–468.
21. Zimmerman, R. and Cerutti, P. (1984) Active oxygen acts as a promoter of transformation in mouse embryo C3H/10T1/2/C18 fibroblasts. *Proc. Natl. Acad. Sci. USA* **81,** 2085–2087.
22. Crawford, D., Zbinden, I., Amstad, P. A., et al. (1988) Oxidant stress induces the proto-oncogenes c-fos and c-myc in mouse epidermal cells. *Oncogene* **3,** 27–32.
23. Rao, G. N. and Berk, B. C. (1992) Active oxygen species stimulate vascular smooth muscle cell growth and proto-oncogene expression. *Circ. Res.* **70,** 593–599.
24. Thannickal, V. J. and Fanburg, B. L. (2000) Reactive oxygen species in cell signaling. *Am. J. Physiol.* **279,** L1005–L1028.
25. Jones, S. A., O'Donnell, V. B., Wood, J. D., et al. (1996) Expression of phagocyte NADPH oxidase components in human endothelial cells. *Am. J. Physiol.* **271,** H1626–H1634.
26. Bayraktutan, U., Draper, N., Lang, D., et al. (1998) Expression of functional neutrophil-type NADPH oxidase in cultured rat coronary microvascular endothelial cells. *Cardiovasc. Res.* **38,** 256–262.
27. Wedgwood, S., Dettman, R. W., Black, S. M. (2001) ET-1 stimulates pulmonary arterial smooth muscle cell proliferation via induction of reactive oxygen species. *Am. J. Physiol.* **281,** L1058–L1067.
28. Ushio-Fukai, M., Alexander, R. W., and Akers, M. (1998) p38 Mitogen-activated protein kinase is a critical component of the redox-sensitive signaling pathways activated by angiotensin II. Role in vascular smooth muscle cell hypertrophy. *J. Biol. Chem.* **273,** 15,022–15,029.
29. Ushio-Fukai, M., Zafari, A. M., Fukui, T., et al. (1996) p22phox is a critical component of the superoxide-generating NADH/NADPH oxidase system and regulates angiotensin II-induced hypertrophy in vascular smooth muscle cells. *J. Biol. Chem.* **271,** 23,317–23,321.

30. Lassegue, B., Sorescu, D., Szocs, K., et al. (2001) Novel gp91^{phox} homologues in vascular smooth muscle cells: nox1 mediates angiotensin II-induced superoxide formation and redox-sensitive signaling pathways. *Circ. Res.* **88,** 888–894.

31. Yamakawa, T., Tanaka, S., Numaguchi, K., et al. (2000) Involvement of Rho-kinase in angiotensin II-induced hypertrophy of rat vascular smooth muscle cells *Hypertension* **35,** 313–318.

32. Schmitz, U., Thommes, K., Beier, I., et al. (2001) Angiotensin II-induced stimulation of p21-activated kinase and c-Jun NH$_2$-terminal kinase is mediated by Rac1 and Nck. *J. Biol. Chem.* **276,** 22,003–22,010.

33. Lee, S. L., Wang, W. W., and Fanburg, B. L. (1998) Superoxide as an intermediate signal for serotonin-induced mitogenesis. *Free Radic. Biol. Med.* **24,** 855–858.

34. Lee, S. L., Simon, A. R., Wang, W. W., et al. (2001) H$_2$O$_2$ signals 5-HT-induced ERK MAP kinase activation and mitogenesis of smooth muscle cells. *Am. J. Physiol.* **281,** L646–L652.

35. Sulciner, D. J., Irani, K., Yu, Z. X., et al. (1996) Rac1 regulates a cytokine-stimulated, redox-dependent pathway necessary for NF-kappaB activation. *Mol. Cell. Biol.* **16,** 7115–7121.

36. Davis, R. J. (1993) The mitogen-activated protein kinase signal transduction pathway. *J. Biol. Chem.* **268,** 14,553–14,556.

37. Kyriakis, J. M., App, H., Zhang, X. F., et al. (1992) Raf-1 activates MAP kinase-kinase. *Nature* **358,** 417–421.

38. Abe, M. K., Chao, T. S., Solway, J., et al. (1994) Hydrogen peroxide stimulates mitogen-activated protein kinase in bovine tracheal myocytes: implications for human airway disease. *Am. J. Respir. Cell. Mol. Biol.* **11,** 577–585.

39. Guyton, K. Z., Liu, Y., Gorospe, M., et al. (1996) Activation of mitogen-activated protein kinase by H$_2$O$_2$. Role in cell survival following oxidant injury. *J. Biol. Chem.* **271,** 4138–4142.

40. Sundaresan, M., Yu, Z. X., Ferrans, V. J., et al. (1995) Requirement for generation of H$_2$O$_2$ for platelet-derived growth factor signal transduction. *Science* **270,** 296–299.

41. Viedt, C., Soto, U., Krieger-Brauer, H. I., et al. (2000) Differential activation of mitogen-activated protein kinases in smooth muscle cells by angiotensin II: involvement of p22phox and reactive oxygen species. *Arterioscler. Thromb. Vasc. Biol.* **20,** 940–948.

42. Karandikar, M. and Cobb, M. H. (1999) Scaffolding and protein interactions in MAP kinase modules. *Cell Calcium* **26,** 219–226.

43. Lee, S. L., Wang, W. W., Finlay, G. A., et al. (1999) Serotonin stimulates mitogen-activated protein kinase activity through the formation of superoxide anion. *Am. J Physiol.* **277,** L282–L291.

44. Griendling, K. K., Sorescu, D., Lassegue, B., et al. (2000) Modulation of protein kinase activity and gene expression by reactive oxygen species and their role in vascular physiology and pathophysiology. *Arterioscler. Thromb. Vasc. Biol.* **20,** 2175–2183.

45. Brivanlou, A. H. and Darnell, J. E. (2002) Jr. Signal transduction and the control of gene expression. *Science* **295,** 813–818.

46. Suzuki, Y. J., Tan, C. C., Sandven, T. H., et al. (2003) Activation of GATA-4 by serotonin in pulmonary artery smooth muscle cells. *J. Biol. Chem.* **28,** 17,525–17,531.

47. Simon, A. R., Rai, U., Fanburg, B. L., et al. (1998 Activation of the JAK-STAT pathway by reactive oxygen species. *Am. J. Physiol.* **44,** C1640–C1652.

48. Schreck, R., Rieber, P., and Baeuerle, P. A. (1991) Reactive oxygen intermediates as apparently widely used messengers in the activation of the NF-κB transcription factor and HIV-1. *EMBO J.* **10,** 2247–2258.

49. Naftilan, A. J., Gilliland, G. K., Eldridge, C. S., et al. (1990) Induction of the proto-oncogene c-jun by angiotensin II. *Mol. Cell. Biol.* **10,** 5536–5540.

50. Duff, J. L., Marrero, M. B., Paxton, W. G., et al. (1995) Angiotensin II signal transduction and the mitogen-activated protein kinase pathway. *Cardiovasc. Res.* **30,** 511–517.

51. Suzuki, Y. J., Shi, S. S., and Blumberg, J. B. (1999) Modulation of angiotensin II signaling for GATA4 activation by homocysteine. *Antioxid. Redox Signal.* **1,** 233–238.

52. McWhinney, C. D., Dostal, D., and Baker, K. (1998) Angiotensin II activates Stat5 through Jak2 kinase in cardiac myocytes. *J. Mol. Cell. Cardiol.* **30,** 751–761.

53. Fei, J., Viedt, C., Soto, U., et al. (2000) Endothelin-1 and smooth muscle cells: induction of jun amino-terminal kinase through an oxygen radical-sensitive mechanism. *Arterioscler. Thromb. Vasc. Biol.* **20,** 1244–1249.

54. Kitta, K., Clement, S. A., Remeika, J., et al. (2001) Endothelin-1 induces phosphorylation of GATA-4 transcription factor in the HL-1 atrial-muscle cell line. *Biochem. J.* **359,** 375–380.

55. Browatzki, M., Schmidt, J., Kubler, W., and Kranzhofer, R. (2000) Endothelin-1 induces interleukin-6 release via activation of the transcription factor NF-kappaB in human vascular smooth muscle cells. *Basic Res. Cardiol.* **95,** 98–105.

56. Guillet-Deniau, I., Burnol, A. F., and Girard, J. (1997) Identification and localization of a skeletal muscle serotonin 5-HT2A receptor coupled to the Jak/STAT pathway. *J. Biol. Chem.* **272,** 14825–14829.

57. Wilcox, C. B., Weisberg, E., Dumin, J. A., et al. (2000) Serotonin-dependent collagenase transcription in myometrial cells requires extended AP-1 site. *Mol. Cell. Endocrinol.* **170,** 41–56.

58. Huang, T. T., Vinci, J. M., Lau, L., et al. (1999) Serotonin-inducible transcription of interleucukin-1alpha in uterine smooth muscle cells requires an AP-1 site: cloning and partial characterization of the rat IL-1alpha promoter. *Mol. Cell. Endocrinol.* **152,** 21–35.

59. Meyyappan, M., Wheaton, K., and Riabowol, K. T. (1999) Decreased expression and activity of the immediate-early growth response (Egr-1) gene product during cellular senescence. *J. Cell. Physiol.* **179,** 29–39.

60. Gashler, A. L., Swaminathan, S., and Sukhatme, V. P. (1993) A novel repression module, and extensive activation domain, and a bipartite nuclear localization signal defined in the immediate-early transcription factor Egr-1. *Mol. Cell Biol.* **13,** 4556–4571.

61. Lim, C. P., Jain, N., and Cao, X. (1998) Stress-induced immediate-early gene egr-1, involves activation of p38/JNK1. *Oncogene* **16,** 2915–2926.
62. Kawai-Kowase, K., Kurabayashi, M., Hoshino, Y., et al. (1999) Transcriptional activation of the zinc finger transcription factor BTEB2 gene by Egr-1 through mitogen-activated protein kinase pathways in vascular smooth muscle cells. *Circ. Res.* **85,** 787–795.
63. Lundberg, A. S. and Weinberg, R. A. (1999) Control of the cell cycle and apoptosis. *Eur. J. Cancer* **35,** 1886–1894.
64. Lee, S. L., Wang, W. W., Lanzillo, J. J., et al. (1994) Serotonin produces both hyperplasia and hypertrophy of bovine pulmonary artery smooth muscle cells in culture. *Am. J. Physiol.* **266,** L46–L52.
65. Nebigil, C. G., Launay, J. M., Hickel, P., et al. (2000) 5-hydroxytryptamine 2B receptor regulates cell-cycle progression: cross-talk with tyrosine kinase pathways. *Proc. Natl. Acad. Sci. USA* **97,** 2591–2996.
66. Ito, T., Ikeda, U., Shimpo, M., Yamamoto, K., and Shimada, K. (2000) Serotonin increases interleukin-6 synthesis in human vascular smooth muscle cells. *Circulation* **102,** 2522–2527.
67. Funakoshi, Y., Ichiki, T., Ito, K., and Takeshita, A. (1999) Induction of interleukin-6 expression by angiotensin II in rat vascular smooth muscle cells. *Hypertension* **34,** 118–125.
68. Han, Y., Runge, M. S., and Brasier, A. R. (1999) Angiotensin II induces interleukin-6 transcription in vascular smooth muscle cells through pleiotropic activation of nuclear factor-kappa B transcription factors. *Circ. Res.* **84,** 695–703.

13

Reactive Oxygen Species and Cell Signaling in Lung Ischemia

Aron B. Fisher

SUMMARY

This chapter presents a new paradigm for the response to ischemia in the pulmonary circulation. The ischemic response depends on the sensing of decreased shear stress by the endothelial cell, resulting in the activation of membrane-associated NADPH oxidase, generation of O_2^-, and activation of a signaling cascade. The initial response of the endothelium leading to NADPH oxidase activation is depolarization of the endothelial cell membrane, possibly a result of inactivation of membrane K_{ATP} channels (K_{IR} 6.2). ROS signaling leads to NO generation and cell proliferation. Thus, the K_{ATP} channel may function as a "flow sensor" with the ability to initiate signaling subsequent to flow cessation. This response to altered shear stress may represent a physiological attempt to promote both vasodilation and the generation of new capillaries as mechanisms to restore blood perfusion.

Key Words: Endothelial cells; mechanotransduction; shear stress; superoxide generation; NADPH oxidase; K_{ATP} channel; eNOS activation; Ca^{2+} influx; cell proliferation.

1. INTRODUCTION TO ISCHEMIA/REPERFUSION INJURY

Recent years have seen a rapid increase in our understanding of the phenomenon of tissue injury mediated by reperfusion following a period of ischemia (I/R). Ischemia is defined as the loss of blood flow and in most instances is accompanied by anoxia, which accounts for the major manifestations. Thus, the pathophysiology of I/R essentially represents the effects of anoxia/reoxygenation. The basic observation is that tissues that "survive" an ischemic episode show increased damage during the subsequent reperfusion period. This paradoxical response to restoration of blood flow has been described in the intestine, kidneys, heart, brain, skeletal muscle, and other organs, including the lung (1,2). The major pulmonary manifestations include increased lung permeability, fluid accumulation, hemorrhage, and increased pulmonary vascular resistance (3–7). With intact dogs, lung fluid accumulation occurred with 2–4 h of ischemia and 0.5–5 h of reperfusion, although additional stress, such as positive end-expiratory pressure (PEEP) or increased left atrial pressure, sometimes was required to elicit the injury (8–12). A longer protocol (48 h of ischemia with 4 h of reperfusion) resulted in greater injury, including ultrastructural alterations of capillary endothelial and alveolar epithelial cells (13).

These in vivo studies have been supplemented by studies with isolated perfused lung preparations. With the perfused lung model, the direct effects of ischemia-reperfusion can be evaluated without the confounding variables of neuroendocrine effects, altered cardiac output, secondary effects on the control lung, and other systemic manifestations. Evidence of altered endothelial permeability and/or lung edema was seen after 3 h of ischemia and 1 h of reperfusion in the isolated dog lung (14), after

From: *Cell Signaling in Vascular Inflammation*
Edited by: J. Bhattacharya © Humana Press Inc., Totowa, NJ

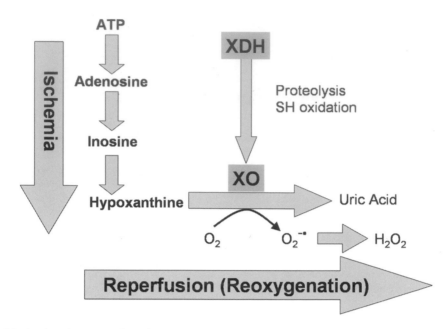

Fig. 1. Mechanism for generation of reactive oxygen species with ischemia reperfusion. Ischemia (anoxia) results in breakdown of ATP to hypoxanthine and proteolytic conversion of xanthine dihydrogenase (XDH) to xanthine oxidase (XO). With reperfusion and re-introduction of oxygen, XO converts hypoxanthine to uric acid and generates O_2^-, which can dismute to H_2O_2.

0.5–2 h of ischemia followed by 1 h of reperfusion in the isolated rabbit lung *(15–18)*, after 3 h ischemia plus short reperfusion in the isolated ferret lung *(19)*, and with varying periods of ischemia (45–90 min) and reperfusion (30–105 min) in isolated rat lung models *(20–30)*. The increased filtration coefficient associated with I/R in the rat lung was reversible by treatment with enhancers of cAMP activity, indicating that edema was not just a terminal event *(17,23,25)*.

It is widely accepted that tissue damage with I/R represents an oxidative injury associated with increased generation of reactive oxygen species (ROS). I usually will refer generically to ROS in this chapter, because differentiation of the individual species using chemical traps is difficult and generally has not been clearly delineated in the literature. Although ROS may be generated during reperfusion from more than one source, a widely accepted pathway is via xanthine oxidase, which is produced during the ischemic period by proteolytic conversion of xanthine dexydrogenase *(1)*. The major substrates for this pathway are derived from breakdown of ATP during anoxia; O_2 is necessary and is supplied by reperfusion (**Fig. 1**).

ROS generation has been demonstrated with I/R in isolated lung models and appears to correlate with subsequent pathophysiology. With I/R in isolated rabbit lungs, production of $^*OH$ was demonstrated by the salicylate trap (hydroxylation) method *(18)*, and release of O_2^- into the perfusate was shown by reduction of succinylated ferricytochrome c *(20)*. Reperfusion lung edema in this model was partially blocked by a xanthine oxidase inhibitor, allopurinol, providing evidence that this enzyme has a role in the generation of ROS. ROS scavengers also protect against the (patho) physiological manifestations of injury with I/R; superoxide dismutase (SOD), catalase, and thiols all have been effective *(14,20,31,32)*. Pretreatment of isolated rat lungs with Fe chelators such as U74500A or U74389G (21 amino steroids), transferrin, or desferrioxamine also inhibited lung edema formation with I/R, providing evidence that Fe^{2+} in addition to ROS is required for oxidant injury *(20,33,34)*.

Table 1
ATP Content and Tissue Oxidation in Isolated Rat Lung During Anoxia/Reoxygenation

	ATP mmol/g dry wt	TBARS pmol/mg prot.	Protein carbonyls nmol/mg prot.	DCF fluorescence arbitrary units
Control perfusion	9.4 ± 0.5	34.7 ± 3.6	3.7 ± 0.1	10.6 ± 0.7
Ischemia, 1 h	8.9 ± 0.6	$134 \pm 3.4^*$	$10.1 \pm 0.7^*$	$84.6 \pm 1.7^*$
N_2, 1 h	$3.9 \pm 0.6^*$	40.1 ± 3.8	3.9 ± 0.2	10.6 ± 1.3
$N_2 \rightarrow O_2$	$5.6 \pm 0.5^*$	$132 \pm 17^*$	$5.4 \pm 0.1^*$	$38.1 \pm 2.5^*$

Data are mean $\pm$ SE for n = 4-7. $N_2 \rightarrow O_2$ indicates 1 h anoxia followed by 1 h reoxygenation. TBARS, thiobarbituric acid reactive substances, an index of lipid peroxidation. Protein carbonyls are an index of oxidatively modified proteins. All parameters were measured in the lung homogenate. $^*p < 0.05$ vs control.

In contrast to the biochemical effects in systemic organs, the response of the lung to acute ischemia is unique, since continued ventilation is expected to maintain adequate tissue oxygenation. Stated another way, O_2 diffuses from the airspaces to the capillaries, and the function of the pulmonary circulation is to *accept* O_2 for systemic delivery, not to *deliver* it to the lung parenchyma. Thus, acute ischemia, such as that seen with a pulmonary thromboembolus, does not result in lung anoxia, and reperfusion is not accompanied by reoxygenation. (Over the longer term, ischemia may lead to atelectasis and resultant tissue hypoxia.) Despite these differences between the lung and systemic organs with respect to tissue oxygenation, I/R is associated with lung tissue injury as described above.

2. ROS PRODUCTION WITH ISCHEMIA BY THE INTACT LUNG

We have used the isolated perfused rat lung preparation as an intact organ model for studying the response to I/R and for comparison to the effects of anoxia/reoxygenation. Lungs were isolated under surgical anesthesia, cleared of blood, placed in a perfusion apparatus maintained at 37°C, perfused at 8- 10 mL/min with artificial medium (Krebs-Ringer bicarbonate solution containing glucose and either albumin or dextran to maintain osmolality) and continuously ventilated with air. Global ischemia was produced by cessation of perfusion while ventilation continued; anoxia/reoxygenation was produced by ventilation of lungs with N_2 and then subsequently with O_2 while perfusion continued. All ventilation gases contained 5% CO_2 to maintain pH homeostasis. As expected, tissue ATP was unchanged with ischemia but decreased significantly with anoxia (**Table 1**) *(35,36)*. The major finding of this study was that generation of ROS occurs during the ischemic period itself, provided that tissue oxygenation is maintained by ventilation *(36–39)*. (By definition, oxygen must be present for generation of ROS.) In our isolated rat lung model, oxidative tissue injury as indicated by lipid peroxidation and protein oxidation was detected at approx 15–30 min of ischemia, with a significant further increase at 60 min of ischemia (**Table 1**) *(35,40)*.

To detect ROS generation during ischemia, lungs were preperfused with a fluorescent dye that serves as a trap for radical species. We used a light guide placed against the pleural surface to excite the fluorophore and to record the reflected light at specific wavelengths *(35)*. The ROS indicator utilized for this study was dihydroethidine, a fluorophore that is oxidized by ROS to ethidium, which intercalates into cellular DNA. Dihydroethidine and ethidium have very different fluorescence spectra, which can be clearly differentiated. The pleural surface fluorescence signals during ischemia showed a marked increase in ethidium and parallel decrease in hydroethidine, indicating the generation of ROS (**Fig. 2**). A recent study of rat lungs using an enhanced chemiluminescence method has provided evidence for the generation of ROS in vivo with lung ischemia *(41)*.

In order to determine the cellular origin of ROS, we used an inverted epifluoresence microscope and a charge-coupled device (CCD) or digital camera for high-resolution digital imaging of the sub-

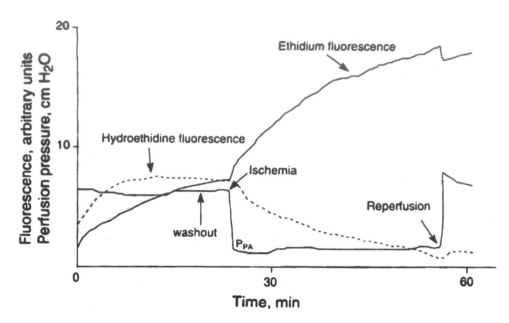

Fig. 2. Effect of ischemia on hydroethidine and ethidium fluorescence from the lung surface. Ischemia is indicated by the abrupt decrease in pulmonary artery (P_{PA}) perfusion pressure. Note the increase in ethidium fluorescence and corresponding decrease in hydroethidine fluorescence, indicating oxidation of hydroethidine by reactive oxygen species (ROS). From ref. *39*, with permission of the American Physiological Society.

pleural microvascular endothelial cells *(37)*. Deconvolution of fluorescence images was obtained using a graphic software program (Metamorph Imaging System, Universal Imaging Corp., West Chester, PA). For these studies, we used as fluorophore dichlorofluorescein (DCF) diacetate, a cell-membrane-permeable probe that becomes less permeable following deacetylation. A marked increase in DCF fluorescence with ischemia indicated endothelial ROS generation. Localization of DCF to microvascular endothelium was confirmed by imaging the cell association of diI-acetylated low-density lipoprotein (diI-LDL), an endothelial-specific marker *(37)*.

Additional studies of ROS generation utilized amplex red, a fluorophore that gives increased fluorescence primarily after reaction with H_2O_2 (in the presence of peroxidase). This fluorophore remains in the pulmonary vascular space and is not taken up by the endothelial cells. Increased ROS generation with ischemia was indicated by a marked increase in amplex red fluorescence, which was abolished by the addition of catalase *(38)*. With video imaging of the pulmonary microvasculature, we could determine the temporal relationship between ischemia and ROS generation *(38)*. Increased fluorescence of amplex red was detected at approx 2–4 s after abrupt cessation of perfusion, with a progressive increase during a 30-min observation period. Thus, ROS generation with ischemia is initiated rapidly and is continuous. The generation of ROS continuously over a period of 30 min or longer provides a mechanism for the oxidative injury to rat lung detected at 15–30 min of ischemia by our assays for lipid peroxidation and protein oxidation *(39,40)*. At a still later time, approx 180 min of ischemia in the ferret lung, physiological derangement, i.e., increased microvascular permeability, can be demonstrated *(19)*.

3. MECHANOTRANSDUCTION AND ENDOTHELIAL ROS GENERATION

The basic mechanism(s) for the initiation of ROS production during lung ischemia is not immediately obvious. That is, what is the trigger, or how does the lung "know" that it is ischemic? With other tissues, either decreased delivery of O_2 or other substrates, or decreased metabolite removal could

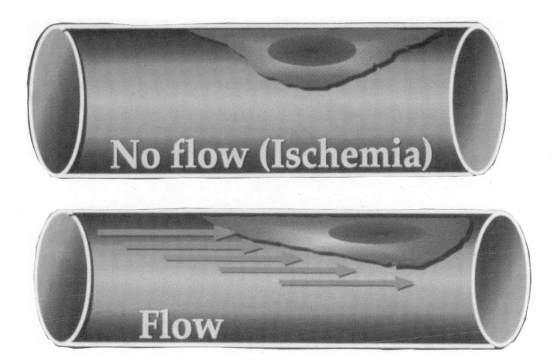

Fig. 3. Schematic representation of the effect of flow on the endothelial cell. This figure indicates the distortion of the endothelial cell membrane and cell contents that results with changes in shear stress.

theoretically be the mechanisms(s) for initiation of ROS generation. With the ventilated lung model, oxygen lack (anoxia) is not a factor. The lack of change in ATP during ischemia in the isolated lung model provides support for this conclusion (35,39). Likewise, we found that changes in pH (either acidosis or alkalosis) or change in substrate supply (glucose) did not significantly alter the extent of oxidant-mediated ischemic injury in the perfused lung model (39). Our conclusion is that metabolic alterations commonly associated with ischemia in other organs are unlikely to be primary initiators of lung ROS generation with ischemia.

Another possibility is that a mechanical, e.g., decreased flow, rather than a metabolic component of ischemia is responsible for initiation of the events leading to oxidative lung injury. Pulsatile blood flow evokes physical forces such as pressure, stretch, and shear-stress, which act on the vessel wall, specifically on the endothelium, which transforms the mechanical stimuli into electrical and biochemical signals (mechanotransduction). These physical factors and the concept of their role in endothelial regulation have come under study relatively recently (42–46). Although the precise mechanism(s) of cellular mechanotransduction have yet to be elucidated, ion channels and cytoskeletal elements responsive to stretch and shear-stress appear to be involved. We have put particular emphasis on the effects of shear stress, since the endothelial cell is in a unique position to sense this physical force associated with blood flow (Fig. 3).

Prior studies of mechanotransduction in endothelium have evaluated the effect of increased shear in endothelial cells cultured under static conditions that then are subjected to shear. Time-dependent responses with aortic endothelial cells include hyperpolarization of the cell membrane and activation of G proteins within 1 min, activation of MAP kinases and NFκβ and cytoskeletal rearrangement in 1–60 min, induction of connexin 43 and cell adhesion protein realignment of focal adhesions in 1–6 h, and a reorganized cell surface and cellular alignment in the direction of flow in 6–24 h (47). These cells are then considered "flow adapted." In seeking an explanation for the effect of ischemia on cell

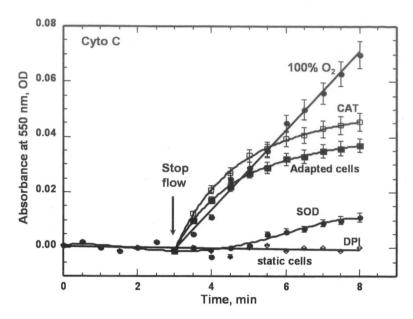

Fig. 4. Extracellular production of O_2^- by bovine pulmonary artery endothelial cells during simulated is-ischemia. Absorbance was measured in a spectrophotometer in the presence of cytochrome c as an indicator for O_2^- production. Simulated ischemia is indicated by "stop flow," resulting in increased O_2^- production by flow-adapted cells that is inhibited by superoxide dismutase (SOD) and diphenyleneiodonium (DPI). Catalase (CAT) or equilibration of medium with 100% oxygen had no significant effect on the initial rate of O_2^- production. There was no O_2^- production in cells that were cultured under static conditions and were not flow adapted (static cells). Adapted from ref. *48*, with permission of the American Physiological Society.

function, we recognized that endothelial cells may sense loss of shear in an analogous fashion to their ability to sense increased shear.

4. SIMULATED ISCHEMIA IN FLOW-ADAPTED ENDOTHELIAL CELLS IN VITRO

Mechanotransduction as the basis for the response to ischemia was further investigated with an in vitro model. Bovine pulmonary artery endothelial cells (BPAEC) were first flow adapted and then studied for their response to acute cessation of flow ("simulated ischemia"). A parallel-plate flow chamber was designed so that endothelial cells could be flow adapted and then placed in a standard cuvette holder for continuous monitoring of cellular fluorescence *(48)*. This design permitted the real-time detection of the cellular response to acute ischemia. BPAEC cultured under flow for 24 h in this apparatus demonstrated cellular realignment in the direction of flow indicating adaptation to a laminar shear stress *(48)*.

The generation of ROS was evaluated with this model during simulated ischemia by measuring changes in absorbance of cytochrome c added to the perfusing medium. There was no change in absorbance with cells that had been cultured under static conditions and then subjected to 30 min of flow immediately before the experiment (**Fig. 4**). However, cells that had been flow adapted for 24 h demonstrated a rapid increase in absorbance at 550 nm shortly after stopping perfusate flow, indicat-ing cytochrome c reduction. The reaction was inhibited by superoxide dismutase but was unaffected by catalase (a slight increase in absorbance with catalase is compatible with reoxidation of reduced cytochrome c by H_2O_2) (**Fig. 4**). The reaction also was inhibited by the presence of diphenyleneiodonium (DPI), an inhibitor of flavoprotein oxidases. These results are compatible with ischemia-induced generation of O_2^- into the extracellular space, where its dismutation would pro-duce freely diffusible H_2O_2. The calculated O_2^- production with ischemia accounted for approx 70%

of the O_2 consumption of "ischemic" BPAEC and was similar in magnitude (approx 6 nmol/min/10^6 cells) to the respiratory burst of stimulated polymorphonuclear leukocytes *(48)*.

5. SOURCE OF ROS WITH LUNG ISCHEMIA

Based on these observations, we postulated that the enzymatic source of endothelial O_2^- with ischemia was a membrane NADPH oxidase similar to the enzyme in phagocytes. Phagocyte-type NADPH oxidase is a multi-component system that is activated by the translocation of three cytosolic protein components (p47[phox], p67[phox], and p21[rac1]) to the plasma membrane, where they associate with the cytochrome b558 heterodimer (gp91[phox] and p22[phox]); other components may be involved in transport and stability of the complex *(49,50)*. Recently published results indicate the presence in endothelial cells of many of the components of the phagocyte-type NADPH oxidase enzyme system *(37,51–53)*. Activity of this enzyme in phagocytes is inhibited by DPI and produces superoxide into the extracellular milieu, properties that echo the results described above for ischemia in flow-adapted endothelial cells.

The results obtained with isolated cells were confirmed with the isolated perfused rat lung. As mentioned above, oxidation of amplex red in the isolated lung suggests extracellular generation of oxidants *(38)*, although diffusion of H_2O_2 from intracellular sources cannot be excluded. Like the observations with cells, there was marked inhibition of ischemia-mediated ROS production (DCF oxidation) by the presence of DPI *(36,37)*. DCF oxidation with ischemia also was prevented by pre-perfusion with PR-39, a polypeptide that inhibits src homology 3 (SH3) domains; the NADPH complex is known to utilize these domains for activation of the enzyme complex *(37)*. Confirmation of a role for NADPH oxidase was obtained by the study of mice that were deficient (knockout) in gp91[phox], the flavoprotein component of the complex responsible for O_2^- production *(37)*. Lungs from the knockout animals showed no increase in DCF fluorescence after ischemia, in contrast to the effects of ischemia in lungs from wild-type mice. Further, we showed that lung tissue oxidative injury also occurs with anoxia/reoxygenation as well as ischemia (**Table 1**); however, distinctly different biochemical pathways are responsible for ROS generation during ischemia (inhibited by DPI, but not allopurinol) vs anoxia/reoxygenation (inhibited by allopurinol but not DPI) (**Fig. 5**) *(36)*.

6. ROS-MEDIATED SIGNALING IN RESPONSE TO ISCHEMIA

These results indicating a rapid onset of ROS generation associated with ischemia led us to investigate the physiological significance of the response. We focused on signaling pathways, since recent studies have demonstrated an important role for ROS as signaling molecules *(54)*. In order to generate a sufficient number of cells for study, flow adaptation was accomplished utilizing a commercially available artificial capillary system, which simulates the pulmonary microvasculature *(55)*. BPAEC were seeded in the capillaries and allowed to attach while oxygenation of the medium was maintained by the flow of medium through abluminal ports. Following attachment, flow adaptation was obtained by switching flow to the lumen of the capillaries. Simulated ischemia was produced by again switching perfusion to the abluminal ports, abolishing shear stress but providing continued oxygenation of the medium during the ischemic period. BPAEC cultured in the artificial capillary system either could be adapted to continuous laminar flow or cultured under static conditions.

Flow-adapted BPAEC, when subjected to simulated ischemia (cessation of flow with continued oxygenation), showed ROS production that was inhibited by pretreatment with DPI. This effect was in clear contrast to the cells cultured under static conditions, which showed no change in ROS production when flow was discontinued after a 30-min perfusion period *(55)*. We measured extracellular signal-regulated kinases 1and 2 (ERK1/2), nuclear factor (NF)-κB, and activator protein-1 (AP-1) with ischemia in flow-adapted cells. ERK1/2 was activated (i.e., phosphorylated) during the first 10 min of ischemia and reached a plateau of activity at 20–30 min *(56)*. NF-*k*B showed activation when studied at 1 h of ischemia, with increase in both the p65/p65 and p65/p50 dimers *(55)*. AP-1, also studied at 1 h of ischemia, showed activation of c-jun/c-fos heterodimer *(55)*. These changes in sig-

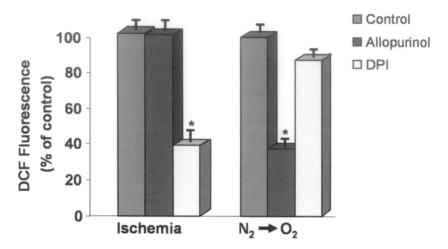

Fig. 5. Differential effects of reactive oxygen species (ROS) inhibitors with ischemia vs anoxia/ reoxygenation ($N_2 \rightarrow O_2$) in isolated rat lungs. Dichlorofluorescein (DCF) fluorescence in the lung homogenate, used as an index of ROS production, was measured at the end of 1 h ischemia or following 1 h anoxia followed by 1 h reoxygenation. Control indicates the fluorescence value in the absence of inhibitors. ROS production with ischemia was inhibited by diphenyleneiodonium (DPI) but not allopurinol. ROS production with anoxia/ reoxygenation was inhibited by allopurinol but not by DPI. $*p < 0.05$ vs control. Adapted from ref. *36,* with permission of the American Phyiological Society.

naling molecules required prior flow adaptation of the cells and were inhibited by pretreatment of cells with either of the antioxidants *N*-acetylcysteine or DPI. Thus, generation of ROS by the endothelial cells with ischemia appears to represent a cell signaling mechanism.

7. THE ENDOTHELIAL RESPONSE TO ISCHEMIA

These studies present a new paradigm for the response to ischemia in the pulmonary circulation. The ischemic response depends on the sensing of decreased shear stress by the endothelial cell, resulting in the activation of membrane-associated NADPH oxidase, generation of O_2^-, and activation of a signaling cascade (**Fig. 6**). Evidence gathered during these investigations has indicated that the initial response of the endothelium leading to NADPH oxidase activation is depolarization of the endothelial cell membrane, possibly due to inactivation of membrane K_{ATP} channels (K_{IR} 6.2) *(38,57,58)*. Additional studies have provided evidence that ROS signaling leads to NO generation *(56,59)* and cell proliferation, as indicated by increased DNA synthesis with entry of cells into the cell cycle *(55)*. Thus, the K_{ATP} channel may function as a "flow sensor" with the ability to initiate signaling subsequent to flow cessation. This response to altered shear stress may represent a physiological attempt to promote both vasodilation and the generation of new capillaries as mechanisms to restore blood perfusion.

ACKNOWLEDGMENTS

I thank the many collaborators who have made this research possible with special thanks to Drs. Abu Al-Mehdi (**Figs. 1–3** and **5**), Yefim Manevich (**Fig. 4**), and Zhihua Wei and Shampa Chatterjee for their invaluable contributions. The research reported herein was supported from grants from the NHLBI (HL 41939 and HL 60290).

REFERENCES

1. McCord, J. M. (1985) Oxygen-derived free radicals in postischemic tissue injury. *N. Engl. J. Med.* **312,** 159–163.
2. Cross, C. E., Halliwell, B., Borish, E. T., et al. (1987) Oxygen radicals and human disease. *Ann. Intern. Med.* **107,** 526–545.

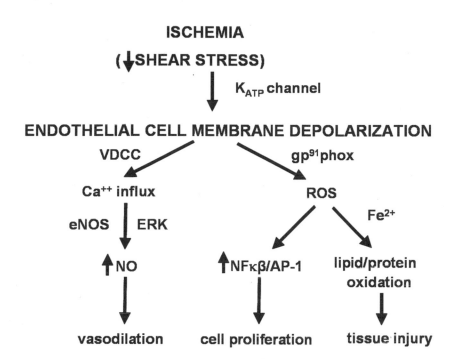

Fig. 6. Scheme for response of the pulmonary endothelium to ischemia (loss of shear stress). The indicated pathways result in generation of nitric oxide (NO), activation of transcription factors, and tissue injury (lipid peroxidation/protein oxidation).

3. Horgan, M. J., Lum, H., and Malik, A. B. (1989) Pulmonary edema after pulmonary artery occlusion and reperfusion. *Am. Rev. Respir. Dis.* **140,** 1421–1428.
4. Bishop, M. J., Lamm, W., Guidotti, S. M., and Albert, R. K. (1992) Pulmonary artery occlusion is sufficient to increase pulmonary vascular permeability in rabbits. *J. Appl. Physiol.* **73,** 272–275.
5. Murata, T., Nakazawa, H., Mori, I., Ohta, Y., and Yamabayashi, H. (1992) Reperfusion after a two-hour period of pulmonary artery occlusion causes pulmonary necrosis. *Am. Rev. Respir. Dis.* **146,** 1048–1053.
6. Gilroy, R. J., Jr., Bhatte, M. J., Wickersham, N. E., Pou, N. A., Loyd, J. E., and Overholser, K. A. (1993) Postischemic hypoperfusion during unilateral lung reperfusion in vivo. *Am. Rev. Respir. Dis.* **147,** 276–282.
7. Eppinger, M. J., Deeb, G. M., Bolling, S. F., and Ward, P. A. (1997) Mediators of ischemia-reperfusion injury of rat lung. *Am. J. Pathol.* **150,** 1773–1784.
8. Johnson, R. L., Jr., Cassidy, S. S., Haynes, M., Reynolds, R. L., and Schulz, W. (1981) Microvascular injury distal to unilateral pulmonary artery occlusion. *J. Appl. Physiol.* **51,** 845–851.
9. Barie, P. S., Hakim, T. S., and Malik, A. B. (1981) Effect of pulmonary artery occlusion and reperfusion on extravascular fluid accumulation. *J. Appl. Physiol.* **50,** 102–106.
10. Ide, H., Ino, T., Hasegawa, T., and Matsumoto, H. (1990) The role of leukocyte depletion by in vivo use of leukocyte filter in lung preservation after warm ischemia. *Angiology* **41,** 318–327.
11. Palazzo, R., Hamvas, A., Shuman, T., Kaiser, L., Cooper, J., and Schuster, D. P. (1992) Injury in nonischemic lung after unilateral pulmonary ischemia with reperfusion. *J. Appl. Physiol.* **72,** 612–620.
12. Horiguchi, T. and Harada, Y. (1993) The effect of protease inhibitor on reperfusion injury after unilateral pulmonary ischemia. *Transplantation* **55,** 254–258.
13. Bishop, M. J., Chi, E. Y., and Cheney, F. W., Jr. (1987) Lung reperfusion in dogs causes bilateral lung injury. *J. Appl. Physiol.* **63,** 942–950.
14. Allison, R. C., Kyle, J., Adkins, W. K., Prasad, V. R., McCord, J. M., and Taylor, A. E. (1990) Effect of ischemia reperfusion or hypoxia reoxygenation on lung vascular permeability and resistance. *J. Appl. Physiol.* **69,** 597–603.
15. Adkins, W. K. and Taylor, A. E. (1990) Role of xanthine oxidase and neutrophils in ischemia-reperfusion injury in rabbit lung. *J. Appl. Physiol.* **69,** 2012–2018.
16. Zamora, C. A., Baron, D., and Heffner, J. E. (1991) Washed human platelets prevent ischemia-reperfusion edema in isolated rabbit lungs. *J. Appl. Physiol.* **70,** 1075–1084.
17. Adkins, W. K., Barnard, J. W., May, S., Seibert, A. F., Haynes, J., and Taylor, A. E. (1992) Compounds that increase cAMP prevent ischemia-reperfusion pulmonary capillary injury. *J. Appl. Physiol.* **72,** 492–497.
18. Fisher, P. W., Huang, Y. C., Kennedy, T. P., and Piantadosi, C. A. (1993) PO2-dependent hydroxyl radical production during ischemia-reperfusion lung injury. *Am. J. Physiol.* **265,** L279–L285.

19. Becker, P. M., Pearse, D. B., Permutt, S., and Sylvester, J. T. (1992) Separate effects of ischemia and reperfusion on vascular permeability in ventilated ferret lungs. *J. Appl. Physiol.* **73,** 2616–2622.
20. Kennedy, T. P., Rao, N. V., Hopkins, C., Pennington, L., Tolley, E., and Hoidal, J. R. (1989) Role of reactive oxygen species in reperfusion injury of the rabbit lung. *J. Clin. Invest.* **83,** 1326–1335.
21. Ljungman, A. G., Grum, C. M., Deeb, G. M., Bolling, S. F., and Morganroth, M. L. (1991) Inhibition of cyclooxygenase metabolite production attenuates ischemia-reperfusion lung injury. *Am. Rev. Respir. Dis.* **143,** 610–617.
22. Eckenhoff, R. G., Dodia, C., Tan, Z., and Fisher, A. B. (1992) Oxygen-dependent reperfusion injury in the isolated rat lung. *J. Appl. Physiol.* **72,** 1454–1460.
23. Seibert, A. F., Thompson, W. J., Taylor, A., Wilborn, W. H., Barnard, J., and Haynes, J. (1992) Reversal of increased microvascular permeability associated with ischemia-reperfusion: role of cAMP. *J. Appl. Physiol.* **72,** 389–395.
24. Okuda, M., Furuhashi, K., Nakai, Y., and Muneyuki, M. (1993) Decrease of ischaemia-reperfusion related lung oedema by continuous ventilation and allopurinol in rat perfusion lung model. *Scand. J. Clin. Lab. Invest.* **53,** 625–631.
25. Barnard, J. W., Seibert, A. F., Prasad, V. R., et al. (1994) Reversal of pulmonary capillary ischemia-reperfusion injury by rolipram, a cAMP phosphodiesterase inhibitor. *J. Appl. Physiol.* **77,** 774–781.
26. Das, K. C. and Misra, H. P. (1994) Amelioration of postischemic reperfusion injury by antiarrhythmic drugs in isolated perfused rat lung. *Environ. Health Perspect.* **102 Suppl. 10,** 117–121.
27. Hsu, K., Wang, D., Wu, S. Y., Shen, C. Y., and Chen, H. I. (1994) Ischemia-reperfusion lung injury attenuated by ATP-MgCl2 in rats. *J. Appl. Physiol.* **76,** 545–552.
28. Imai, T. and Fujita, T. (1994) Unilateral lung injury caused by ischemia without hypoxia in isolated rat lungs perfused with buffer solution. *J. Lab. Clin. Med.* **123,** 830–836.
29. Reignier, J., Mazmanian, M., Detruit, H., et al. (1994) Reduction of ischemia-reperfusion injury by pentoxifylline in the isolated rat lung. Paris-Sud University Lung Transplantation Group. *Am. J. Respir. Crit. Care Med.* **150,** 342–347.
30. Moore, T. M., Khimenko, P., Adkins, W. K., Miyasaka, M., and Taylor, A. E. (1995) Adhesion molecules contribute to ischemia and reperfusion-induced injury in the isolated rat lung. *J. Appl. Physiol.* **78,** 2245–2252.
31. Jurmann, M. J., Dammenhayn, L., Schaefers, H. J., and Haverich, A. (1990) Pulmonary reperfusion injury: evidence for oxygen-derived free radical mediated damage and effects of different free radical scavengers. *Eur. J. Cardiothorac. Surg.* **4,** 665–670.
32. Ayene, I. S., al-Mehdi, A. B., and Fisher, A. B. (1993) Inhibition of lung tissue oxidation during ischemia/reperfusion by 2-mercaptopropionylglycine. *Arch. Biochem. Biophys.* **303,** 307–312.
33. Haynes, J., Jr., Seibert, A., Bass, J. B., and Taylor, A. E. (1990) U74500A inhibition of oxidant-mediated lung injury. *Am. J. Physiol.* **259,** H144–H148.
34. Takeyoshi, I., Iwanami, K., Kamoshita, N., et al. (2001) Effect of lazaroid U-74389G on pulmonary ischemia-reperfusion injury in dogs. *J. Invest. Surg.* **14,** 83–92.
35. Fisher, A. B., Dodia, C., Tan, Z. T., Ayene, I., and Eckenhoff, R. G. (1991) Oxygen-dependent lipid peroxidation during lung ischemia. *J Clin. Invest.* **88,** 674–679.
36. Zhao, G., al-Mehdi, A. B., and Fisher, A. B. (1997) Anoxia-reoxygenation versus ischemia in isolated rat lungs. *Am. J. Physiol.* **273,** L1112–L1117.
37. Al-Mehdi, A. B., Zhao, G., Dodia, C., et al. (1998) Endothelial NADPH oxidase as the source of oxidants in lungs exposed to ischemia or high K+. *Circ. Res.* **83,** 730–737.
38. Song, C., Al-Mehdi, A. B., and Fisher, A. B. (2001) An immediate endothelial cell signaling response to lung ischemia. *Am. J. Physiol. Lung Cell Mol. Physiol.* **281,** L993–L1000.
39. Al-Mehdi, A. B., Shuman, H., and Fisher, A. B. (1997) Intracellular generation of reactive oxygen species during nonhypoxic lung ischemia. *Am. J. Physiol.* **272,** L294–L300.
40. Ayene, I. S., Dodia, C., and Fisher, A. B. (1992) Role of oxygen in oxidation of lipid and protein during ischemia/reperfusion in isolated perfused rat lung. *Arch. Biochem. Biophys.* **296,** 183–189.
41. Midorikawa, J., Maehara, K., Yaoita, H., et al. (2001) Continuous observation of superoxide generation in an in-situ ischemia-reperfusion rat lung model. *Jpn. Circ. J.* **65,** 207–212.
42. Lansman, J. B. (1988) Endothelial mechanosensors. Going with the flow. *Nature* **331,** 481–482.
43. Riley, D. J., Rannels, D. E., Low, R. B., Jensen, L., and Jacobs, T. P. (1990) NHLBI Workshop Summary. Effect of physical forces on lung structure, function, and metabolism. *Am. Rev. Respir. Dis.* **142,** 910–914.
44. Watson, P. A. (1991) Function follows form: generation of intracellular signals by cell deformation. *FASEB J.* **5,** 2013–2019.
45. Davies, P. F. and Tripathi, S. C. (1993) Mechanical stress mechanisms and the cell. An endothelial paradigm. *Circ. Res.* **72,** 239–245.
46. Fisher, A. B., Chien, S., Barakat, A. I., and Nerem, R. M. (2001) Endothelial cellular response to altered shear stress. *Am. J. Physiol. Lung Cell Mol. Physiol.* **281,** L529–L533.
47. Davies, P. F., Barbee, K. A., Volin, M. V., et al. (1997) Spatial relationships in early signaling events of flow-mediated endothelial mechanotransduction. *Annu. Rev. Physiol.* **59,** 527–549.
48. Manevich, Y., Al-Mehdi, A., Muzykantov, V., and Fisher, A. B. (2001) Oxidative burst and NO generation as initial response to ischemia in flow-adapted endothelial cells. *Am. J. Physiol. Heart Circ. Physiol.* **280,** H2126–H2135.
49. DeLeo, F. R. and Quinn, M. T. (1996) Assembly of the phagocyte NADPH oxidase: molecular interaction of oxidase proteins. *J. Leukoc. Biol.* **60,** 677–691.
50. Babior, B. M., Lambeth, J. D., and Nauseef, W. (2002) The neutrophil NADPH oxidase. *Arch. Biochem. Biophys.* **397,** 342–344.
51. Zulueta, J. J., Sawhney, R., Yu, F. S., Cote, C. C., and Hassoun, P. M. (1997) Intracellular generation of reactive oxygen species in endothelial cells exposed to anoxia-reoxygenation. *Am. J. Physiol.* **272,** L897–L902.

52. Jones, S. A., O'Donnell, V. B., Wood, J. D., Broughton, J. P., Hughes, E. J., and Jones, O. T. (1996) Expression of phagocyte NADPH oxidase components in human endothelial cells. *Am. J. Physiol.* **271**, H1626–H1634.
53. Babior, B. M. (2000) The NADPH oxidase of endothelial cells. *IUBMB Life* **50**, 267–269.
54. Forman, H. J. and Torres, M. (2001) Signaling by the respiratory burst in macrophages. *IUBMB Life* **51**, 365–371.
55. Wei, Z., Costa, K., Al-Mehdi, A. B., Dodia, C., Muzykantov, V., and Fisher, A. B. (1999) Simulated ischemia in flow-adapted endothelial cells leads to generation of reactive oxygen species and cell signaling. *Circ. Res.* **85**, 682–689.
56. Wei, Z., Al-Mehdi, A. B., and Fisher, A. B. (2001) Signaling pathway for nitric oxide generation with simulated ischemia in flow-adapted endothelial cells. *Am. J. Physiol. Heart Circ. Physiol.* **281**, H2226–H2232.
57. Al-Mehdi, A. B., Zhao, G., and Fisher, A. B. (1998) ATP-independent membrane depolarization with ischemia in the oxygen-ventilated isolated rat lung. *Am. J. Respir. Cell Mol. Biol.* **18**, 653–661.
58. Chatterjee, S., Al-Mehdi, A. B., Levitan, I., Stevens, T., and Fisher, A. B. (2003) Shear stress increases expression of a KATP channel in rat and bovine pulmonary vascular endothelial cells. *Am. J. Physiol. Cell Physiol.* **285**, C959–C967.
59. Al-Mehdi, A. B., Song, C., Tozawa, K., and Fisher, A. B. (2000) Ca2+- and phosphatidylinositol 3-kinase-dependent nitric oxide generation in lung endothelial cells in situ with ischemia. *J. Biol. Chem.* **275**, 39,807–39,810.

Pulmonary Vascular Barrier Regulation by Thrombin and Edg Receptors

Jeffrey R. Jacobson and Joe G. N. Garcia

SUMMARY

Lung vascular permeability is directly determined by the integrity of the endothelial cell (EC) monolayer, which involves dynamic regulation by the actomyosin cytoskeleton with subsequent effects on cell–cell and cell–matrix interactions. Although the list of biochemical and biophysical agonists that alter EC barrier regulation is extensive, in this chapter we consider two in particular—the barrier-disruptive serine protease thrombin and barrier-enhancing sphingosine-1-phosphate, an activator of the Edg receptor. Both agonists, via elaborate receptor-specific and tightly orchestrated signaling pathways, offer important insights into lung vascular barrier regulation with respect to the role of individual cellular components and signaling events that target the endothelial cytoskeleton. Additionally, we detail the combined effect of thrombin and cyclic stretch, mechanistically distinct agonists, to provide further insight into lung vascular regulation. Our understanding of EC barrier regulation and lung vascular permeability has advanced remarkably in only a short time and, with the use of newly available technologies, will undoubtedly continue to rapidly evolve.

Key Words: Thrombin; sphingosine-1-phosphate; PAR1; endothelial; permeability; vascular leak; mechanical stretch; cytoskeleton; actin; transendothelial electrical resistance.

1. OVERVIEW OF LUNG ENDOTHELIAL CELL BARRIER REGULATION

The pulmonary vasculature exists as a dynamically regulated, semipermeable barrier between the lung interstitium and the pulmonary circulation. This endothial cell barrier is maintained by multiple components, including the negatively charged glycocalyx, comprised of membrane-bound proteoglycans and glycoproteins, which coat the luminal surface. Specific members of the glycocalyx include a number of bioactive elements, such as various cell-adhesion molecules as well as mediators of coagulation and fibrinolysis, including tissue factor and plasminogen (1). A second major contributor to the intact cellular barrier is the tight apposition of individual endothelial cells with neighboring cells via intercellular junctions (quasi "tight junctions," adherens junctions, PECAM), which collectively contribute to basal endothelial barrier function. Finally, specific components of the focal adhesion complex, i.e., the integrin-based linkage between the extracellular matrix and the endothelial cytoskeleton, provide strong tethering of the endothelium to the vessel wall and thus enhanced barrier integrity. Although once perceived as a passive cellular barrier, endothelial cells are now recognized as highly dynamic and are responsive to a number of barrier promoting effectors. For example, our studies and others have separately characterized the effects of growth factors such as hepatocyte growth factor (2), mechanical shear stress (3), and novel angiogenic factors such as angiopoietin (4) and sphingosine-1-phosphate (Sph-1-P) (5), a product of platelets, in this respect (**Fig. 1**).

From: *Cell Signaling in Vascular Inflammation*
Edited by: J. Bhattacharya © Humana Press Inc., Totowa, NJ

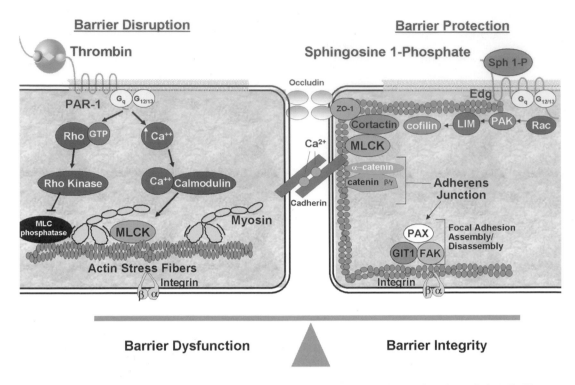

Fig. 1. Endothelial cell (EC) barrier regulation by thrombin and sphingosine-1-phosphate (Sph-1-P). Thrombin cleavage of the PAR-1 receptor on the surface of EC activates both heterotrimeric G proteins (Gq, Gi, G12/13) as well as small GTPases such as Rho. Activated Rho, Rho-GTP, induces Rho kinase which via phosphorylation of the phosphatase regulatory subunit inhibits the myosin light chain (MLC) phosphatase. Rho kinase and myosin light chain kinase (MLCK) activation occurs via independent pathways (left panel). Separately, increased cytosolic Ca^{++} activates the Ca^{++}/calmodulindependent MLCK with conformational changes allowing the enzyme to access the preferred substrate (MLC). Rho kinase and MLCK activation both culminate in increased MLC phosphorylation which, in turn, enables actomyosin contraction resulting in increased cellular contraction, paracellular gap formation, and ultimately barrier dysfunction. Conversely, Sph-1-P enhances EC barrier function via activation of a signaling cascade which involves Rac, MLCK, cortactin, and various components of adherens junctions and focal adhesions (right). Sph-1-P activates specific G protein-coupled EC Edg receptors leading to activation of the small GTPase Rac. Subsequently, Rac activation initiates intracellular events dependent on Pak, LIM kinase, and the actin severing protein, cofilin which contribute to increased cortical actin (left).

It is, therefore, intuitive that any increases in vascular permeability must ultimately be attributed to a loss or disruption of endothelial intercellular junctions, in combination with a breakdown of the tethering forces characteristic of cell–cell or cell–matrix interactions, which result in paracellular vascular leakage. Similar to barrier enhancement, this loss of barrier integrity appears to also occur as a result of adhesive biophysical forces, as with the cyclic lung stretch associated with ventilator-induced lung injury, or as a consequence of receptor ligation by specific inflammatory mediators, such as thrombin (**Fig. 1**).

It has now been well established that a key common element to vascular barrier regulation is the deep integration of both barrier-enhancing and integrity-reducing responses, with dynamic cytoskeletal elements driven primarily by actin and myosin but also with contributions of the microtubule scaffolding complex *(6,7)*. Consistent with a central role for the endothelial cytoskeleton as a key effector in barrier regulation, our lab has examined in detail the activation of the EC contractile apparatus, a critical determinant of vascular permeability characterized by increased myosin light

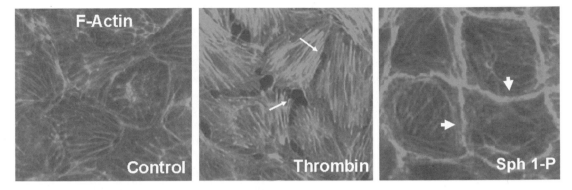

Fig. 2. Endothelial cell (EC) cytoskeletal rearrangement induced by thrombin and sphingosine-1-phosphate (Sph-1-P). These immunofuorescent images utilizing Texas red-conjugated phalloidin to identify polymerized actin filaments demonstrate that relative to controls, human pulmonary artery EC stimulated with thrombin demonstrate a prominent increase in actin stress fibers associated with cell contraction and evidence of paracellular gaps (small arrows) *(5)*. In contrast, EC stimulated with Sph-1-P reveal prominent cortical actin enhancement (large arrows), a relative paucity of central stress fibers, and no paracellular gaps.

chain (MLC) phosphorylation mediated by rho kinase and the Ca^{2+}/calmodulin (CaM)-dependent MLC kinase (MLCK). These events culminate in the formation of actin stress fibers and resultant increased intracellular tension *(7)*.

In this chapter, regulation of pulmonary vascular barrier properties will be discussed, with specific focus on cytoskeletal rearrangements that occur after endothelial cell (EC) activation with thrombin, the central regulatory molecule of hemostasis and coagulation. These results will be discussed and contrasted with the specific signaling pathways evoked by Sph-1-P, an activator of the Edg receptor, which potentially enhances EC barrier function.

2. THROMBIN

The serine protease thrombin represents an ideal model for the examination of agonist-mediated EC activation and barrier dysfunction. Thrombin evokes numerous endothelial cell responses that regulate hemostasis, thrombosis, and vessel wall pathophysiology, and is recognized as a potentially important mediator in the pathogenesis of acute lung injury. Our prior studies and work detailed the events that followed thrombin infusion into the pulmonary artery of the chronically instrumented lung lymph sheep model. The result is profound lung microembolization by proteolytic conversion of fibrinogen to fibrin, initiating a cascade of events that culminate in intravascular coagulation, inflammation, and vascular leak *(8–11)*. In this awake sheep model, thrombin increases both pulmonary lymph flow and lung weight gain, and reduces the sigma reflective coefficient in the isolated perfused lung, consistent with enhanced permeability *(12–14)*.

We have also previously investigated the ability of thrombin to activate the endothelium directly and to increase albumin permeability across endothelial cell monolayers in vitro *(15)*. Thrombin induced a concentration-dependent increase in I125-albumin clearance that was independent of its interaction with fibrinogen and appeared to be due to a reversible change in EC shape with the formation of intercellular gaps (**Fig. 2**). This observation provided a blueprint for the mechanistic examination of EC barrier properties, with subsequent studies reporting that the direct activation of ECs by thrombin is dependent upon the ability of thrombin to proteolytically cleave the extracellular NH2-terminal domain of the PAR-1 receptor, a member of the family of proteinase-activated receptors (PARs) *(16–19)* (**Fig. 1**). The cleaved NH2-terminus, acting as a tethered ligand, activates the receptor and initiates a number of downstream effects, including the activation of phospholipases A2, C, and D, increases in cytosolic Ca++, and increased permeability *(18–23)*. Activation of the EC thrombin receptor also induces the release of various products, including von Willebrand factor, endothelin, NO, and PGI2 *(24–26)*.

Our work has elucidated specific components of the contractile apparatus as the target for thrombin-mediated barrier regulatory signaling pathways. For example, activation of the thrombin receptor induces rapid activation of a Gq protein-coupled phospholipase C, leading to inositol 1,4,5-triphosphate3 (IP_3)-mediated increases in cyotsolic Ca^{++}. In turn, increased cytosolic Ca^{++} leads to the coordinate activation of the small GTPase Rho and Ca^{++}/CaM-dependent MLCK *(27–31)* (**Fig. 1**), which phosophorylates MLC at Thr-18 and Ser-19. Activation of the thrombin receptor also induces G12/13-mediated Rho activation and, via its target effector, Rho kinase, inhibits MLC phosphatase activity by myosin phosphatase phosphorylation, thus attenuating dephosphorylation of MLC *(28)*. This potent increase in MLCK/Rho kinase-mediated MLC phosphorylation results in a dramatic increase in intracellular force development and tension, a diminution of the cortical actin ring, and a prominent increase in F-actin stress fibers that traverse the cell (**Fig. 2**).

The resultant increases in actin stress fiber formation and actomyosin cellular contraction disrupt the barrier regulatory balance with tethering forces unable to maintain the paracellular space, culminating in increased EC barrier permeability *(27,32)*. Indeed, the morphologic cellular changes observed in the setting of thrombin-induced endothelial cell permeability are associated with the formation of intercellular gaps with the disruption of adherens junctions and reorganization of focal adhesion plaques *(15,33–35)*. Evidence as to the critical importance of these changes in the regulation of barrier function is provided by the ability of NBD-phallacidin, a stabilizer of actin filaments, to prevent thrombin-induced increases in EC permeability *(36)*. Consistent with this, we have previously reported that both direct inhibition of either MLCK or Rho kinase as well as Ca^{++}/calmodulin antagonism attenuate thrombin-induced MLC phosphorylation and barrier dysfunction *(34,37)*.

The endothelial MLCK isoform was initially cloned by our lab, and we have demonstrated its involvement in regulating EC apoptosis, leukocyte diapedesis, EC migration, and redox signaling. The regulation of the MLCK isoform in the endothelium is complex and differs significantly from the smooth-muscle MLCK isoform (for review, see Dudek *[7]*). EC MLCK is a high-molecular-mass (214 kDa) protein and has a unique NH_2 terminus containing multiple sites for protein–protein interactions as well as sites for p60src-catalyzed tyrosine phosphorylation, which regulates enzyme activity *(38–40)*. Protein tyrosine phosphorylation appears to play an important role in regulation of EC permeability, as evidenced by the modest enhancement of barrier function with the nonspecific tyrosine kinase inhibitor genistein *(41)*. We found that diperoxovanadate, both an activator of tyrosine kinase and an inhibitor of tyrosine phosphatase, stimulates EC MLCK phosphotyrosine accumulation and promotes the stable association of p60src and cortactin, an 80-kDa actin-binding protein, with MLCK and the actin cytoskeleton *(7)*. The importance of these components (p60src and cortactin, along with Ca^{++}/calmodulin, MLC, and actin) in the regulation of EC barrier function by MLCK is now well recognized, although a full understanding of their coordinate activity remains an area of ongoing investigation.

3. EFFECT OF THROMBIN ON CYCLIC STRETCH-CONDITIONED LUNG ENDOTHELIUM

Our work indicates that the attenuation of thrombin-induced EC permeability by MLCK inhibition may have significant clinical implications. Specifically, there is evidence to suggest that such a strategy may be able to improve outcomes in ventilator-induced lung injury (VILI), a condition characterized by increased vascular permeability *(42)*. In our lab, employing the Flexercell® Tension Plus™ (FX-4000T™) system, we have studied EC subjected to cyclic stretch as an in vitro model of VILI (**Fig. 3**). This apparatus allows for EC to be grown in a monolayer overlying a flexible substrate under which a vacuum can be applied, thus inducing stretch proportional to the degree of vacuum

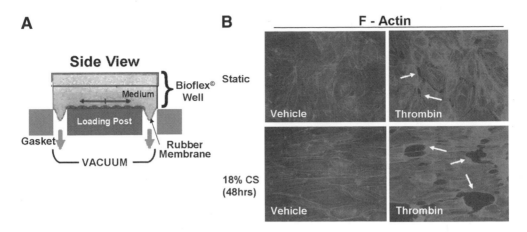

Fig. 3. Thrombin-induced barrier dysfunction in cyclic-stretched endothelial cells (EC). Employing the Flexercell® Tension Plus™ system, human pulmonary artery EC were grown in a monolayer on a flexible substrate overlying a fixed loading post around which a vacuum was applied (**A**). Cells were subjected to 18% radial stretch with a frequency of 0.5 hz for 48 h prior to thrombin stimulation (**B**). Relative to controls, stretched cells demonstrated reorientation of the cytoskeleton and exhibited a more pronounced response to thrombin stimulation characterized by prominent paracellular gaps (arrows).

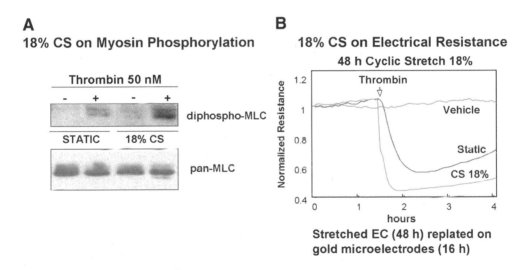

Fig. 4. Effect of cyclic stretch on thrombin-induced MLC phosphorylation and barrier dysfunction. Human pulmonary artery endothelial cells (EC) exposed to 18% radial stretch, 0.5 hz for 48 h exhibit an increased MLC phosphorylation relative to controls after thrombin stimulation (50 nm, 5 min) consistent with activated cytoskeletal rearrangement (**A**). Transmonolayer electrical resistance (TER) measured 16 h after stretching in cells replated on gold microelectrodes demonstrate a more pronounced response to thrombin consistent with increased barrier dysfunction and a slower recovery relative to static controls (**B**).

pressure. EC exposed to 18% radial stretch for 48 h did not demonstrate any breach in monolayer integrity evaluated histologically or by measurements of transmonolayer electrical resistance (TER) under basal conditions. However, cyclic stretch-preconditioned EC demonstrated greater paracellular gap formation, with increase gap surface area in response to thrombin (**Fig. 3**) that correlated with increased levels of MLC phosphorylation (**Fig. 4**) *(43)*. Likely determinants of this heightened re-

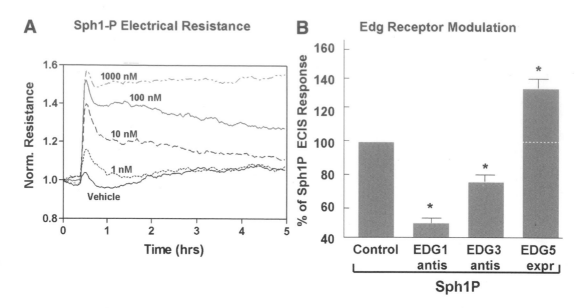

Fig. 5. Effect of sphingosine-1-phosphate (Sph-1-P) on endothelial cell (EC) barrier function: dependence on Edg receptor ligation. EC treated with Sph-1-P show a rapid, dose-response effect with respect to barrier enhancement as measured by transmonolayer electrical resistance via Electric Cell-substrate Impedance Sensing (ECIS™, Applied Biophysics, Troy, NY) (**A**). This effect is significantly attenuated by expression of both an Edg-1 and Edg-3 antisense oligonucleotide (**B**). Conversely, overexpression of Edg-5, an Edg receptor not normally present in vascular endothelium, leads to an increased barrier enhancing response to Sph-1-P (left). Reprinted from ref. 5, with permission.

sponse include increased intracellular signaling events via mechanical transduction, priming of the activated cytoskeleton, and the resultant concurrent effects of increased contractile and decreased tethering forces. Additionally, our findings were associated with significant changes in the expression of genes related to regulation of the cytoskeleton (including MLCK) as determined by Affymetrix microarray experiments *(43,44)*.

4. SPHINGOSINE-1-PHOSPHATE

Our lab has been interested in the integration between EC barrier regulation and angiogenesis. Our initial studies determined that sphingosine-1-phosphate (Sph-1-P), a platelet-derived phospholipid, is the most potent EC chemotactic agent present in serum and is ultimately involved in angiogenesis and vascular hemostasis through its ability to evoke various cell-specific responses *(45–51)*. In the setting of coagulation, Sph-1-P is abundantly released from platelets and, via its pleiotropic effects, potentially contributes to new blood-vessel formation. This is evidenced by in vivo studies that establish Sph-1-P as remarkably effective in avian chorioallantoic membranes *(52)*, in Matrigel-implanted plugs in mice *(48)*, and in the avascular mouse cornea *(46)*.

Direct activation of EC by Sph-1-P is dependent in part on its binding to G protein (Gi and Gi2/i3)-coupled receptors encoded by members of the endothelial differentiation gene (Edg) family of receptors *(48,49,53)*. Of this family, Edg-1 and -3, found on the surface of EC, as well as Edg-5 and -6, are high-affinity Edg receptors for Sph-1-P *(5,50,54)*. We recently described Sph-1-P as a potent enhancer of barrier function in vitro *(5)*, and more recently in vivo *(55)*. Sph-1-P strongly enhances transmonolayer electrical resistance (TER) across both bovine and human EC monolayers (**Fig. 5**). In addition, Sph-1-P significantly attenuates thrombin-induced barrier disruption and is able to rapidly restore barrier integrity when added subsequent to thrombin stimulation *(5)*. Preincubation with Edg-

1 or Edg-3 antisense oligonucleotides to deplete the Sph-1-P receptor expression leads to decreased barrier protection in response to Sph-1-P as measured by TER, whereas overexpression of Edg-5, not normally expressed in EC, accentuates the protective effects of Sph-1-P (**Fig. 5**). Furthermore, we are now confident that Sph-1-P is a major component of platelet releasates that nurture the microcirculation *(56)*.

We investigated several potential mediators of intercellular signaling events instigated by Sph-1-P and identified an important role for Rho family GTPases. Specifically, Rac GTPase, recognized as playing an important role in lamellipodial formation and cortical cytoskeletal reorganization *(57)*, is rapidly activated by Sph-1-P *(5)*. Evidence suggests that the p21-associated Ser/Thr kinase 1 (PAK1) may be an important downstream Rac target in this setting *(5)*, as its binding to Rac results in the phosphorylation and activation of LIM kinase and the subsequent inactivation of the LIM kinase target cofilin, an actin-severing protein *(58)*, events that are consistent with EC barrier enhancement. Additionally, we recently reported that Sph-1-P induces rapid redistribution of focal adhesions, attachment sites for actin filaments, via Rac and G protein-coupled receptor kinase interacting proteins (GITs) *(59,60)*.

Interestingly, both cortactin and MLCK appear to participate in Sph-1-P-induced cortical actin thickening and lamellipodia formation *(61)*, although their interaction in the context of Sph-1-P remains to be elucidated.

5. CONCLUSION

Our understanding of pulmonary vascular permeability and EC barrier regulation continues to evolve. There is little doubt that the specific features of thrombin-induced barrier disruption and Sph-1-P-mediated barrier enhancement have helped identify critically important effectors of EC cytoskeletal regulation. Further investigation of these and other agonists, relying on thoughtful experimental design and employing powerful tools such as cDNA microarray analysis and proteomic approaches, will ultimately allow us to fine-tune our current working model of EC barrier regulation. Realization of a detailed and accurate model will be of enormous significance and has the potential to lead to novel approaches in the management of many clinical conditions in which aberrant EC barrier function is a prominent feature.

ACKNOWLEDGMENTS

This work was supported by grants from the National Heart, Lung, and Blood Institute (F32 HL 71411, R01 HL 68034, and R01 58604) and the Dr. David Marine Endowment. Special thanks to Konstantin Birukov, Nicholas Shank, and Steven Dudek for their assistance in preparing this manuscript.

REFERENCES

1. Pries, A. R., Secomb, T. W., and Gaehtgens, P. (2000) The endothelial surface layer. *Pflugers Arch.* **440,** 653–666.
2. Liu, F., Schaphorst, K. L., Verin, A. D., et al. (2002) Hepatocyte growth factor enhances endothelial cell barrier function and cortical cytoskeletal rearrangement: potential role of glycogen synthase kinase-3beta. *FASEB J.* **16,** 950–962.
3. Birukov, K. G., Birukova, A. A., Dudek, S. M., et al. (2002) Shear stress-mediated cytoskeletal remodeling and cortactin translocation in pulmonary endothelial cells. *Am. J. Respir. Cell Mol. Biol.* **26,** 453–464.
4. Iizasa, H., Bae, S. H., Asashima, T., et al. (2002) Augmented expression of the tight junction protein occludin in brain Endothelial cell line TR-bBB by rat angiopoietin-1 expressed in baculovirus-infected sf plus insect cells. *Pharm. Res.* **19,** 1757–1760.
5. Garcia, J. G., Liu, F., Verin, A. D., et al. (2001) Sphingosine 1-phosphate promotes endothelial cell barrier integrity by Edg-dependent cytoskeletal rearrangement. *J. Clin. Invest.* **108,** 689–701.
6. Verin, A. D., Birukova, A., Wang, P., et al. (2001) Microtubule disassembly increases endothelial cell barrier dysfunction: role of MLC phosphorylation. *Am. J. Physiol. Lung Cell Mol. Physiol.* **281,** L565–L574.
7. Dudek, S. M. and Garcia, J. G. (2001) Cytoskeletal regulation of pulmonary vascular permeability. *J. Appl. Physiol.* **91,** 1487–1500.
8. Saldeen, T. (1976) Trends in microvascular research. The microembolism syndrome. *Microvasc. Res.* **11,** 227–259.
9. Johnson, A., Tahamont, M. V., Kaplan, J. E., et al. (1982) Lung fluid balance after pulmonary embolization: effects of thrombin vs. fibrin aggregates. *J. Appl. Physiol.* **52,** 1565–1570.

10. Malik, A. B. and Horgan, M. J. (1987) Mechanisms of thrombin-induced lung vascular injury and edema. *Am. Rev. Respir. Dis.* **136,** 467–470.
11. Garcia, J. G., Perlman, M. B., Ferro, T. J., et al. (1988) Inflammatory events after fibrin microembolization. Alterations in alveolar macrophage and neutrophil function. *Am. Rev. Respir. Dis.* **137,** 630–635.
12. Horgan, M. J., Fenton, J. W., 2nd, and Malik, A. B. (1987) Alpha-thrombin-induced pulmonary vasoconstriction. *J. Appl. Physiol.* **63,** 1993–2000.
13. Lo, S. K., Garcia-Szabo, R. R., and Malik, A. B. (1990) Leukocyte repletion reverses protective effect of neutropenia in thrombin-induced increase in lung vascular permeability. *Am. J. Physiol.* **259,** H149–H155.
14. Lo, S. K., Perlman, M. B., Niehaus, G. D., et al. (1985) Thrombin-induced alterations in lung fluid balance in awake sheep. *J. Appl. Physiol.* **58,** 1421–1427.
15. Garcia, J. G., Siflinger-Birnboim, A., Bizios, R., et al. (1986) Thrombin-induced increase in albumin permeability across the endothelium. *J. Cell Physiol.* **128,** 96–104.
16. Vogel, S. M., Gao, X., Mehta, D., et al. (2000) Abrogation of thrombin-induced increase in pulmonary microvascular permeability in PAR-1 knockout mice. *Physiol. Genomics* **4,** 137–145.
17. Vu, T. K., Hung, D. T., Wheaton, V. I., et al. (1991) Molecular cloning of a functional thrombin receptor reveals a novel proteolytic mechanism of receptor activation. *Cell* **64,** 1057–1068.
18. Garcia, J. G., Patterson, C., Bahler, C., et al. (1993) Thrombin receptor activating peptides induce Ca2+ mobilization, barrier dysfunction, prostaglandin synthesis, and platelet-derived growth factor mRNA expression in cultured endothelium. *J, Cell Physiol.* **156,** 541–549.
19. Garcia, J. G. (1992) Molecular mechanisms of thrombin-induced human and bovine endothelial cell activation. *J. Lab. Clin. Med.* **120,** 513–519.
20. Garcia, J. G., Fenton, J. W., 2nd, and Natarajan, V. (1992) Thrombin stimulation of human endothelial cell phospholipase D activity. Regulation by phospholipase C, protein kinase C, and cyclic adenosine 3'5'-monophosphate. *Blood* **79,** 2056–2067.
21. Tiruppathi, C., Lum, H., Andersen, T. T., et al. (1992) Thrombin receptor 14-amino acid peptide binds to endothelial cells and stimulates calcium transients. *Am. J. Physiol.* **263,** L595–L601.
22. Pollock, W. K., Wreggett, K. A., and Irvine, R. F. (1988) Inositol phosphate production and Ca2+ mobilization in human umbilical-vein endothelial cells stimulated by thrombin and histamine. *Biochem. J.* **256,** 371–376.
23. Hong, S. L. and Deykin, D. (1982) Activation of phospholipases A2 and C in pig aortic endothelial cells synthesizing prostacyclin. *J. Biol. Chem.* **257,** 7151–7154.
24. Bartha, K., Muller-Peddinghaus, R., and Van Rooijen, L. A. (1989) Bradykinin and thrombin effects on polyphosphoinositide hydrolysis and prostacyclin production in endothelial cells. *Biochem. J.* **263,** 149–155.
25. Schini, V. B., Hendrickson, H., Heublein, D. M., et al. (1989) Thrombin enhances the release of endothelin from cultured porcine aortic endothelial cells. *Eur. J. Pharmacol.* **165,** 333–334.
26. Garcia, J. G., Painter, R. G., Fenton, J. W., 2nd, et al. (1990) Thrombin-induced prostacyclin biosynthesis in human endothelium: role of guanine nucleotide regulatory proteins in stimulus/coupling responses. *J. Cell Physiol.* **142,** 186–193.
27. Amano, M., Chihara, K., Kimura, K., et al. (1997) Formation of actin stress fibers and focal adhesions enhanced by Rho-kinase. *Science* **275,** 1308–1311.
28. Essler, M., Amano, M., Kruse, H. J., et al. (1998) Thrombin inactivates myosin light chain phosphatase via Rho and its target Rho kinase in human endothelial cells. *J. Biol. Chem.* **273,** 21,867–21,874.
29. Goeckeler, Z. M. and Wysolmerski, R. B. (1995) Myosin light chain kinase-regulated endothelial cell contraction: the relationship between isometric tension, actin polymerization, and myosin phosphorylation. *J. Cell. Biol.* **130,** 613–627.
30. van Nieuw Amerongen, G. P., Draijer, R., Vermeer, M. A., et al. (1998) Transient and prolonged increase in endothelial permeability induced by histamine and thrombin: role of protein kinases, calcium, and RhoA. *Circ. Res.* **83,** 1115–1123.
31. Vouret-Craviari, V., Boquet, P., Pouyssegur, J., et al. (1998) Regulation of the actin cytoskeleton by thrombin in human endothelial cells: role of Rho proteins in endothelial barrier function. *Mol. Biol. Cell* **9,** 2639–2653.
32. Chrzanowska-Wodnicka, M., and Burridge, K. (1996) Rho-stimulated contractility drives the formation of stress fibers and focal adhesions. *J. Cell. Biol.* **133,** 1403–1415.
33. Laposata, M., Dovnarsky, D. K., and Shin, H. S. (1983) Thrombin–induced gap formation in confluent endothelial cell monolayers in vitro. *Blood* **62,** 549–556.
34. Rabiet, M. J., Plantier, J. L., Rival, Y., et al. (1996) Thrombin-induced increase in endothelial permeability is associated with changes in cell-to-cell junction organization. *Arterioscler. Thromb. Vasc. Biol.* **16,** 488–496.
35. Schaphorst, K. L., Pavalko, F. M., Patterson, C. E., et al. (1997) Thrombin-mediated focal adhesion plaque reorganization in endothelium: role of protein phosphorylation. *Am. J. Respir. Cell. Mol. Biol.* **17,** 443–455.
36. Phillips, P. G., Lum, H., Malik, A. B., et al. (1989) Phallacidin prevents thrombin-induced increases in endothelial permeability to albumin. *Am. J. Physiol.* **257,** C562–567.
37. Garcia, J. G., Davis, H. W., and Patterson, C. E. (1995) Regulation of endothelial cell gap formation and barrier dysfunction: role of myosin light chain phosphorylation. *J. Cell. Physiol.* **163,** 510–522.
38. Birukov, K. G., Csortos, C., Marzilli, L., et al. (2001) Differential regulation of alternatively spliced endothelial cell myosin light chain kinase isoforms by p60(Src). *J. Biol. Chem.* **276,** 8567–8573.
39. Garcia, J. G., Lazar, V., Gilbert-McClain, L. I., et al. (1997) Myosin light chain kinase in endothelium: molecular cloning and regulation. *Am. J. Respir. Cell. Mol. Biol.* **16,** 489–494.
40. Shi, S., Verin, A. D., Schaphorst, K. L., et al. (1998) Role of tyrosine phosphorylation in thrombin-induced endothelial cell contraction and barrier function. *Endothelium* **6,** 153–171.

41. Carbajal, J. M. and Schaeffer, R. C., Jr. (1998) H2O2 and genistein differentially modulate protein tyrosine phosphorylation, endothelial morphology, and monolayer barrier function. *Biochem. Biophys. Res. Commun.* **249**, 461–466.
42. Parker, J. C. (2000) Inhibitors of myosin light chain kinase and phosphodiesterase reduce ventilator-induced lung injury. *J. Appl. Physiol.* **89**, 2241–2248.
43. Birukov, K. G., Jacobson, J. R., Flores, A. F., et al. (2003) Magnitude-dependent regulation of pulmonary endothelial cell barrier function by cyclic stretch. *Am. J. Physiol. Lung Cell Mol. Physiol.* **285(4)**, L785–L797.
44. Birukov, K. G., Shikata, Y., Ye, S. Q., et al. (2003) Differential effects of cyclic stretch and shear stress on pulmonary endothelial cell cytoskeleton, cell adhesions, and barrier function. *Am. J. Respir. Crit. Care Med.* **167**, A568 (Abstract).
45. English, D., Kovala, A. T., Welch, Z., et al. (1999) Induction of endothelial cell chemotaxis by sphingosine 1-phosphate and stabilization of endothelial monolayer barrier function by lysophosphatidic acid, potential mediators of hematopoietic angiogenesis. *J. Hematother. Stem Cell Res.* **8**, 627–634.
46. English, D., Welch, Z., Kovala, A. T., et al. (2000) Sphingosine 1-phosphate released from platelets during clotting accounts for the potent endothelial cell chemotactic activity of blood serum and provides a novel link between hemostasis and angiogenesis. *FASEB J.* **14**, 2255–2265.
47. Kovala, A. T., Harvey, K. A., McGlynn, P., et al. (2000) High-efficiency transient transfection of endothelial cells for functional analysis. *FASEB J.* **14**, 2486–2494.
48. Lee, M. J., Thangada, S., Claffey, K. P., et al. (1999) Vascular endothelial cell adherens junction assembly and morphogenesis induced by sphingosine-1-phosphate. *Cell* **99**, 301–312.
49. Wang, F., Van Brocklyn, J. R., Hobson, J. P., et al. (1999) Sphingosine 1-phosphate stimulates cell migration through a G(i)-coupled cell surface receptor. Potential involvement in angiogenesis. *J. Biol. Chem.* **274**, 35,343–35,350.
50. Pyne, S. and Pyne, N. J. (2000) Sphingosine 1-phosphate signalling in mammalian cells. *Biochem. J.* **349**, 385–402.
51. Liu, F., Verin, A. D., Wang, P., et al. (2001) Differential regulation of sphingosine-1-phosphate- and VEGF-induced endothelial cell chemotaxis. Involvement of G(ialpha2)-linked Rho kinase activity. *Am. J. Respir. Cell Mol. Biol.* **24**, 711–719.
52. English, D., Garcia, J. G., and Brindley, D. N. (2001) Platelet-released phospholipids link haemostasis and angiogenesis. *Cardiovasc. Res.* **49**, 588–599.
53. Lee, M. J., Van Brocklyn, J. R., Thangada, S., et al. (1998) Sphingosine-1-phosphate as a ligand for the G protein-coupled receptor EDG-1. *Science* **279**, 1552–1555.
54. Zondag, G. C., Postma, F. R., Etten, I. V., et al. (1998) Sphingosine 1-phosphate signalling through the G-protein-coupled receptor Edg-1. *Biochem. J.* **330 (Pt 2)**, 605–609.
55. Peng, X., Hassoun, P. M., Sammani, S., et al. (2004) Protective effects of sphingosine 1-phosphate in murine endotoxin-Induced inflammatory lung injury. *Am. J. Respir. Crit. Care Med.* **169(11)**, 1245–1251.
56. Schaphorst, K. L., Chiang, E. T., Jacobs, K. N., et al. (2003) Role of sphingosine 1-phosphate in the enhancement of endothelial barrier integrity by platelet-released products. *Am. J. Phys.* **285(1)**, L258–L267.
57. Edwards, D. C., Sanders, L. C., Bokoch, G. M., et al. (1999) Activation of LIM-kinase by Pak1 couples Rac/Cdc42 GTPase signalling to actin cytoskeletal dynamics. *Nat. Cell. Biol.* **1**, 253–259.
58. Yang, N., Higuchi, O., Ohashi, K., et al. (1998) Cofilin phosphorylation by LIM-kinase 1 and its role in Rac-mediated actin reorganization. *Nature* **393**, 809–812.
59. Shikata, Y., Birukov, K. G., and Garcia, J. G. (2002) S1P induces FA remodeling in human pulmonary endothelial cells: role of Rac, GIT1, FAK and paxillin. *J. Appl. Physiol.* **94(3)**, 1193–1203.
60. Shikata, Y., Birukov, K. G., Birukova, A. A., et al. (2003) Involvement of site-specific FAK phosphorylation in sphingosine 1 phosphate- and throbin-induced focal adhesion remodeling: role of Src and GIT. *FASEB J.* **17(15)**, 2240–2249.
61. Dudek, S. M., Jacobson, J. R., Chaing, E. T., et al. (2004) Pulmonary endothelial barrier enhancement by sphingosine 1-phosphate: role of cortactin and myosin light chain kinase. *J. Biol. Chem.* **279(23)**, 24,692–24,700.

15

Second-Messenger Signaling in Lung Capillaries

Kaushik Parthasarathi

SUMMARY

In the lung, several endothelial cell (EC) processes are regulated by an increase in EC cytosolic Ca^{2+}. However, the role of EC cytosolic Ca^{2+} in mediating capillary proinflammatory processes is not clear. Mainly, it is not clear to what extent EC cytosolic Ca^{2+} increases activate other second messengers, which in turn might play a direct role in initiating proinflammatory responses. We determined this in intact lung capillaries using videomicroscopy and image analysis. We subjected the lungs to stressors including increased vascular pressure and tumor necrosis factor α. Our studies indicate that the primary response to these lung stresses is an increase in EC cytosolic Ca^{2+}. These stresses induce proinflammatory responses in these capillaries, as indicated by the increase in P-selectin expression. However, determination of the signaling pathways underlying the Ca^{2+}-induced P-selectin expression indicates a role for mitochondrial mechanisms. The lung stressors induce cytosolic Ca^{2+}-dependent increases in mitochondrial Ca^{2+} and reactive oxygen species, which in turn regulate exocytosis of P-selectin. Hence, mitochondrial reactive oxygen species act as signaling intermediates in Ca^{2+}-induced P-selectin exocytosis in lung capillaries. Thus, second messengers Ca^{2+} and mitochondrial reactive oxygen species are critical in the regulation of lung proinflammatory responses.

Key Words: Arachidonate; endothelial; mitochondria; P-selectin; reactive oxygen species; TNF-α.

1. INTRODUCTION

Lung stressors, including sepsis *(1)*, pneumonia *(2)*, and high vascular pressure *(3)*, lead to endothelial cell (EC) activation. Activated EC exhibit increased cytosolic calcium (Ca^{2+}_{CYT}), which mediates several cellular processes, including secretion *(4)*, nuclear factor (NF)-κB activation *(5)* and gene transcription *(5,6)*, and other proinflammatory responses. Regulation of Ca^{2+}_{CYT} may underlie the extent to which proinflammatory responses are regulated. In addition, Ca^{2+}_{CYT} modulates other cellular messengers *(7,8)* that might play a role in regulating specific proinflammatory responses, like an increase in EC P-selectin expression. This chapter addresses the role of Ca^{2+}_{CYT} in coordinating other second-messenger activation and, finally, P-selectin expression in lung capillaries.

2. Ca^{2+}_{CYT} REGULATION

Regulation of Ca^{2+}_{CYT} is characterized by mechanisms that cause an influx of Ca^{2+} and those that extrude Ca^{2+} to maintain Ca^{2+}_{CYT} at resting levels. The balance between these two opposing sets of mechanisms determines Ca^{2+}_{CYT} homeostasis in lung capillaries.

2.1. Receptor-Mediated Mechanisms

Ligand binding activates phospholipase C leading to release of inositol 1,4,5-trisphosphate (InsP3) *(9–11)*. Receptor ligation of InsP3 on the endoplasmic reticulum (ER) *(12,13)* leads to formation of

From: *Cell Signaling in Vascular Inflammation*
Edited by: J. Bhattacharya © Humana Press Inc., Totowa, NJ

an ion channel on the ER membrane *(14)*. As Ca^{2+} concentration in ER is higher than that in cytosol (1 mM vs 100 nM) *(15)*, the ER ion channel formation leads to release of ER store Ca^{2+} into the cytosol, resulting in a rapid increase in Ca^{2+}_{CYT} *(16,17)*. This increase in Ca^{2+}_{CYT} acts in a negative feedback loop to limit the sensitivity of InsP3 receptors, leading to a reduction in Ca^{2+} release from ER *(17)*.

Release of Ca^{2+} from the ER activates compensatory replenishment mechanisms that serve to maintain ER Ca^{2+} levels. Sarcoplasmic/endoplasmic reticulum Ca^{2+}-ATPase (SERCA) pumps on the ER membrane refill the ER through rapid re-uptake of Ca^{2+} from the cytosol *(13,18,19)*. This re-uptake entails a transient nature to the InsP3-mediated Ca^{2+}_{CYT} responses. Further, the resulting decrease in Ca^{2+}_{CYT} restores the sensitivity of the ER InsP3 receptors and a repeated Ca^{2+} release *(13,17)*. Continuation of this negative-feedback-regulated process leads to the generation of Ca^{2+}_{CYT} oscillations *(17,20,21)*, which may mediate cellular processes *(22–25)*.

In addition, depletion of ER Ca^{2+} stores also activates plasma membrane Ca^{2+} channels that induce entry of external Ca^{2+} into the cytosol. This mechanism is termed *capacitative Ca2+ entry* (CCE) and serves to further amplify the InsP3-induced Ca^{2+}_{CYT} increase *(14,26,27)*. This increase in Ca^{2+}_{CYT} leads to activation of proteins in the cytosol *(28)*. Because a prolonged increase in Ca^{2+}_{CYT} is detrimental to cellular survival, an increase in Ca^{2+}_{CYT} also activates Ca^{2+}-ATPase pumps on the plasma membrane *(13,29,30)* that extrude calcium out into the extracellular space and return Ca^{2+}_{CYT} to resting levels.

2.2. Direct Entry of External Ca^{2+}

A second mechanism of Ca^{2+}_{CYT} regulation is through direct entry of external Ca^{2+} into the cytosol. This mechanism is invoked by agents that act directly on plasma membrane ion channels and induce Ca^{2+} entry from outside the cell, where the Ca^{2+} concentration is higher. For example, arachidonate activates plasma membrane channels that are different from those that are activated during CCE *(31)*. This mechanism bypasses both generation of InsP3 and release of ER Ca^{2+} from stores.

3. Ca^{2+} OSCILLATIONS

Modulations in frequency and amplitude of Ca^{2+} oscillations may be important factors controlling cellular responses to agonists in EC. Ca^{2+} oscillations are inherently advantageous over an increase in mean Ca^{2+} in that the message may be conveyed through changes in amplitude and frequency *(22)*, thus sparing the cell from detrimental increases in Ca^{2+} *(32)*. Both physiological and pathological stimuli, including shear stress, tumor necrosis factor (TNF)-α, ATP, vascular pressure, and histamine, have been reported to increase Ca^{2+} oscillations *(15,33)*. EC exposed to shear stress exhibit Ca^{2+} oscillations that vary with varying flow patterns *(34)*. Keubler et al. *(35)* reported that in EC of lung venular capillaries, Ca^{2+} oscillations increase in response to capillary infusion of TNF-α. In addition, it has been indicated that in lung capillaries, increased vascular pressure increases both the frequency and amplitude of EC Ca^{2+} oscillations *(36)*. Glucose and ATP increased the frequency of Ca^{2+} oscillations in the bovine arotic EC *(37)*. Ca^{2+} oscillations have been reported to regulate several processes in both EC and other nonexcitable cells. In pancreatic acinar cells, Ca^{2+} oscillations closely regulate exocytosis *(38)*. Ca^{2+} oscillations lower the threshold for activating transcription factors NF-AT and NF-κB *(22)*. In EC, changes in Ca^{2+} oscillation frequency modulated NF-κB activity in histamine-stimulated human aortic EC *(28)*. Transcription factor regulation then appropriately regulates the cellular responses in EC subjected to either physiological or pathological stimuli.

4. REACTIVE OXYGEN SPECIES

Reactive oxygen species (ROS) commonly denotes the group of oxygen-derived reactive species including the superoxide radical and its derivatives hydrogen peroxide (H_2O_2) and hydroxyl radical.

Superoxide is produced by the univalent reduction of oxygen, and the major sources include the plasma membrane-bound NADPH oxidase, xanthine oxidase, and the electron transport chain of the mitochondria. Dismutation of superoxide by mitochondrial manganese superoxide dismutase (Mn-SOD) or cytosolic cupric superoxide dismutase (Cu-SOD) in the cytosol yields the nonradical H_2O_2. H_2O_2 is converted to the highly reactive hydroxy radical in the presence of Fe^{3+} or Cu^{2+} ions or to water in the presence of catalase or glutathione peroxidase. Leukocytes are major producers of ROS that is secreted at sites of inflammation and used in phagocytosis. Activated EC also produce increased amounts of ROS. Although this increased EC ROS production is widely considered cytotoxic through oxidative damage of proteins *(39,40)*, several recent findings have increasingly implicated ROS as second messengers involved in EC signaling. In EC subjected to hypoxia, generation of EC ROS regulated proinflammatory cytokine secretion leading to altered EC permeability *(41)*. ROS augments as well as reduces several EC secretions. For example, H_2O_2 reduced endothelin-1 secretion by pulmonary artery EC *(42)* while it increased the secretion of vasodilators C-type natriuretic peptide and adrenomedullin from carotid EC *(43)*. H_2O_2 also mediated cyclic-strain-induced increase in endothelin secretion *(44)*, whereas superoxide mediated low-density lipoprotein component-induced secretion of matrix metalloprotcinases *(45)*. ROS mediate thrombin-induced rapid exocytosis of P-selectin in human umblical vein EC *(46)*. In lung, our studies indicate that exocytosis of P-selectin induced by physiological stimuli is also regulated by ROS.

5. LUNG EC STRESSORS

Lung capillary EC are subjected to several pathological stimuli that elicit responses through evoking Ca^{2+} as the second messenger. An increase in capillary pressure increases shear stress on lung EC and also increases vascular distension. These mechano-stresses induce increases of Ca^{2+}_{CYT} *(47)*, activation of transcription factors *(48)*, and suppression of mRNA levels *(49)*. In sepsis, the lung capillary EC are the target of cytokines, such as TNF-α. Alveolar macrophages secrete TNF-α and other cytokines in response to bacterial invasion of the alveoli. The target of these alveolar secretions is the capillary EC, which responds through an increase in Ca^{2+}. These responses might underlie induction of vascular pathological responses such as inflammation *(50)* or permeability increases *(51)*. Studies using cultured EC have attempted to address these issues, but the difficulty is in delineating these issues at the single EC level *in situ*. Our studies using the isolated blood-perfused rat lung have permitted us to determine EC responses to pathological stimuli *in situ*. We herein describe responses to lung stressors including high vascular pressure and TNF-α in EC of lung capillaries.

5.1. Vascular Pressure

Increases in microvascular pressure are pathogenic in the lung vasculature. The cellular mechanisms that underlie this pathogenesis are poorly understood and are only currently beginning to be delineated. Because EC subjected to high pressure undergo both high shear stress and high stretch, quantification of EC responses in intact capillaries reflects the *in situ* responses more closely than in vitro. Hence, EC responses to increased vascular pressure were determined in the intact blood-perfused rat lung preparation. The description of the lung preparation is detailed elsewhere *(52)*. In brief, rat lungs were isolated and artificially perfused with autologous blood through cannulas connected to the pulmonary artery and left atrium. The lungs were maintained at constant inflation. Agents and dyes were infused into lungs using a left atrial catheter. Fluorescence images of surface capillaries were visualized using a epifluorescence microscope and recorded.

In the first study, Kuebler et al. *(53)* increased left atrial pressure from a 5 cmH_2O baseline and maintained at 20 cmH_2O for 30 min *(53)*. EC Ca^{2+}_{CYT} responses were determined using the ratiometric indicator fura 2. In response to the increased vascular pressure, both the mean and oscillations of venular capillary EC Ca^{2+}_{CYT} rapidly increased twofold from baseline levels. The Ca^{2+} responses were abolished both in the presence of gadolinium, an inhibitor of mechano-gated plasma membrane channels, and under external Ca^{2+}-depleted conditions, indicating that entry of external Ca^{2+} induced these cytosolic responses. Elevated vascular pressure also increased fusion pore formation, as determined by the fluorescence of FM1-43, which localizes to specific exocytotic sites *(53)*. Fusion pore formation was a Ca^{2+}-dependent process, indicating that Ca^{2+} increases were necessary for exocytosis in EC. Because P-selectin is stored in Weibel-Palade bodies *(54)* and is exocytosed in response to inflammatory stimuli, Kuebler et al. *(53)* determined P-selectin expression using indirect immunofluorescence *(53)*. Elevated vascular pressure upregulated P-selectin expression in these capillaries. As P-selectin induces neutrophil rolling *(55)* as part of the early inflammatory response, the increase in P-selectin expression indicated that moderate increases in vascular pressure initiates proinflammatory processes in the lung capillaries. In addition, the P-selectin expression was Ca^{2+}_{CYT}-dependent, suggesting that Ca^{2+} is a second messenger that mediates proinflammatory responses to elevated vascular pressure.

Ichimura et al. *(56)* determined lung capillary responses to a vascular pressure increase from 5 to 15 cmH_2O and maintained the higher pressure for 10 min. This stimulus also increased EC Ca^{2+}_{CYT} oscillations and capillary P-selectin expression. To determine the intermediate mechanisms, Ichimura et al. *(56)* measured Ca^{2+}_{MIT} responses in these capillaries. Elevation of vascular pressure increased both the mean and amplitude of Ca^{2+}_{MIT}, which was concomitant with the Ca^{2+}_{CYT} increase. Both mitochondrial and endoplasmic reticulum inhibitors blocked the Ca^{2+}_{MIT} response, indicating that vascular pressure increase induced ER Ca^{2+} release and subsequent Ca^{2+}_{MIT} increase. Further, the EC ROS production measured using the fluorescent indicator dichloro fluorescin (DCFH) also increased in response to the pressure stress. Inhibiting either the cytosolic or the mitochondrial Ca^{2+} increase abolished the ROS response, suggesting its mitochondrial origin. Increases in mitochondrial ROS production were spatially predominant at capillary branch-point EC, implying a spatial distribution of these responses. Mitochondrial ROS increase was upstream of the P-selectin responses, indicating that the vascular pressure-induced proinflammatory responses were mediated by Ca^{2+}-regulated mitochondrial mechanisms.

5.2. Alveolar TNF-α

In lung, pathogens and other airborne particles that lodge in alveolar spaces activate alveolar macrophages and stimulate the upregulation of cytokines such as TNF-α *(57)*. This leads to increased recruitment of leukocytes from the adjoining capillaries *(58)* and their subsequent transmigration into the interstitial and alveolar compartments. The role of cellular second messengers in mediating this crosstalk between the alveolar and vascular compartments was explored in experiments by Kuebler et al. *(59)*. A main reason for targeting second messengers as the mediator of this communication is that the alveolar barrier is impermeable to the passage of macromolecules, and hence limits direct cytokine access to the vasculature. Instillation of TNF-α in the alveolar compartment increased Ca^{2+} in both alveolar epithelium and capillary EC. These increases were abolished by ligation of the epithelial TNF-α receptor, but not the EC TNF-α, confirming that the EC Ca^{2+} response was not as a result of TNF-α diffusion into the vascular segment. Alveolar TNF-α also increased EC P-selectin expression, indicating a possible mechanism for inducing leukocyte adhesion in the vasculature. Epithelial Ca^{2+} induced activation of cytosolic phospholipase A2 and its subsequent translocation to the perinuclear EC. Ca^{2+} responses were inhibited by blocking activation of cytosolic phospholipase A2, a precursor of arachidonate *(60)*, indicating a second-messenger role for arachidonate. In addition, this also abolished the EC P-selectin expression, indicating that arachidonate mediates capillary proinflammatory responses to alveolar TNF-α. Hence, Ca^{2+}_{CYT} increases in both epithelial and endothelial cells acts as the second messenger in mediating proinflammatory responses in lung capillaries to alveolar stresses.

5.3. Capillary TNF-α

Impairment of pulmonary function is commonly referred to as acute respiratory distress syndrome (ARDS). One of the major causes of ARDS is an increase in levels of TNF-α in the blood. Pathologi-

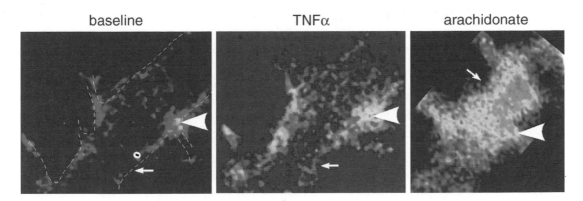

Fig. 1. Endothelial cell (EC) reactive oxygen species (ROS) responses in lung capillaries. Capillaries were loaded with the cell-permeable form of the ROS indicator, dichloro fluorescin (DCFH). Arrowheads indicate branch point EC, whereas arrows indicate mid-segmental EC. Fluorescence was sparse at baseline (left), indicating very low ROS production. Both tumor necrosis factor (TNF)-α (200 ng/mL) (center) and arachidonate (10 μM) increased capillary ROS production. Note that the TNF-α-induced ROS production was uneven and predominated at branch points, while that by arachidonate was more spatially extensive (right).

cal conditions such as sepsis increase levels of TNF-α in the circulation (61,62). A concurrent event is an increase in leukocyte recruitment (62). It has been reported that the increased level of TNF-α might be responsible for this increased recruitment (63–64) through expression of endothelial cell adhesion molecules, including P- and E-selectin (63–65). To determine the EC signaling pathways, we conducted experiments in the isolated blood-perfused intact lung (66). Infusion of TNF-α through a microcatheter into venular capillaries of the lung increased EC Ca^{2+}_{CYT}. Concomitantly, the mitochondrial Ca^{2+} (Ca^{2+}_{MIT}) also increased. To determine whether the increase in Ca^{2+}_{MIT} was dependent on the mechanism of Ca^{2+}_{CYT} increase, the ER store Ca^{2+} was determined. In response to TNF-α infusion, store Ca^{2+} levels decreased. Blocking the store Ca^{2+} release by previously emptying store Ca^{2+} using the SERCA pump blocker tert-butyl hydroquinone (t-BHQ) completely abolished this increase. In addition, the ER InsP3 blocker xestospongin C also prevented the store Ca^{2+} release and the Ca^{2+}_{CYT} increase, indicating that the TNF-α-induced Ca^{2+}_{CYT} increase was mediated by InsP3. To test the mechanism of Ca^{2+}_{MIT} increase further, we infused venular capillaries with the inflammatory product arachidonate. Arachidonate also caused an equipotent increase in EC Ca^{2+}_{CYT} that was dependent on external Ca^{2+}, but not release of ER store Ca^{2+}. This mechanism of Ca^{2+}_{CYT} increase also did not increase Ca^{2+}_{MIT}, indicating that in EC of lung capillaries, store Ca^{2+} release determines Ca^{2+}_{MIT} increase. This functional coupling of ER and mitochondria could be as a result of the close proximity of ER to mitochondria (67). To determine whether an increase in Ca^{2+}_{MIT} could increase ROS production in mitochondria, we determined ROS using the indicator dichlorofluorescin (DCFH). DCFH is converted to fluorescent dichlorofluorescein (DCF) by ROS. In response to TNF-α infusion, EC ROS production increased (**Fig. 1**). Inhibition of mitochondrial Ca^{2+} uptake prevented this ROS increase, indicating that the TNF-α-induced ROS production was dependent on mitochondrial Ca^{2+} increases. Further, the ROS responses were abolished by inhibitors of the mitochondrial electron transport chain, indicating that the TNF-α-induced ROS originated in mitochondria. In contrast to the TNF-α-induced ROS response, arachidonate-induced ROS (**Fig. 1**) originated from nonmitochondrial sources. However, the arachidonate-induced ROS production was also dependent on Ca^{2+}_{CYT} increases. Hence, we conclude that Ca^{2+}_{CYT} increases mediate the augmentation of EC ROS, the origin of which is dependent on the Ca^{2+} increase mechanism.

To determine whether TNF-α-induced ROS acted as a second messenger in mediating downstream events, we quantified P-selectin expression in venular capillaries. TNF-α infusion markedly increased P-selectin expression in capillaries, indicating that TNF-α induced proinflammatory responses in lung capillaries. These responses were abolished by both increases in Ca^{2+}_{CYT} as well as ROS inhibitors. These results support the commonly held view that Ca^{2+}_{CYT} acts as a signaling mediator to increase P-selectin expression in EC. However, these results also introduce the new signaling concept that an increase in Ca^{2+}_{CYT} is not a sufficient condition to induce P-selectin expression, but a downstream induction of ROS is required.

Another aspect of this study was that it highlighted spatial heterogeneity in EC to responses evoked by the two Ca^{2+} mobilization mechanisms. ROS responses induced by TNF-α were predominantly higher at branch-point EC than at mid-segment EC (**Fig. 1**). However, ROS responses by arachidonate were more extensive (**Fig. 1**). The spatial distributions of P-selectin responses were similar to those of the ROS responses. In addition, the spatial patterning of the TNF-α-induced responses were similar to those of the mitochondrial distributions, that predominated at branch-point EC. Hence, the spatial patterning of the TNF-α-induced ROS and P-selectin responses could be attributed to their being mediated by mitochondrial mechanisms. In contrast, the extensive spatial distribution of the arachidonate-induced responses could be attributed to their nonmitochondrial mechanisms, whose distributions may define the spatial distributions to arachidonate.

In summary, our findings with vascular pressure increase and capillary TNF-α reveal the new insight that in EC, mitochondrial ROS may act as diffusible messengers to induce proinflammatory signaling. The branch-point dominance of vascular pressure and TNF-α-induced proinflammatory responses may reflect a mechanism that protects capillary mid-segments from deleterious inflammatory effects that could interfere with gas exchange and reduce blood flow. By contrast, the spatially extensive effects of arachidonate may exemplify the pattern of a more fulminant response. These considerations may be relevant to the understanding of the extent to which the spatial profile of vascular inflammation determines lung injury. In addition, the differences in the signaling mechanisms mediated by ER-derived Ca^{2+} increases and direct Ca^{2+} increases might represent that the Ca^{2+} mobilization pathway may determine the extent to which EC participate in vascular inflammation.

ACKNOWLEDGMENTS

Supported by HL57556, HL64896, and HL075503.

REFERENCES

1. Czermak, B. J., Breckwoldt, M., Ravage, Z. B., et al. (1999) Mechanisms of enhanced lung injury during sepsis. *Am. J. Pathol.* **154**, 1057–1065.
2. Sato, S., Ouellet, N., Pelletier, I., Simard, M., Rancourt, A., and Bergeron, M. G. (2002) Role of galectin-3 as an adhesion molecule for neutrophil extravasation during streptococcal pneumonia. *J. Immunol.* **168(4)**, 1813–1822.
3. Frank, J. A., Gutierrez, J. A., Jones, K. D., Allen, L., Dobbs, L., and Matthay, M. A. (2002) Low tidal volume reduces epithelial and endothelial injury in acid-injured rat lungs. *Am. J. Respir. Crit. Care Med.* **165**, 242–249.
4. Vischer, U. M. and Wollheim, C. B. (1998) Purine nucleotides induce regulated secretion of von Willebrand factor: involvement of cytosolic Ca^{2+} and cyclic adenosine monophosphate-dependent signaling in endothelial exocytosis. *Blood* **91(1)**, 118–127.
5. Quinlan, K. L., Naik, S. M., Cannon, G., et al. (1999) Substance P activates coincident NF-AT- and NF-kappa B-dependent adhesion molecule gene expression in microvascular endothelial cells through intracellular calcium mobilization. *J. Immunol.* **163(10)**, 5656–5665.
6. Murase, T., Kume, N., Korenaga, R., et al. (1998) Fluid shear stress transcriptionally induces lectin-like oxidized LDL receptor-1 in vascular endothelial cells. *Circ. Res.* **83(3)**, 328–333.
7. Stevens, T., Nakahashi, Y., Cornfield, D. N., McMurtry, I. F., Cooper, D. M. and Rodman, D. M. (1995) Ca^{2+}-inhibitable adenylyl cyclase modulates pulmonary artery endothelial cell cAMP content and barrier function. *Proc. Natl. Acad. Sci. USA* **92(7)**, 2696–2700.
8. Wei, Z., Al-Mehdi, A. B. and Fisher, A. B. (2001) Signaling pathway for nitric oxide generation with simulated ischemia in flow-adapted endothelial cells. *Am. J. Physiol. Heart Circ. Physiol.* **281(5)**, H2226–H2232.
9. Resink, T. J., Grigorian, G. Yu., Moldabaeva, A. K., Danilov, S. M., and Buhler, F. R. (1987) Histamine-induced phosphoinositide metabolism in cultured human umbilical vein endothelial cells. Association with thromboxane and prostacyclin release. *Biochem. Biophys. Res. Commun.* **144(1)**, 438–446.
10. Pirotton, S., Verjans, B., Boeynaems, J. M., and Erneux, C. (1991) Metabolism of inositol phosphates in ATP-stimulated vascular endothelial cells. *Biochem. J.* **277 (Pt 1)**, 103–110.
11. Wu, H. M., Yuan, Y., Zawieja, D. C., Tinsley, J., and Granger, H. J. (1999) Role of phospholipase C, protein kinase C, and calcium in VEGF-induced venular hyperpermeability. *Am. J. Physiol.* **276 (Pt 2)**, H535–H542.

12. Madge, L., Marshall, I. C., and Taylor, C. W. (1997) Delayed autoregulation of the Ca^{2+} signals resulting from capacitative Ca^{2+} entry in bovine pulmonary artery endothelial cells. *J. Physiol.* **498,** 351–369.

13. Moccia, F., Berra-Romani, R., Baruffi, S., et al. (2002) Ca^{2+} uptake by the endoplasmic reticulum Ca^{2+}-ATPase in rat microvascular endothelial cells. *Biochem. J.* **364(1),** 235–244.

14. Luckhoff, A. and Clapham, D. E. (1992) Inositol 1,3,4,5-tetrakisphosphate activates an endothelial Ca^{2+} -permeable channel. *Nature* **355(6358),** 356–358.

15. Shmigol, A. V., Eisner, D. A., and Wray, S. (2001) Simultaneous measurements of changes in sarcoplasmic reticulum and cytosolic. *J. Physiol.* **531 (Pt 3),** 707–713.

16. Wood, P. G. and Gillespie, J. I. (1998) In permeabilised endothelial cells IP3-induced Ca^{2+} release is dependent on the cytoplasmic concentration of monovalent cations. *Cardiovasc. Res.* **37(1),** 263–270.

17. Carter, T. D. and Ogden, D. (1997) Kinetics of Ca^{2+} release by InsP3 in pig single aortic endothelial cells: evidence for an inhibitory role of cytosolic Ca^{2+} in regulating hormonally evoked Ca^{2+} spikes. *J. Physiol.* **504 (Pt 1),** 17–33.

18. Wang, X., Reznick, S., Li, P., Liang, W., and van Breemen, C. (2002) Ca^{2+} removal mechanisms in freshly isolated rabbit aortic endothelial cells. *Cell Calcium* **31(6),** 265–277.

19. Poulsen, J. C., Caspersen, C., Mathiasen, D., et al. (1995) Thapsigargin-sensitive Ca^{2+}-ATPases account for Ca^{2+} uptake to inositol 1,4,5-trisphosphate-sensitive and caffeine-sensitive Ca^{2+} stores in adrenal chromaffin cells. *Biochem. J.* **307,** 749–758.

20. Paltauf-Doburzynska, J., Frieden, M., Spitaler, M., and Graier, W. F. (2000) Histamine-induced Ca^{2+} oscillations in a human endothelial cell line depend on transmembrane ion flux, ryanodine receptors and endoplasmic reticulum Ca^{2+}-ATPase. *J. Physiol.* **524 (Pt 3),** 701–713.

21. Barker, C. J., Nilsson, T., Kirk, C. J., Michell, R. H., and Berggren, P. O. (1994) Simultaneous oscillations of cytoplasmic free Ca2+ concentration and Ins(1,4,5)P3 concentration in mouse pancreatic beta-cells. *Biochem. J.* **297 (Pt 2),** 265–268.

22. Dolmetsch, R. E., Xu, K., and Lewis, R. S. (1998) Calcium oscillations increase the efficiency and specificity of gene expression. *Nature* **392(6679),** 933–936.

23. Maturana, A., Van Haasteren, G., Piuz, I., Castelbou, C., Demaurex, N., and Schlegel, W. (2002) Spontaneous calcium oscillations control c-fos transcription via the serum response element in neuroendocrine cells. *J. Biol. Chem.* **277(42),** 39,713–39,721.

24. Gordo, A. C., Rodrigues, P., Kurokawa, M., et al. (2002) Intracellular calcium oscillations signal apoptosis rather than activation in in vitro aged mouse eggs. *Biol. Reprod.* **66(6),** 1828–1837.

25. Soderblom, T., Laestadius, A., Oxhamre, C., Aperia, A., and Richter-Dahlfors, A. (2002) Toxin-induced calcium oscillations: a novel strategy to affect gene regulation in target cells. *Int. J. Med. Microbiol.* **291(6–7),** 511–515.

26. Li, L., Bressler, B., Prameya, R., Dorovini-Zis, K., and Van Breemen, C. 1999) Agonist-stimulated calcium entry in primary cultures of human cerebral microvascular endothelial cells. *Microvasc. Res.* **57(3),** 211–226.

27. Huser, J., Holda, J. R., Kockskamper, J., and Blatter, L. A. (1999) Focal agonist stimulation results in spatially restricted Ca^{2+} release and capacitative Ca^{2+} entry in bovine vascular endothelial cells. *J. Physiol.* **514 (Pt 1),** 101–109.

28. Hu, Q., Natarajan, V., and Ziegelstein, R. C. (2002) Phospholipase D regulates calcium oscillation frequency and nuclear factor-κB activity in histamine- stimulated human endothelial cells. *Biochem. Biophys. Res. Commun.* **292(2),** 325–332.

29. Snitsarev, V. A. and Taylor, C. W. (1999) Overshooting cytosolic Ca2+ signals evoked by capacitative Ca^{2+} entry result from delayed stimulation of a plasma membrane Ca^{2+} pump. *Cell Calcium* **25(6),** 409–417.

30. Sedova, M. and Blatter, L. A. (1999) Dynamic regulation of $[Ca^{2+}]i$ by plasma membrane Ca^{2+}-ATPase and Na^{+}/Ca^{2+} exchange during capacitative Ca^{2+} entry in bovine vascular endothelial cells. *Cell Calcium* **25(5),** 333–343.

31. Shuttleworth, T. J. (1996) Arachidonic acid activates the noncapacitive entry of Ca^{2+} during $[Ca^{2+}]i$ oscillations. *J. Biol. Chem.* **271,** 21,720.

32. Oshimi, Y., Oshimi, K., and Miyazaki, S. (1996) Necrosis and apoptosis associated with distinct Ca^{2+} response patterns in target cells attacked by human natural killer cells. *J. Physiol.* **495 (Pt 2),** 319–329.

33. Haller, T., Dietl, P., Pfaller, K., et al. (2001) Fusion pore expansion is a slow, discontinuous, and Ca^{2+}-dependent process regulating secretion from alveolar type II cells. *J. Cell. Biol.* **155(2),** 279–289.

34. Helmlinger, G., Berk, B. C., and Nerem, R. M. (1996) Pulsatile and steady flow-induced calcium oscillations in single cultured endothelial cells. *J. Vasc. Res.* **33(5),** 360–369.

35. Kuebler, W. M., Ying, X., and Bhattacharya, J. (2002) Pressure-induced endothelial Ca^{2+} oscillations in lung capillaries. *Am. J. Physiol. Lung Cell Mol. Physiol.* **282,** L917–L923.

36. Kuebler, W. M., Ying, X., Singh, B., Issekutz, A., and Bhattacharya, J. (1999) Pressure is proinflammatory in lung venular capillaries. *J. Clin. Invest.* **104,** 495.

37. Kimura, C., Oike, M., and Ito, Y. (1998) Acute glucose overload abolishes Ca^{2+} oscillation in cultured endothelial cells from bovine aorta: A possible role of superoxide anion. *Circ. Res.* **82,** 677–685.

38. Zhao, X., Shin, D., Liu, L., Shull, G. E., and Muallem, S. (2001) Plasticity and adaptation of Ca^{2+} signaling and Ca^{2+}-dependent exocytosis in SERCA2+/- mice. *EMBO J.* **20(11),** 2680–2689.

39. Ginis, I., Hallenbeck, J. M., Liu, J., Spatz, M., Jaiswal, R., and Shohami, E. (2000) Tumor necrosis factor and reactive oxygen species cooperative cytotoxicity is mediated via inhibition of NF-kappaB. *Mol. Med.* **6(12),** 1028–1041.

40. Lin, C. P., Lynch, M. C., and Kochevar, I. E. (2000) Reactive oxidizing species produced near the plasma membrane induce apoptosis in bovine aorta endothelial cells. *Exp. Cell. Res.* **259(2),** 351–359.

41. Ali, M. H., Schlidt, S. A., Chandel, N. S., Hynes, K. L., Schumacker, P. T., and Gewertz, B. L. (1999) Endothelial permeability and IL-6 production during hypoxia: role of ROS in signal transduction. *Am. J. Physiol.* **277,** L1057–L1065.

42. Love, G. P. and Keenan, A. K. (1998) Cytotoxicity-associated effects of reactive oxygen species on endothelin-1 secretion by pulmonary endothelial cells. *Free Radic. Biol. Med.* **24(9)**, 1437–1445.
43. Chun, T. H., Itoh, H., Saito, T., et al. (2000) Oxidative stress augments secretion of endothelium-derived relaxing peptides, C-type natriuretic peptide and adrenomedullin. *J. Hypertens.* **18(5)**, 575–580.
44. Cheng, T. H., Shih, N. L., Chen, S. Y., et al. (2001) Reactive oxygen species mediate cyclic strain-induced endothelin-1 gene expression via Ras/Raf/extracellular signal-regulated kinase pathway in endothelial cells. *J. Mol. Cell. Cardiol.* **33(10)**, 1805–1814
45. Inoue, N., Takeshita, S., Gao, D., et al. (2001) Lysophosphatidylcholine increases the secretion of matrix metalloproteinase 2 through the activation of NADH/NADPH oxidase in cultured aortic endothelial cells. *Atherosclerosis* **155(1)**, 45–52.
46. Takano, M., Meneshian, A., Sheikh, E., et al. (2002) Rapid upregulation of endothelial P-selectin expression via reactive oxygen species generation. *Am. J. Physiol. Heart Circ. Physiol.* **283(5)**, H2054–H2061.
47. Brakemeier, S., Eichler, I., Hopp, H., Kohler, R., and Hoyer, J. (2002) Up-regulation of endothelial stretch-activated cation channels by fluid shear stress. *Cardiovasc. Res.* **53(1)**, 209–218.
48. Sumpio, B. E., Chang, R., Xu, W. J., Wang, X. J., and Du, W. (1997) Regulation of tPA in endothelial cells exposed to cyclic strain: role of CRE, AP-2, and SSRE binding sites. *Am. J. Physiol.* **273(5 Pt 1)**, C1441–C1448.
49. Kato, H., Uchimura, I., Nawa, C., Kawakami, A., and Numano, F. (2001) Fluid shear stress suppresses interleukin 8 production by vascular endothelial cells. *Biorheology* **38(4)**: 347–353.
50. Maneta-Peyret, L., Kitsiouli, E., Lekka, M., Nakos, G., and Cassagne, C. (2001) Autoantibodies to lipids in bronchoalveolar lavage fluid of patients with acute respiratory distress syndrome. *Crit. Care Med.* **29(10)**, 1950–1954.
51. Parker, J. C, and Yoshikawa S. (2002) Vascular segmental permeabilities at high peak inflation pressure in isolated rat lungs. *Am. J. Physiol. Lung Cell Mol. Physiol.* **283(6)**, L1203–L1209.
52. Ying, X., Minamiya, Y., Fu, C., and Bhattacharya, J. (1996) Ca^{2+} waves in lung capillary endothelium. *Circ. Res.* **79(4)**, 898–908.
53. Kuebler, W. M., Ying, X., Singh, B., Issekutz, A., and Bhattacharya, J. (1999) Pressure is proinflammatory in lung venular capillaries. *J. Clin. Invest.* **104**, 495–502.
54. Smith, C. B. and Betz, W. J. (1996) Simultaneous independent measurement of endocytosis and exocytosis. *Nature* **380**, 531–534.
55. Ley, K., Bullard, D. C., Arbones, M. L., et al. (1995) Sequential contribution of L- and P-selectin to leukocyte rolling in vivo. *J. Exp. Med.* **181**, 669–675.
56. Ichimura, H., Parthasarathi, K., Quadri, S., Issekutz, A. C., and Bhattacharya, J. (2003) Mechano-oxidative coupling by mitochondria induces proinflammatory responses in lung venular capillaries. *J. Clin. Invest.* **111**, 691–699.
57. Nicod, L. P. (1999) Pulmonary defense mechanisms. *Respiration* **66**, 2–11.
58. Strieter, R. M. and Kunkel, S. L.. (1994) Acute lung injury: the role of cytokines in the elicitation of neutrophils. *J. Investig. Med.* **42**, 640–651.
59. Kuebler, W. M., Parthasarathi, K., Wang, P. M., and Bhattacharya, J. (2000) A novel signaling mechanism between gas and blood compartments of the lung. *J. Clin. Invest. 105,* 905.
60. Tithof, P. K., Peters-Golden, M., and Ganey, P. E. (1998) Distinct phospholipases A2 regulate the release of arachidonic acid for eicosanoid production and superoxide anion generation in neutrophils. *J. Immunol.* **160(2)**, 953–960.
61. Mal, H., Dehoux, M., Sleiman, C., et al. (1998) Early release of proinflammatory cytokines after lung transplantation. *Chest* **113(3)**, 645–651.
62. Abraham, E., Carmody, A., Shenkar, R., and Arcaroli, J. (2000) Neutrophils as early immunologic effectors in hemorrhage- or endotoxemia-induced acute lung injury. *Am. J. Physiol. Lung Cell Mol. Physiol.* **279(6)**, L1137–L1145.
63. Wan, M. X., Riaz, A. A., Schramm, R., et al. (2002) Leukocyte rolling is exclusively mediated by P-selectinin colonic venules. *Br. J. Pharmacol.* **135(7)**, 1749–1756.
64. Piccio, L., Rossi, B., Scarpini, E., et al. (2002) Molecular mechanisms involved in lymphocyte recruitment in inflamed brain microvessels: critical roles for P-selectin glycoprotein ligand-1 and heterotrimeric G(i)-linked receptors. *J. Immunol.* **168(4)**, 1940–1949.
65. Issekutz, A. C. and Issekutz, T. B. (2002) The role of E-selectin, P-selectin, and very late activation antigen-4 in T lymphocyte migration to dermal inflammation. *J. Immunol.* **168(4)**, 1934–1939.
66. Parthasarathi, K., Ichimura, H., Quadri, S., Issekutz, A., and Bhattacharya, J. (2002) Mitochondrial reactive oxygen species induced proinflammatory responses in lung capillaries. *J. Immunol.* **169(12)**, 7078–7086.
67. Rizzuto, R., Pinton, P., Carrington, W., et al. (1998) Close contacts with the endoplasmic reticulum as determinants of mitochondrial Ca^{2+} responses. *Science* **280**, 1763.

16

Plasma Membrane-to-Nucleus Calcium Signaling

Giles E. Hardingham

SUMMARY

Calcium is a ubiquitous cellular second messenger that mediates a vast array of cellular processes. Elevation of intracellular calcium activates signaling cascades that are able to target the nucleus, where they modify gene transcription. The eukaryotic cell is wired up in a sophisticated manner to enable it to respond differently to different calcium signals. In this way a single second messenger can exert differing effects within the same cell.

Key Words: Calcium; CaM kinase; MAP kinase; transcription; CREB; CBP; NFAT.

1. INTRODUCTION

Many extracellular stimuli result in an elevation of intracellular calcium concentration. Calcium ions act as messengers, coupling many external events or stimuli to the cell's responses to those stimuli. Calcium has a central role to play in the nervous system, as well as mediating other important processes such as activation of the immune system and fertilization.

As eukaryotic cells evolved, the calcium ion has been selected as an intracellular second messenger in preference to other monatomic ions prevalent in the cellular environment—namely magnesium, sodium, potassium, and chloride ions. The reasons why this is the case are discussed more fully in a review by Carafoli and Penniston (1982) *(1)*, and essentially center around the need for an intracellular messenger to bind tightly and with high specificity to downstream components of the signaling cascade (often enzymes) and for the capacity for the concentration of the messenger to vary considerably between elevated and basal levels in a manner that is as energetically efficient as possible.

The singly charged ions of sodium, potassium, and chlorine would not bind as tightly to the binding site of proteins as doubly charged calcium. In addition, potassium and chloride ions are considerably larger than calcium, meaning even weaker interactions. The doubly charged magnesium ion is smaller than the calcium ion, but rather than creating strong interactions with the protein binding site, it cannot be effectively coordinated by protein binding sites—being too inflexible, the ion ends up forming bonds with water molecules as well as the protein. As the coordination number of magnesium is invariant (six), this means fewer bonds are made with the protein, and so fewer bonds need breaking to free the magnesium. Thus it seems that the calcium ion strikes a happy balance between strength of interaction with electron donating groups on the protein, and a certain level of flexibility that enables it to interact tightly and specifically with the appropriate protein.

In addition, it is energetically favorable to utilize calcium as a second messenger. Basal levels of free calcium in the cell are necessarily very low (approx 10^{-7} M), as higher levels would combine with phosphate ions in the cell to form a lethal precipitate. The very low basal levels of intracellular calcium compared to other ions (approx 10^{-3} M for magnesium) make it energetically efficient to use

From: *Cell Signaling in Vascular Inflammation*
Edited by: J. Bhattacharya © Humana Press Inc., Totowa, NJ

it as a second messenger—a relatively small amount of calcium needs to pass into the cytoplasm to increase the concentration of the ion several fold, and similarly, relatively little energy need be spent pumping it out again to return the concentration to basal levels.

This review will address how calcium acts as a second messenger in mammalian neurons to couple synaptic activity to gene transcription. Such new gene expression has an important role to play in triggering long-term changes to neuronal physiology, function, and fate.

2. CALCIUM AS AN INTRACELLULAR SECOND MESSENGER

Many cell types rely on an elevation of intracellular calcium to activate essential biological functions. This elevation can occur either via influx of calcium through proteinaceous channels into the cell from the extracellular medium, or through the release of calcium from internal stores (typically the endoplasmic reticulum).

Calcium influx is a critical step in communication between neurons. An action potential, traveling the length of a neuron, will arrive at the axon terminal and trigger calcium entry into the terminal through voltage-dependent calcium channels. This in turn results in calcium-dependent neurotransmitter release into the synaptic cleft. This neurotransmitter causes an electrical change in the postsynaptic neuron through the activation of neurotransmitter-gated ion channels. Thus, calcium is responsible for coupling action potentials to neurotransmitter release and enabling information to be passed on from neuron to neuron.

However, as well as contributing to the nuts and bolts of interneuronal communication, synaptically evoked cellular calcium transients activate signaling pathways in the cell and so are responsible for much intracellular communication as well. The predominant excitatory neurotransmitter in the central nervous system is glutamate, and when released at the synapse it acts on glutamate receptors located on the postsynaptic membrane. Calcium influx is mainly mediated by the NMDA subtype of ionotropic glutamate receptors. Although some forms of non-NMDA receptors also pass calcium, it is more often than not NMDA receptors that mediate the calcium influx at the postsynaptic membrane and activate intracellular signaling pathways. This calcium influx can be augmented by release from intracellular stores—for example, release from inositol triphosphate-sensitive stores via the activation of certain metabotropic glutamate receptors or via simple calcium-induced calcium release via ryanodine receptors *(2)*.

3. SYNAPTIC PLASTICITY IN THE NERVOUS SYSTEM

An important characteristic of an animal's nervous system is that it adapts in a structural and functional way in response to certain patterns of synaptic stimulation *(3)*. The mature animal depends on this activity-dependent plasticity to change neuronal connectivity and strength in ways that enable the process of learning and memory. It is therefore a fundamental goal of neurobiologists to understand how electrical activity results in these long-lasting changes.

Synaptic plasticity can be split into two phases. During the early phase, seconds to minutes after electrical activity, changes in neuronal connections take place via the modification of existing proteins, particularly ion channels, for example by phosphorylation or delivery to the postsynaptic membrane *(4,5)*. In the later stage (minutes to hours), new gene expression and subsequent protein synthesis converts these initial transient changes into long-lasting ones. In the mammalian brain, these changes in gene expression are primarily triggered by calcium influx into neurons and involve the activation of intracellular signaling pathways *(6)*.

The hippocampus has long been the focus of studies of memory formation in mammals, since clinicians observed that patients with hippocampal lesions could not form new memory, suffered anterograde and retrograde amnesia, and were deficient in spatial learning tasks *(7,8)*. The phenomenon of hippocampal long-term potentiation (LTP) is an extensively studied model for learning and memory. LTP is an activity-dependent increase in synaptic efficacy that can last for days to weeks in intact animals *(9)*. It is induced in the postsynaptic neuron by repeated high-frequency stimulation of presynaptic afferents. LTP is characterized by an early protein synthesis-independent phase and a late phase whose establishment is blocked by protein synthesis inhibitors *(10)* and requires a critical period of transcription after the LTP-inducing stimuli have been applied *(11)*. Critically, its induction was found to be dependent on an elevation of postsynaptic calcium *(12)*.

The changes in calcium following LTP-inducing stimuli elicit the rapid induction of a number of immediate early genes (IEGs). IEGs are genes whose transcription can be triggered in the absence of *de novo* protein synthesis, and many are transcription factors. These transcription factors likely contribute to secondary waves of transcription, leading to the structural and functional changes to the neuron required for the maintenance of LTP, although the exact mechanisms underlying this are unclear. Since these early studies, many genes upregulated by LTP-inducing stimuli have been implicated in the maintenance phase of LTP, such as tissue plasminogen activator and activity-regulated cytoskeleton-associated protein (ARC), although an analysis of their importance and proposed mode of action falls outside the scope of this review.

Thus, the activation of gene expression in electrically excitable cells has been the subject of much recent research. Below is a brief overview of the essentials of transcriptional activation—the point at which gene expression is most often regulated.

4. CONTROL OF GENE EXPRESSION

The control of gene expression (at the protein level) can occur at many stages in the process; at transcription initiation and elongation, RNA processing (including alternative splicing), mRNA stability, and control of translation and of protein degradation. By far the most common point of regulation is in transcription initiation. The synthesis of mRNA is catalyzed by RNA polymerase (pol) II, but a large number of additional proteins are needed to direct and catalyze initiation at the correct place.

A DNA sequence near the transcription start site, called the core promoter element, is the site for the formation of the pre-initiation complex (PIC), a complex of RNA pol II and proteins called basal transcription factors. RNA pol II and the basal transcription factors are sufficient to facilitate a considerable amount of transcription in vitro (called basal transcription). However, in vivo, basal transcription levels are often extremely low, reflecting the fact that in vivo the DNA containing the core promoter is associated with histones and consequently less accessible to incoming factors. For transcription to take place, other accessory factors, called activating transcription factors (hereafter known as transcription factors), are required. These factors bind to specific DNA promoter elements located upstream of the core promoter, and enhance the rate of PIC formation by contacting and recruiting the basal transcription factors, either directly or indirectly, via adapters or coactivators *(13)*. They can also modify or disrupt the chromatin structure (for example, by histone acetylation) to make it easier for other factors to come in and bind.

The ability of many transcription factors to influence the rate of transcription initiation can be regulated by signaling pathways. This provides a mechanism whereby a stimulus applied to the cell that activates a signaling pathway can result in the specific activation of a subset of transcription factors. These signaling mechanisms often involve regulatory phosphorylation events at the transcription factor level that control, for example, DNA binding affinity, subcellular localization, or its interactions with the basal transcription machinery *(14)*. Genes whose promoters contain binding sites for these signal-inducible transcription factors are transcribed as a result of signal-activating stimuli. There are several well-characterized DNA elements that act as binding sites for transcription factors that are regulated by calcium-activated signaling pathways, some examples of which are listed below.

4.1. Calcium-Responsive DNA Regulatory Elements and Their Transcription Factors

The cyclic-AMP response element (CRE) was first identified in the promoter of the somatostatin gene as the element required to confer cAMP inducibility on the gene *(15,16)*. The CRE was subsequently found in a number of other genes and is an 8-bp palindromic sequence, 5'-TGACGTCA-3'.

Bursts of synaptic activity strongly activate CRE-binding protein (CREB) by triggering synaptic NMDA receptor-dependent calcium transients in hippocampal neurons *(17)*, and the CRE is activated by stimuli that generate long-lasting LTP in area CA1 of the hippocampus *(18)*. The transcription factor that can mediate activation via the CRE, CREB, was isolated as a phosphoprotein that bound the CRE on the mouse somatostatin gene *(19)*. In neurons, calcium activation of CREB is mediated by the CaM kinase and Ras-ERK1/2 signaling pathways (discussed later).

The serum response element (SRE) was identified as an element centered at -310 bp required for serum induction of *c-fos* in fibroblasts *(20)*. The SRE comprises a core element 5'-CC[A/T]6GG-3' that is the binding site for serum response factor, SRF *(21,22)*. In addition, the SRE contains a ternary complex factor (TCF) binding site, 5'-CAGGAT-3', situated immediately 5' to the core SRE, which is bound by TCF. TCF is an umbrella name for a group of Ets domain proteins—SAP-1, Elk-1, and SAP-2. These proteins cannot bind the SRE on their own, but recognize the SRE/SRF complex. Like the CRE, the SRE is a target for calcium signaling pathways, and can confer calcium inducibility onto a minimal *c-fos* promoter in response to activation of L-type calcium channels and NMDA receptors *(6)*. Calcium-dependent synaptic activation of the SRE in hippocampal neurons is mediated by the ERK1/2 pathway *(23)*.

The nuclear factor of activated T-cells (NFAT) response element is another well-characterized calcium-response element *(24)*. NFAT activity is regulated by the calcium-activated phosphatase calcineurin at the level of subcellular localization. Calcineurin dephosphorylates the normally cytoplasmic NFAT, which exposes a nuclear localization signal and leads to its active transport into the nucleus. In the absence of continuing elevated levels of calcium (and calcineurin activity), NFAT becomes rephosphorylated by glycogen synthase kinase 3 (GSK3) and is re-exported to the cytoplasm. While these mechanisms were primarily characterized in T-cells, they also apply to neurons *(25)*.

The next section of this review will focus on the mechanism of calcium-dependent CREB activation. The importance of CREB-dependent transcription on various aspects of neuronal physiology makes it an extensively studied transcription factor.

5. THE PHYSIOLOGICAL IMPORTANCE OF CREB

The study of the calcium activation of CREB-mediated gene expression bears considerable neurophysiological relevance. CREB seems to have an important role in the establishment of long-term memory in a variety of organisms *(26)*. Genetic and molecular studies of learning paradigms in the marine snail *Aplysia californica* and the fruit fly *Drosophila melanogaster* have shown that modulating CREB levels or affecting CREB-dependent transcription severely affects the long-term, protein synthesis-dependent phase of the learning paradigm studied (*see 26*, and references therein). In the mammalian central nervous system, CREB was also found to play a role in information storage. The intrahippocampal perfusion of antisense oligonucleotides designed to bind and trigger degradation of CREB mRNA achieved a transient decrease in CREB levels in the hippocampus, an area of the brain needed for certain spatial memory tasks. This strategy blocked the animal's long-term memory of these spatial tasks without affecting short-term memory *(27)*. Mice deficient in alpha and delta forms of CREB have defective long-term (but not short-term) memory *(28)*.

There is also considerable evidence that CREB has a role in other aspects of neuronal physiology, including drug addiction *(29)*, circadian rhythmicity *(30)*, and neuronal survival *(31)*. Mice deficient in CREB exhibit excess apoptosis in sensory neurons *(32)*, and CREB mediates many of the prosurvival effects of neurotrophins *(31)*.

One mechanism by which the calcium-mediated activation of CREB modulates neuronal functions may involve BDNF, the activation of which is controlled at least in part by a CRE/CREB-dependent mechanism *(33,34)*. BDNF plays an important role in the survival and differentiation of certain classes of neurons during development *(35,36)* and is also implicated in the establishment of neuronal plasticity. Other CREB-regulated genes that are implicated in maintaining changes in synaptic strength and efficacy include nNOS *(37)* and tissue plasminogen activator *(38)*. Apart from

BDNF, other CREB-dependent pro-survival genes include bcl-2, mcl-1, and vasoactive intestinal peptide.

6. THE MECHANISM OF CREB ACTIVATION

6.1. CREB Activation Requires a Crucial Phosphorylation Event

CREB can bind to the CRE even prior to the activation of CRE-dependent gene expression, indicating that regulation of its activity is not via the control of its DNA-binding activity *(39)*. CREB binds the CRE as a dimer, mediated by a leucine zipper motif. To activate CREB-mediated transcription, CREB must become phosphorylated on serine 133 *(40)*.

Sheng et al. showed that elevation of intracellular calcium, following depolarization of PC12 cells, resulted in CREB phosphorylation on serine 133 and activation of CREB-mediated gene expression *(41)*. CREB-mediated gene expression was abolished by mutating serine 133 to an alanine, underlining the importance of the site as a point of control by calcium signaling pathways. These results showed that CREB is a calcium-responsive transcription factor and led to the assumption that CREB-mediated gene expression was triggered solely by phosphorylation of CREB on serine 133. Calcium-activated phosphorylation of CREB was subsequently shown in neurons of several types *(42–44)*.

6.1.1. Calcium-Dependent Signaling Molecules Capable of Phosphorylating CREB on Serine 133

6.1.1.1. CaM Kinases and Their Role in Calcium-Activated, CRE-Dependent Gene Expression

CREB phosphorylation on serine 133 can be mediated by a number of protein kinases, including the multifunctional calcium/calmodulin-dependent protein kinases (CaM kinases) II, IV, and the less well studied CaM kinase I *(41,45,46)*. CaM kinases play a role in diverse biological processes, such as secretion, gene expression, LTP, cell-cycle regulation, and translational control. A role for CaM kinases in the calcium activation of *c-fos* expression (which contains a CRE and a SRE) was indicated by the attenuation of L-type calcium channel–activated *c-fos* expression in neurons by the CaM kinase inhibitor KN-62 *(6)*, and by the blocking of calcium-dependent *c-fos* expression by the calmodulin antagonist calmidazolium *(6)*. CaM kinase II is a protein highly expressed in the nervous system. CaM kinase IV is similar in sequence to CaM kinase II's catalytic domain and is expressed in some cells of the immune system, but also in neuronal cells, including the cerebellum and the hippocampus; it has been shown to be mainly localized to the nucleus *(43)*.

Regulation and structural organization of CaM kinases II and IV are broadly similar *(47–49)*. Both have an N-terminal catalytic domain and a central calcium/calmodulin-binding regulatory domain. Note that the kinase itself does not bind calcium; activation of the enzyme occurs when calcium complexed with a small protein, calmodulin, binds and displaces an auto-inhibitory domain that otherwise occludes the catalytic site. Despite their structural similarities and their ability to phosphorylate CREB on serine 133, CaM kinases II and IV have very different effects on CRE/CREB-mediated gene expression. Matthews et al. *(46)* showed that a constitutively active form of CaM kinase IV, but not an active form of CaM kinase II, could activate CRE-dependent transcription. This is because CaM kinase II also phosphorylates CREB at an inhibitory site, serine 142 *(45)*.

Thus CaM kinase IV appears to be a prime candidate for the activation of CREB-mediated gene expression by nuclear calcium signals, being located largely in the nucleus and able to efficiently activate CREB. Indeed, antisense oligonucleotide-mediated disruption of CaM kinase IV expression suppressed calcium-activated CREB phosphorylation in hippocampal neurons *(43)*, and calcium-activated CREB phosphorylation is impaired in neuron cultures from mice deficient in CaM kinase IV *(50–52)*. As would be predicted from the importance of CREB in long-term synaptic plasticity, CaM kinase IV is critical for long-term hippocampal LTP *(50,51)*.

6.1.1.2. The Ras-ERK1/2 (MAP Kinase) Cascade

The role of the ERK1/2 pathway in signaling to CREB was characterized first in the context of growth-factor stimulation. Growth factors such as nerve growth factor (NGF) can activate CREB phosphorylation by a mechanism mediated by the Ras-ERK1/2 pathway. NGF treatment of PC12 cells resulted in the Ras-ERK1/2-dependent activation of a CREB kinase *(53)* found to be the a member of the previously identified pp90 RSK family, RSK2. RSK2 was able to mediate CREB phosphorylation in vivo and in vitro. The fact that NGF cannot efficiently activate CRE-dependent transcription *(54)* demonstrates that CREB phosphorylation on serine 133 is not sufficient to activate CREB-mediated gene expression—additional activating steps are required (discussed later).

The Ras/MAP kinase (ERK1/2) pathway is also activated by calcium *(55)*, and so RSK2 is activated by calcium signals as well as growth factors. This pathway is involved in both the induction and maintenance of LTP and other memory paradigms *(56)*.

6.1.2. Parallel Activation of CaM Kinase and ERK1/2 Pathways by Synaptic Activity

At first glance, it may appear that there is a certain degree of redundancy in the parallel activation of both the CaM kinase and ERK1/2 pathways when it comes to phosphorylating CREB. However, both pathways have critical roles to play. Whereas CaM kinase IV itself is calcium dependent, ERK1/2 and RSK2 are not (the calcium-dependent activation step is far upstream); they are activated slower than CaM kinases and, importantly, their activity remains long after synaptic activity has ceased. Thus, while the CaM kinase pathway mediates CREB phosphorylation within the first few seconds of calcium influx, and both pathways contribute to CREB phosphorylation at intermediate time points, the ERK1/2 pathway is needed to prolong CREB phosphorylation after activity has ceased *(23,57–59)*, which is important for robust activation of CREB-dependent gene expression *(43,59)*.

The importance of CaM kinase IV comes from its role in not only phosphorylating CREB, but in carrying out a second critical activating step.

6.1.3. Uncoupling of CREB Phosphorylation From CREB-Mediated Transcription

CREB phosphorylation on serine 133, while necessary for CREB to function as a transcriptional activator, is not sufficient for full induction of gene expression. A wide variety of extracellular signals lead to CREB phosphorylation on serine 133, but many of them, including stimulation with NGF or epidermal growth factor (EGF), which rely solely on the ERK1/2 pathway to trigger phosphorylation, are poor activators of CRE-mediated transcription *(60)*. Further experiments demonstrate that serine 133 phosphorylation is not sufficient for calcium-induced CREB-mediated transcription: CaM kinase inhibition blocks CRE-mediated gene expression without inhibiting CREB phosphorylation *(57,61)*, showing that the remaining "CREB kinase" pathway (the ERK1/2 pathway) is unable to activate CREB-dependent gene expression.

Thus, CRE-dependent transcription requires additional activation events that are provided by CaM kinase activity but not, for example, by NGF or EGF treatment, activators of the Ras-ERK1/2 kinase pathway. This fact is further reinforced by the observation that both acutely activated CaM kinase IV and activated Ras trigger CREB phosphorylation, but that only CaM kinase IV could activate CREB-mediated transcription *(61)*.

6.2. The Role of CREB-Binding Protein (CBP) in CREB-Mediated Transcription

6.2.1. Phosphorylated CREB Activates Transcription by Recruiting Its Coactivator, CREB-Binding Protein

As stated earlier, CREB is regulated by modification of its transactivation domain, rather than its subcellular localization or DNA-binding activity. For CREB to activate transcription, it must be associated with its coactivator, CBP, via the inducible part of the CREB transactivation domain, the kinase-inducible domain (KID). CBP and p300 (a closely related protein) function as coactivators for many signal-dependent transcription factors, such as c-Jun, interferon-α signaling through STAT2, Elk-1, p53, and nuclear hormone receptors. The association of CBP with CREB is dependent on CREB being phosphorylated on serine 133 *(62)*.

CBP's ability to stimulate transcription may be due to its ability to recruit to the promoter components of the basal transcription machinery—it has been reported to associate with TFIIB, TATA binding protein (TBP), and RNA polymerase II complex. In addition, CBP has an intrinsic histone acetyl transferase (HAT) activity as well as being able to associate with other HAT proteins, p/CAF and SRC1 (*see* ref. *63* for a thorough review on CBP).

6.2.2. A Model for Nuclear Calcium-Regulated Transcription: Regulation of CBP

The purpose of CREB phosphorylation on serine 133 appears to be to recruit the transcriptional coactivator CREB-binding protein (CBP) to the promoter *(62)*. However, evidence described above suggests that this is insufficient to activate transcription fully. This pointed to the possibility that the second regulatory event critical for transcriptional activation may involve the activation of CBP. This was indeed found to be the case. CBP's transactivating potential is positively regulated by calcium, acting via CaM kinase IV *(57,61,64)*. CaM kinase IV-dependent enhancement of CBPs activity occurs predominantly via a phosphorylation event on serine-301 *(65)*. In addition, recent use of a mutant form of CREB that constitutively binds CBP showed that in hippocampal neurons this mutant, while modestly active, is nowhere near as active as wild-type CREB activated by calcium signals, and could itself be further activated by calcium signals and CaM kinase IV *(65)*. Thus, the critical role for CaM kinase IV in calcium activation of CREB-dependent transcription is in activating CBP, while the ERK1/2 pathway is responsible for ensuring prolonged CREB phosphorylation (and thus association of CREB with CBP) (*see* **Fig. 1**).

As mentioned earlier, CBP/p300 acts as a coactivator for a large number of transcription factors. Thus, the fact that CBP is subject to calcium-dependent regulation means that calcium could potentially regulate transcription mediated by many of these factors, either on its own or in conjunction with other signals. Indeed, the calcium-dependent activation of the CBP-interacting transcription factor c-Jun has been reported *(66)* to be able to occur independently of what were hitherto thought to be crucial regulatory phosphorylation sites (targets of stress-activated protein kinases).

7. DECODING THE CALCIUM SIGNAL

Until a few years ago, there was little evidence to suggest anything other than the idea that elevated levels of intracellular calcium activate a specific set of "calcium-responsive genes" to a greater or lesser extent, depending on the level of calcium concentration in the cell. This was in contrast to the apparent complexity of the processes that calcium was mediating. However, evidence is mounting that intracellular signaling pathways in neurons are laid down in a very sophisticated manner to enable cells to distinguish between calcium signals of differing properties. These properties include the amplitude of the signal *(67)*, its temporal properties (including oscillatory frequency) *(68)*, its spatial properties *(23,67,69)*, and its site of entry *(6,17,57,70)*. The subcellular localization of calcium-responsive signaling molecules points to different spatial requirements for calcium. For example, CaM kinase IV is predominantly nuclear, which reflects the fact that nuclear calcium transients are necessary for the activation of CREB-dependent transcription and sufficient to activate CaM kinases in the neuronal nucleus *(67,68)*. As well as elevation of nuclear calcium being triggered by electrical activity, translocation of the calcium-sensing protein calmodulin into the nucleus has also been described *(71)*. Were this to happen in neurons where nuclear calmodulin concentration is limiting, this would assist in the activation of nuclear CaM kinases. Thus, an elevation of nuclear calcium is necessary for triggering the crucial second CREB-activating step—activation of CBP *(57,61,64,65)*.

In sharp contrast, many components of the Ras-ERK1/2 pathway (including putative calcium-dependent activators of the pathway, PYK2 and synGAP) are contained within a protein complex with the NMDA receptor at the membrane *(72)*. Calcium requirements for activation of this pathway are very different; increased calcium levels just under the membrane near the site of entry are suffi-

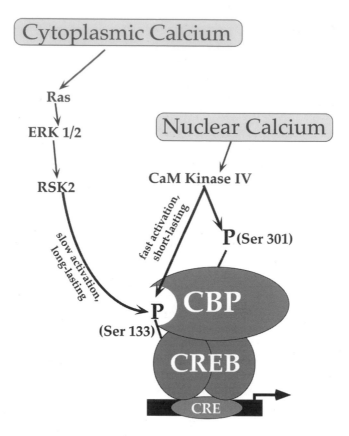

Fig. 1. Calcium-activation of the transcription factor CRE-binding protein (CREB). Synaptically evoked calcium transients trigger two parallel pathways that result in CREB phosphorylation on serine 133 (necessary for CBP recruitment), the Ras-ERK1/2 pathway, and the CaM kinase IV pathway. The Ras-ERK1/2 pathway that activates the CREB kinase RSK2 is in particular responsible for the prolonged phosphorylation of CREB. CaM kinase IV carries out the second critical activation step, targeting CBP; this includes a phosphorylation event on serine 301. Note: the spatial requirements for calcium activation of these pathways is different (*see* **Subheading 7.**).

cient to activate the ERK1/2 pathway *(23)*. Thus, relatively weak or spatially restricted calcium signals would be able to activate this pathway, which acts on the SRF/TCF transcription factor complex and is responsible for prolonged CREB phosphorylation (though it is unable to carry out the crucial second activation step).

Many proteins located to the cytoplasm are of course not tethered near the membrane. For the freely diffusible cytoplasmic signaling molecule calcineurin, submembranous calcium elevation is not enough—it requires a global increase in cytoplasmic calcium concentration to be appreciably activated in order to trigger NFAT nuclear translocation *(23)*. Continued nuclear localization would then rely on active calcineurin in the nucleus (and therefore an elevation in nuclear calcium).

The ability of spatially distinct calcium signals to differentially activate transcription naturally has relevance only if scenarios exist in the neuron whereby nuclear, cytoplasmic, and submembranous calcium levels change to differing degrees. In neurons, isolated synaptic inputs can yield extremely spatially restricted calcium transients *(73)*. However, where synaptic inputs are stronger or repetitive, global calcium transients can result *(74)*. Also, where synaptic inputs contribute to causing the postsynaptic cell to fire action potentials, synaptic inputs can cooperate with back propagating action potentials to yield global calcium transients *(75)*. Thus, differing patterns of electrical activity can in theory recruit different calcium-dependent signaling modules, which would have a qualitative effect on the resulting transcriptional output.

Differing buffering capacities or calcium clearance mechanisms of different areas of the cell can also lead to transient subcellular differences in calcium. The nucleus appears to be particularly suited to the propagation and prolongation of calcium signals. The absence of calcium-buffering ATPases (which take calcium up into the ER/intermembrane space) on the inner nuclear membrane *(76)* is thought to be behind the striking ability of elementary calcium-release events proximal to the nucleus to trigger global increases in nuclear calcium concentration that last long after the cytoplasmic elementary trigger has died away *(77,78)*. This property of nuclei applies to primary neurons, where the nucleus is able to integrate synaptically evoked global calcium transients of quite low frequencies to give an elevated calcium plateau *(68)* ideal for the activation of nuclear events (for example, via CaM kinase IV).

8. CONCLUDING REMARKS

Activation of transcription by synaptic activity is an important adaptive response in the mammalian central nervous system. The neuron is wired in a sophisticated way to respond differently to different calcium signals. Although much remains undiscovered, the molecular mechanisms of transcription-factor activation and the basis for differential genomic responses to different calcium signals are becoming clearer. Such knowledge, coupled with an understanding of the physiological role of synaptically evoked transcription, means that a bridge between molecular and cellular events and physiological behavior is slowly being built.

ACKNOWLEDGMENTS

I would like to apologize to all those whose work I have failed to cite owing to restrictions on reference numbers. The author is supported by the Royal Society.

REFERENCES

1. Carafoli, E. and Penniston, J. (1985) The calcium signal. *Sci. Am.* **253,** 50–58.
2. Verkhratsky, A. J. and Petersen, O. H. (1998) Neuronal calcium stores. *Cell Calcium* **24,** 333–343.
3. Bliss, T. V. P. and Collingridge, G. L. (1993) A synaptic model of memory: long-term potentiation in the hippocampus. *Nature* **361,** 31–38.
4. Robertson, E. D., English, J. D., and Sweatt, J. D. (1996) A biochemists view of LTP. *Learning and Memory* **3,** 1–24.
5. Malinow, R., Mainen, Z. F., and Hayashi, Y. (2000) LTP mechanisms: from silence to four-lane traffic. *Curr. Opin. Neurobiol.* **10,** 352–357.
6. Bading, H., Ginty, D. D., and Greenberg, M. E. (1993) Regulation of gene expression in hippocampal neurons by distinct calcium signaling pathways. *Science* **260,** 181–186.
7. Milner, B., Corkin, S., and Teurber, H. (1968) Further analysis of the hippocampal amnesic syndrome: 14 year follow-up study of H.M. *Neurophysiologia* **6,** 215–234.
8. Nadel, L. and Moscovitch, M. (1997) Memory consolidation, retrograde amnesia and the hippocampal complex. *Curr. Opin. Neurobiol.* **7,** 217–227.
9. Bliss, T. V. P. and Lomo, T. (1973) Long-lasting potentiation of synaptic transmission in the dentate area of the anaesthetized rabbit following stimulation of the perforant path. *J. Physiol.* **232,** 331–356.
10. Frey, U., Huang, Y-Y., and Kandel, E. R. (1993) Effects of cAMP simulate a late stage of LTP in hippocampal CA1 Neurons. *Science* **260,** 1661–1664.
11. Nguyen, P. V., Abel, T., and Kandel, E. R. (1994) Requirement of a critical period of transcription for induction of a late phase of LTP. *Science* **265,** 1104–1107.
12. Lynch, G., Larson, J., Kelso, S., Barrionuevo, G., and Schottler, F. (1983) Intracellular injections of EGTA block induction of hippocampal long-term potentiation. *Nature* **305,** 719–721.
13. Ptashne, M. and Gann, A. (1997) Transcriptional activation by recruitment. *Nature* **386,** 569–577.
14. Whitmarsh, A. J. and Davis, R. (2000) Regulation of transcription factor function by phosphorylation. *Cell. Mol. Life Sci.* **57,** 1172–1183.
15. Montminy, M. R., Sevarino, K. A., Wagner, J. A., Mandel, G., and Goodman, R. H. (1986) Identification of a cyclic-AMP-responsive element within the rat somatostatin gene. *Proc. Natl. Acad. Sci. USA* **83,** 6682–6686.
16. Comb, M., Birnberg, N. C., Seasholtz, A., Herbert, E., and Goodman, H. M. (1986) A cyclic AMP and phorbol ester-inducible DNA element. *Nature* **323,** 353–356.
17. Hardingham, G. E., Fukunaga, Y., and Bading, H. (2002) Extrasynaptic NMDARs oppose synaptic NMDARs by triggering CREB shut-off and cell death pathways. *Nat. Neurosci.* **5,** 405–414.

18. Impey, S., Mark, M., Villacres, E. C., Poser, S., Chavkin, C., and Storm, D. R. (1996) Induction of CRE-medaited gene expression by stimuli that generate long-lasting LTP in Area CA1 of the hippocampus. *Neuron* **16,** 973–982.

19. Montminy, M. R., and Bilezikjian, L. M. Binding ofa nuclear protein to the cyclic-AMP response element of the somatostatin gene. *Nature* (1987) **328,** 175–178.

20. Treisman, R. (1985) Transient accumulation of *c-fos* RNA following serum stimulation requires a conserved 5' element and *c-fos* 3' sequences. *Cell* **42,** 889–902.

21. Treisman, R. (1987) Identification and purification of a polypeptide that binds to the c-*fos* serum response element. *EMBO J.* **6,** 2711–2717.

22. Schröter, H., Shaw, P. E., and Nordheim, A. (1987) Purification of intercalator-released p67, a polypeptide that interacts specifically with the *c-fos* serum response element. *Nucleic Acids Res.* **15,** 10,145–10,157.

23. Hardingham, G. E., Arnold, F., and Bading, H. (2001) Calcium microdomain near NMDA receptors: on-switch of ERK-dependent synapse-to-nucleus communication. *Nat. Neurosci.* **4,** 565–566.

24. Rao, A., Luo, C., and Hogan, P. G. (1997) Transcription factors of the NFAT family: regulation and function. *Annu. Rev. Immunol.* **15,** 707–47.

25. Graef, I. A., Mermelstein, P. G., Stankunas, K., et al. (1999) L-type calcium channels and GSK-3 regulate the activity of NF-ATc4 in hippocampal neurons. *Nature* **401,** 703–708.

26. Silva, A. J., Kogan, J. H., Frankland, P. W., and Kida, S. (1998) CREB and memory. *Annu. Rev. Neurosci.* **21,** 127–148.

27. Guzowski, G. A. and McGaugh, J. L. (1997) Antisense oligodeoxynucleotide-mediated disruption of hippocampal CREB protein levels impairs memory of a spatial task. *Proc. Natl. Acad. Sci. USA* **94,** 2693–98.

28. Bourtchuladze, R., Frenguelli, B., Blendy, J., Cioffi, D., Schutz, G., and Silva, A. J. (1994) Deficient long-term memory in mice with a targeted mutation of the cAMP-responsive element-binding protein. *Cell* **79,** 59–68.

29. Blendy, J. A. and Maldonado, R. (1998) Genetic analysis of drug addiction: the role of cAMP response element binding protein. *J. Mol. Med.* **76,** 104–110.

30. King, D. P. and Takahashi, J. S. (2000) Molecular genetics of circadian rhythms in mammals. *Annu. Rev. Neurosci.* **23,** 713–742.

31. Walton, M. R. and Dragunow, M. (2000) Is CREB a key to neuronal survival? *Trends Neurosci.* **23,** 48–53.

32. Lonze, B. E., Riccio, A., Cohen, S., and Ginty, D. D. (2002) Apoptosis, axonal growth defects, and degeneration of peripheral neurons in mice lacking CREB. *Neuron* **34,** 371–385.

33. Shieh, P. B., Hu, S-C., Bobb, K., Timmusk, T., and Ghosh, A. (1998) Identification of a signaling pathway involved in calcium regulation of BDNF expression. *Neuron* **20,** 727–740.

34. Tao, X., Finkbeiner, S., Arnold, D. B., Shaywitz, A. J., and Greenberg, M. E. (1988) Calcium influx regulates BDNF transcription by a CREB family transcription factor-dependent mechanism. *Neuron* **20,** 709–726.

35. Ghosh, A., Carnahan, J., and Greenberg, M. E. (1994) Requirement for BDNF in activity-dependent survival of cortical neurons. *Science* **263,** 1618–1623.

36. Schwartz, P. M., Borghesani, P. R., Levy, R. L., Pomeroy, S. L., and Segal, R. A. (1997) Abnormal cerebellar development and foliation in BDNF -/- mice reveals a role for neurotrophins in CNS patterning. *Neuron* **19,** 269–281.

37. Sasaki, M., Gonzalez-Zulueta, M., Huang, H., et al. (2000) Dynamic regulation of neuronal NO synthase transcription by calcium influx through a CREB family transcription factor-dependent mechanism. *Proc. Natl. Acad. Sci. USA* **97,** 8617–8622.

38. Baranes, D., Lederfein, D., Huang, Y. Y., Chen, M., Bailey, C. H., and Kandel, E. R. (1998) Tissue plasminogen activator contributes to the late phase of LTP and to synaptic growth in the hippocampal mossy fiber pathway. *Neuron* **21,** 813–825.

39. Sheng, M., McFadden, G., and Greenberg, M. E. (1990) Membrane depolarization and calcium induce *c-fos* transcription via phosphorylation of transcription factor CREB. *Neuron* **4,** 571–582.

40. Gonzalez, G. A. and Montminy, M. R. (1989) Cyclic AMP stimulates somatostatin gene transcription by phosphorylation of CREB at serine 133. *Cell* **59,** 675–680.

41. Sheng, M., Thompson, M. A., and Greenberg, M. E. (1991) CREB: a Ca^{2+}-regulated transcription factor phosphorylated by calmodulin-dependent kinases. *Science* **252,** 1427–1430.

42. Ginty, D. D., Kornhauser, J. M., Thompson, M. A., et al. (1993) Regulation of CREB phosphorylation in the suprachiasmatic nucleus by light and a circadian clock. *Science* **260,** 238–241.

43. Bito, H., Deisseroth, K., and Tsien, R. W. (1996) CREB phosphorylation and dephosphorylation: a calcium and stimulus dependent switch for hippocampal gene expression. *Cell* **87,** 1203–1214.

44. West, A. E., Chen, W. G., Dalva, M. B., et al. (2001) Calcium regulation of neuronal gene expression. *Proc. Natl. Acad. Sci. USA* **98,** 11024–31.

45. Sun, P., Enslen, H., Myung, P. S., and Maurer, R. A. (1994) Differential activation of CREB by Ca^{2+}/calmodulin-dependent protein kinases type II and type IV involves phosphorylation of a site that negatively regulates activity. *Genes Dev.* **8,** 2527–2539.

46. Matthews, R. P., Guthrie, C. R., Wailes, L. M., Zhao, X., Means, A. R., and McKnight, G. S. (1994) Calcium/calmodulin-dependent protein kinase types II and IV differentially regulate CREB-dependent gene expression. *Mol. Cell. Biol.* **14,** 6107–6116.

47. Heist, E. and Schulman, H. (1998) The role of Ca2+/calmodulin dependent protein kinases within the nucleus. *Cell Calcium* **23,** 103–114.

48. Hook, S. S. and Means, A. R. (2001) Ca2+/CaM-dependent kinases: From activation to function. *Annu. Rev. Pharmacol. Toxicol.* **41,** 471–505.

49. Soderling, T. R. and Stull, J. T. (2001) Structure and regulation of calcium/calmodulin-dependent protein kinases. *Chem. Rev.* **101,** 2341–2351.

50. Kang, H., Sun, L. D., Atkins, C. M., Soderling, T. R., Wilson, M. A., and Tonegawa, S. (2001) An important role of neural activity-dependent CaMKIV signaling in the consolidation of long-term memory. *Cell* **106,** 771–783.
51. Ho, N., Liauw, J. A., Blaeser, F. W., et al. (2000) Impaired synaptic plasticity and cAMP response element-binding protein activation in Ca2+/calmodulin-dependent protein kinase type IV/Gr-deficient mice. *J. Neurosci.* **20,** 6459–6472.
52. Ribar, T. J., Rodriguiz, R. M., Khiroug, L., Wetsel, W. C., Augustine, G. J., and Means, A. R. (2000) Cerebellar defects in Ca2+/calmodulin kinase IV-deficient mice. *J. Neurosci.* **20,** RC107.
53. Ginty, D. D., Bonni, A., and Greenberg, M. E. (1994) Nerve growth factor activates a Ras-dependent protein kinase that stimulates *c-fos* transcription via phosphorylation of CREB. *Cell* **77,** 713–725.
54. Bonni, A., Ginty, D. D., Dudek, H., and Greenberg, M. E. (1995) Serine 133-phosphorylated CREB induces transcription via a cooperative mechanism that may confer specificity to neurotrophin signals. *Mol. Cell. Neurosci.* **6,** 168–183.
55. Bading, H. and Greenberg, M. E. (1991) Stimulation of protein tyrosine phosphorylation by NMDA receptor activation. *Science* **253,** 912–914.
56. Adams, J. P. and Sweatt, J. D. (2002) Molecular psychology: Roles for the ERK MAP kinase cascade in memory. *Annu. Rev. Pharmacol. Toxicol.* **42,** 135–163.
57. Hardingham, G. E., Chawla, S., Cruzalegui, F. H., and Bading, H. (1999) Control of recruitment and transcription-activating function of CBP determines gene regulation by NMDA receptors and L-type calcium channels. *Neuron* **22,** 789–798.
58. Wu, G. Y., Deisseroth, K., and Tsien, R. W. (2001) Activity-dependent CREB phosphorylation: convergence of a fast, sensitive calmodulin kinase pathway and a slow, less sensitive mitogen-activated protein kinase pathway. *Proc. Natl. Acad. Sci. USA* **98,** 2808–2813.
59. Impey, S. and Goodman, R. H. (2001) CREB signaling—timing is everything. *Science-STKE* PE1.
60. Xing, J., Ginty, D. D., and Greenberg, M. E. (1996) Coupling of the RAS-MAPK pathway to gene activation by RSK2, a growth factor-regulated CREB kinase. *Science* **273,** 959–963.
61. Chawla, S., Hardingham, G. E., Quinn, D. R., and Bading, H. (1998) CBP: a signal-regulated transcriptional coactivator controlled by nuclear calcium and CaM kinase IV. *Science* **281,** 1505–1509.
62. Chrivia, J. C., Kwok, R. P. S., Lamb, N., Hagiwara, M., Montminy, M. R., Goodman, R. H. (1993) Phosphorylated CREB binds specifically to the nuclear protein CBP. *Nature* **365,** 855–859.
63. Goldman, P. S., Tran, V. K., and Goodman, R. H. (1997) The multifunctional role of the co activator CBP in transcriptional regulation. *Recent Prog. Horm. Res.* **52,** 103–120.
64. Hu, S. C., Chrivia, J., and Ghosh, A. (1999) Regulation of CBP-mediated transcription by neuronal calcium signaling. *Neuron* **22,** 799–808.
65. Impey, S., Fong, A. L., Wang, Y., et al. (2002) Phosphorylation of CBP mediates transcriptional activation by neural activity and CaM kinase IV. *Neuron* **34,** 235–244.
66. Cruzalegui, F. H., Hardingham, G., and Bading, H. (1999) c-Jun functions as a calcium-regulated transcriptional activator in the absence of JNK/SAPK1 activation. *EMBO J.* **18,** 1335–1344.
67. Hardingham, G. E., Chawla, S., Johnson, C. M., and Bading, H. (1997) Distinct functions of nuclear and cytoplasmic calcium in the control of gene expression. *Nature* **385,** 260–265.
68. Hardingham, G. E., Arnold, F. A., and Bading, H. (2001) Nuclear calcium signaling controls CREB-mediated gene expression triggered by synaptic activity. *Nat. Neurosci.* **4,** 261–267.
69. Hardingham, G. E. and Bading, H. (1998) Nuclear calcium: a key regulator of gene expression. *Biometals* **11,** 345–358.
70. Sala, C., Rudolph-Correia, S., and Sheng, M. (2000) Developmentally regulated NMDA receptor-dependent dephosphorylation of cAMP response element-binding protein (CREB) in hippocampal neurons. *J. Neurosci.* **20,** 3529–3536.
71. Deisseroth, K., Heist, E. K., and Tsien, R. W. (1998) Translocation of calmodulin to the nucleus supports CREB phosphorylation in hippocampal neurons. *Nature* **392,** 198–202.
72. Husi, H., Ward, M. A., Choudhary, J. A., Blackstock, W. P., and Grant, S. G. N. (2000) Proteomic analysis of NMDA receptor-adhesion protein signaling complexes. *Nat. Neurosci.* **3,** 661–669.
73. Emptage, N., Bliss, T. V. P., and Fine, A. (1999) Single synaptic events evoke NMDA receptor-mediated release of calcium from internal stores in hippocampal dendritic spines. *Neuron* **22,** 115–124.
74. Alford, S., Frenguelli, B. G., Schofield, J. G., and Collingridge, G. L. (1993) Characterization of Ca2+ signals induced in hippocampal CA1 neurones by the synaptic activation of NMDA receptors. *J. Physiol.* **469,** 693–716.
75. Emptage, N. (1999) Calcium on the up: supralinear calcium signaling in central neurons. *Neuron* **24,** 727–737.
76. Humbert, J. P., Matter, N., Artault, J. C., Koppler, P., and Malviya, A. N. (1996) Inositol 1,4,5-trisphosphate receptor is located to the inner nuclear membrane vindicating regulation of nuclear calcium signaling by inositol 1,4,5-trisphosphate—Discrete distribution of inositol phosphate receptors to inner and outer nuclear membranes. *J. Biol. Chem.* **271,** 478–485.
77. Lipp, P., Thomas, D., Berridge, M. J., and Bootman, M. D. (1997) Nuclear calcium signalling by individual cytoplasmic calcium puffs. *EMBO J.* **16,** 7166–7173.
78. Nakazawa, H. and Murphy, T. H. (1999) Activation of nuclear calcium dynamics by synaptic stimulation in cultured cortical neurons. *J. Neurochem.* **73,** 1075–1083.

17

Signaling by Mitochondria

Navdeep S. Chandel

SUMMARY

A resurgence of interest in mitochondrial physiology has recently developed as a result of new experimental data demonstrating that mitochondria function as important participants in a diverse collection of novel intracellular signaling pathways. Recent data demonstrate that mitochondria regulate molecular and cellular responses to low oxygen levels (hypoxia). Hypoxic conditions between 1 and 2% oxygen typically elicit an increase in transcription of over 100 genes. By contrast, oxygen levels close to 0% initiate programmed cell death. Mitochondria release free radicals that are necessary and sufficient to initiate the increase in gene transcription during hypoxia. Mitochondria also regulate the initiation of programmed cell death during anaerobic conditions by releasing cytochrome c, which results in the activation of caspases. Thus, mitochondria serve to integrate changes in environmental conditions such as changes in oxygen levels to the activation of diverse events, such as gene transcription and programmed cell death

Key Words: Mitochondria; oxygen sensing; HIF-1; Bax; apoptosis; hypoxia; anoxia.

1. INTRODUCTION

The mitochondrion has long been referred to as the "power-house" of the cell because of its ability to generate adenosine-5'-triphosphate (ATP) from adenosine-5'-diphosphate (ADP) and inorganic phosphate (P_i) via respiratory chain phosphorylation. However, the classical viewpoint that mitochondria simply function as organelles responding to changes in ATP demand has recently given way to a more complex portrait. Data have emerged indicating that mitochondria also function as active signaling organelles in a number of important intracellular signaling pathways.

This chapter focuses on the role that mitochondria play in the intracellular signaling mechanisms involved in regulating cellular and molecular responses to low oxygen levels (i.e., hypoxia), such as cellular oxygen sensing and programmed cell death (apoptosis).

2. CELLULAR RESPONSES TO HYPOXIA

Oxygen is necessary for cellular processes, most notably the production of ATP by cellular respiration. The major source of this energy comes from a process known as oxidative phosphorylation, which occurs in the mitochondria of aerobic organisms. Tissue oxygen tension is normally in the range of 20–40 torr. However, cells can encounter oxygen tensions less than 1 torr under a variety of pathological states associated with diseases such as cancer, myocardial infarction, and stroke. Cells deprived of oxygen ultimately undergo death. Cells encounter two different types of oxygen deprivation states. One type of oxygen deprivation is ischemia/reperfusion or hypoxia/reoxygenation (1–3). Briefly, this involves a short period of time (minutes) where oxygen is removed from cells or tissues, followed by a period of time (hours) where oxygen is supplied to the same cells or tissues. This occurs in vivo by stopping blood flow to a perfused tissue bed or in vitro by placing cells in chambers

From: *Cell Signaling in Vascular Inflammation*
Edited by: J. Bhattacharya © Humana Press Inc., Totowa, NJ

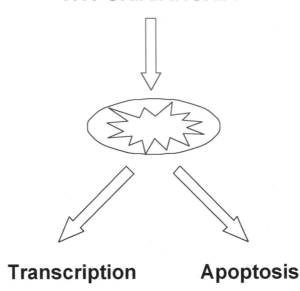

Fig. 1. Mitochondria regulate transcription and apoptosis during hypoxia. We propose that the mitochondrial electron-transport chain is required for hypoxic induction of the electron-transport chain as well as the initiation of apoptosis during hypoxia.

that allow precision control of oxygen tensions. This transient change in oxygen levels is more specific to a stroke and/or a myocardial infarction model. A second type of oxygen deprivation involves a more sustained decrease or absence of oxygen over many hours. This often occurs during disease states characterized by microcirculatory disturbances that result in hypoperfused tissues *(4)*. However, cells have developed an adaptive response to counteract the conditions that lead to the development of a severe deficit of oxygen. Cells respond to hypoxia by activating a multitude of responses designed to prevent cells from reaching 0% oxygen. The best-characterized cellular response is the activation of the transcription factor HIF-1. HIF-1 is a dimeric transcription factor composed of HIF-1α and HIF-1β subunits. HIF-1 is a transcriptional activator that is required for the upregulation of gene expression, such as vascular endothelial growth factor, erythropoietin, glycolytic enzymes, and endothelin-1 in response to low oxygen concentration *(5)*. HIF-1 plays important roles in normal development, physiological responses to hypoxia, and the pathophysiology of common human diseases. In mice, complete HIF-1α deficiency results in embryonic lethality at mid-gestation because of cardiac and vascular malformations *(6)*. Mice that are partially HIF-1α deficient as a result of the loss of one allele (heterozygous) develop normally. However, when these mice are subjected to long-term hypoxia (10% O_2 for 3 wk), they have impaired hypoxia-induced pulmonary hypertension, as indicated by a diminished medial-wall hypertrophy in small pulmonary arterioles *(7)*. Thus, understanding how hypoxia activates HIF-1 is important for understanding the pathology of diseases such as pulmonary hypertension. This chapter explores mechanisms by which mitochondria regulate the activation of HIF-1 during hypoxia, and mechanisms by which the complete absence of oxygen elicits a mitochondria-dependent apoptotic pathway (*see* **Fig. 1**).

3. MITOCHONDRIA REGULATE HYPOXIC STABILIZATION OF HIF-1

HIF-1 is a heterodimer of two basic helix loop–helix/PAS proteins: HIF-1α and the aryl hydrocarbon nuclear translocator (ARNT or HIF-1β) *(8)*. ARNT protein levels are constitutively expressed and not significantly affected by oxygen. In contrast, HIF-1α protein is present only in hypoxic cells.

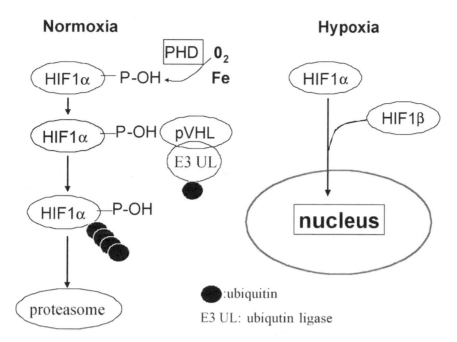

Fig. 2. Hypoxic regulation of HIF-1α. HIF-1α is hydroxylated at two different proline residues under normoxia. The proline residues reside in the oxygen-dependent domain (ODD residues 401–603) of HIF-1α. The hydroxylation of proline residues occurs by a family of prolyl hydroxylases (PHD1-3). The hydroxylation of proline residues serves as a recognition motif for pVHL. The binding of pVHL targets the HIF-1α protein for ubiquitin-mediated degradation.

During normoxia (21% O_2), HIF-1α undergoes polyubiquitination by an E3 ubiquitin ligase complex that contains the von Hippel-Lindau tumor-suppressor protein (pVHL), elongin B, elongin C, Cul2, and Rbx1 *(9,10)*. The binding of pVHL to the oxygen-dependent degradation (ODD) domain is located in the central region of HIF-1α. pVHL binding to HIF-1α is dependent on the hydroxylation of proline residues within HIF-1α (*see* **Fig. 2**) *(11,12)*. This hydroxylated prolyl residue forms two critical hydrogen bonds with pVHL side chains present within the β domain. This constitutes the pVHL substrate recognition unit. The enzymatic hydroxylation reaction is inherently oxygen dependent since the oxygen atom of the hydroxy group is derived from molecular oxygen. In addition, prolyl hydroxylation requires 2-oxoglutarate and iron as cofactors. 2-Oxoglutarate is required because the hydroxylation reaction is coupled to the decarboxylation of 2-oxoglutarate to succinate, which accepts the remaining oxygen atom. In mammalian cells, HIF prolyl hydroxylation is carried out by one of three homologs of *C. elegans* Egl-9 (EGLN1, EGLN2, and EGLN3; also called PHD2, PHD1, and PHD3, respectively, or HPH-2, HPH-3, and HPH-1, respectively) *(13)*. Presumably, the prolyl hydroxylation-mediated degradation of HIF-1α protein is suppressed under hypoxic conditions ranging from 0 to 5% O_2.

A fundamental question for understanding HIF-1α regulation involves the mechanism by which cells sense the lack of oxygen and initiate a signaling cascade that results in the stabilization of HIF-1α protein. Early progress in understanding molecular mechanisms underlying mammalian oxygen sensing came from the observation that erythropoietin mRNA can be induced under normoxic conditions in the human hepatoma Hep3B cell line by incubation with transition metals such as cobalt and iron chelators such as desferrioxamine (DFO) *(14)*. This led to the proposal that a rapidly turning over heme protein capable of interacting with O_2 is a putative oxygen sensor. However, studies using heme synthesis inhibitors failed to show any effect on the hypoxia activation of HIF-1, suggesting that rapidly turning over heme proteins are not involved in hypoxia sensing *(15)*. Subsequently, the

NADPH oxidase was proposed as a possible oxygen sensor, acting by decreasing reactive oxygen species (ROS) generation during hypoxia *(16)*. The decrease in ROS triggers the stabilization of HIF-1. However, this model is confounded by the observation that diphenylene iodonium (DPI), a wide-ranging inhibitor of flavoprotein-containing enzymes including NAD(P)H oxidase, does not trigger HIF-1 stabilization during normoxia. Rather, DPI inhibits the hypoxic induction of HIF-1-dependent genes *(17)*. Because mitochondria are the main site of oxygen consumption, they have long been considered as a possible site of O_2 sensing. As a postdoctoral fellow in the lab of Paul Schumacker, I began to explore whether mitochondria could serve as oxygen sensors by regulating the hypoxic activation of HIF-1. These experiments were done as a collaborative effort between Paul Schumacker's lab and Celeste Simon's lab. We proposed a model in which the increased generation of reactive oxygen species at complex III of the mitochondrial electron transport chain serves as the oxygen sensor for HIF-1α protein stabilization during hypoxia. In support of this model, hypoxia increased ROS generation, HIF-1α protein accumulation, and the expression of a luciferase reporter construct under the control of a hypoxic response element in wild-type cells, but not in cells depleted of their mitochondrial DNA (ρ° cells) *(18,19)*. The ρ° cells do not have a functional electron transport chain. Furthermore, catalase overexpression abolished the luciferase expression in response to hypoxia. Hydrogen peroxide was able to stabilize HIF-1α protein levels and activate luciferase expression under normoxic conditions in both wild-type and ρ° cells. Thus, ROS are both necessary and sufficient to trigger HIF-1 activation. The site of ROS generation during hypoxia is localized to complex III within the mitochondrial electron transport chain. Mitochondrial complex I inhibitors, such as rotenone, that prevent electron flux upstream of complex III ablate ROS generation during hypoxia and subsequently the hypoxic stabilization of HIF-1α protein stabilization. These results have been corroborated by Lamanna and colleagues, who have demonstrated that the neurotoxin 1-methyl-4-phenyl-1,2,3,6-tetrahydropyridine (MPTP), a complex-I inhibitor, prevents the hypoxic stabilization of HIF-1α protein in PC12 cells *(20)*. These investigators have also shown that hypoxic stabilization of HIF-1 protein is severely reduced in human xenomitochondrial cybrids harboring a partial (40%) complex-I deficiency. Further evidence that mitochondria regulate HIF-1 activation comes from Stratford and colleagues, who demonstrated that the complex-IV inhibitor cyanide is sufficient to activate HIF-1-dependent transcription in wild-type Chinese hamster ovary (CHO) cells and HT1080 cells under normoxic conditions *(21)*. Cyanide inhibits the electron transport chain downstream of complex III, thus eliciting an increase in ROS generation.

Recently, Ratcliffe and colleagues have challenged the role of mitochondria as a potential oxygen sensor. These investigators have demonstrated that ρ° cells are able to stabilize HIF-1α protein levels at an oxygen concentration of 0.1% O_2 *(22)*. They have proposed that the prolyl hydroxylases are oxygen sensors that regulate hypoxic stabilization of HIF-1α protein. This model is based on the observation that prolyl hydroxylases require molecular oxygen and iron to catalyze the hydroxylation of proline residues within HIF-1α. In the absence of oxygen or iron, HIF-1α would not undergo proline hydroxylation and subsequent pVHL-mediated ubiquitin-targeted degradation. The hydroxylation inhibition due to anoxia or iron chelation would indicate prolyl hydroxylases as the sensor. However, it is not known whether prolyl hydroxylase would intrinsically be inhibited at an oxygen concentration of 1–2% O_2, where HIF-1 is activated. My lab recently investigated the response of ρ° cells to both hypoxia and anoxia, because Ratcliffe and colleagues used conditions close to anoxia in examining their hypoxic response to ρ° cells. Our results demonstrate that the stabilization of HIF-1α protein at oxygen concentrations of 1–2% did not occur in ρ° cells. However, ρ° cells were able to stabilize HIF-1α protein at 0% O_2 or in the presence of an iron chelator under normoxic conditions *(23)*. This observation is consistent with the requirement of proline hydroxylation as a mechanism for HIF-1α protein degradation under normal oxygen conditions. In the absence of oxygen, hydroxylation of proline residues within HIF-1α by prolyl hydroxylases cannot occur, and intracellular signaling events are not required for the stabilization of HIF-1α protein. Thus, prolyl hydroxylases would effectively serve directly as the oxygen sensors during anoxia or during iron chelation under

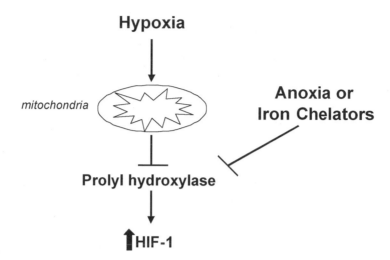

Hypoxia

mitochondria

**Anoxia or
Iron Chelators**

Prolyl hydroxylase

↑HIF-1

Fig. 3. Mitochondria regulate HIF-1α protein stability during hypoxia. Prolyl hydroxylases catalyze hydroxylation of proline residues in HIF-1α under normal oxygen conditions. Prolyl hydroxylation is required to target HIF-1α for ubiquitination and subsequent protein degradation by the 26S proteasome. In the absence of oxygen (anoxia), proline hydroxylation cannot occur because oxygen is a required substrate for hydroxylation. Thus anoxia would directly inhibit prolyl hydroxylases, thereby stabilizing HIF-1α. In contrast, hypoxia requires a functional mitochondrial electron-transport chain to initiate oxidant-dependent signaling that ultimately inhibits prolyl hydroxylases and stabilizes HIF-1α.

normoxia. Furthermore, if prolyl hydroxylase is by itself the oxygen sensor for both hypoxia- and anoxia-induced HIF-1, then there would be no signaling required upstream of prolyl hydroxylase, i.e., kinases/ROS upstream of prolyl hydroxylase. However, other investigators have shown that that hypoxia (1% O_2) stimulates Rac1 activity, and Rac1 is required for the hypoxic stabilization of HIF-1α protein *(24)*. Both the hypoxic activation of Rac1 and the stabilization of HIF-1α protein were abolished by the complex-I inhibitor rotenone. These results indicate that Rac1 is downstream of mitochondrial signaling. Moreover, mitochondria-dependent oxidant signaling has been shown to regulate HIF-1α protein accumulation following exposure to tumor necrosis factor (TNF)-α *(25)*. Non-mitochondria-dependent oxidant signaling has also been shown to stabilize HIF-1α protein under normoxia. For example, thrombin or angiotensin II stabilizes HIF-1α under normoxia through an increase in ROS generation from nonmitochondrial sources *(26)*. Further support for the idea that hypoxic signaling is distinct from anoxia or iron chelation comes from the observation that DPI, an inhibitor of a wide range of flavoproteins including complex I, prevents stabilization of HIF-1α protein and HIF-1 target genes at oxygen levels of 1% *(10)*. However, DPI fails to affect stabilization of HIF-1 in response to the iron chelator desferrioxamine (DFO). This observation is consistent with the notion that iron chelators or lack of oxygen directly inhibit prolyl hydroxylase activity due to substrate limitations, and stabilize HIF-1α protein (*see* **Fig. 3**). Interestingly, DPI can prevent a variety of other hypoxic responses, such as pulmonary vasoconstriction and carotid body nerve firing *(16)*. We speculate that the ultimate target of the oxidant-dependent signaling pathway originating from mitochondria during hypoxia or nonmitochondrial sources such as angiotensin II during normoxia is to inhibit proline hydroxylation (*see* **Fig. 3**).

4. OXYGEN DEPRIVATION INDUCES MITOCHONDRIA-DEPENDENT CELL DEATH

Cells can activate an intracellular death program and "commit suicide" in a controlled process, known as *apoptosis*, or cells can die by an uncontrolled process known as *necrosis (27–30)*. Apoptosis is a morphologically distinct form of programmed cell death that plays essential roles in development, tissue homeostasis, and a wide variety of diseases including cancer, AIDS, stroke, myopathies, and various neurodegenerative disorders *(31)*. Apoptosis, or programmed cell death, can be induced by a variety of factors, including ligand activation of death receptors, growth-factor deprivation, oncogenes, cancer drugs, and staurosporine. The apoptosis pathway is dependent upon caspase activation. Caspases comprise an expanding family of cysteine proteases that exist as inactive pro-enzymes in viable cells *(32,33)*. Upon activation, caspases acquire the ability to cleave key intracellular substrates as well as activate other caspases, resulting in the induction of a protease cascade that can induce cell death. Caspase activation is an ATP-dependent process and is sufficient to induce all of the morphological features of apoptosis. In contrast, necrosis does not involve the activation of caspases and is not an energy-dependent process *(34)*. Apoptotic cells display intranucleosomal DNA cleavage, shrink, and are rapidly engulfed by neighboring cells *(35)*. In contrast, necrotic cells tend to swell and burst, resulting in the spillage of their intracellular contents, triggering an inflammatory response.

Extrinsic and intrinsic apoptotic pathways have been identified by which cells can initiate and execute the cell death process *(see* **Fig. 4**) *(36,37)*. The critical regulators of the intrinsic pathway are the Bcl-2 family members *(38)*. In response to a variety of apoptotic stimuli, pro-apoptotic Bcl-2 family members such as Bax or Bak initiate the mitochondria-dependent apoptotic pathway by causing a loss of outer mitochondrial membrane integrity *(39–41)*. This releases apoptogenic proteins located in the intermembrane space of mitochondria, such as cytochrome c, Smac/Diablo, and apoptosis-inducing factor (AIF) into the cytosol *(41–47)*. Cytochrome c is an electron carrier within the respiratory chain that interacts directly with Apaf-1 in the cytoplasm, leading to the ATP-dependent formation of a macromolecular complex known as the apoptosome. This complex recruits and activates the aspartyl-directed protease caspase-9. Activated caspase-9 can activate additional caspase-9 molecules, as well as the downstream caspases, such as caspase-3 or -7, resulting in morphological features of apoptosis. Smac/DIABLO, another mitochondrial protein released into the cytosol in response to apoptotic stimuli, promotes caspase activation by eliminating the function of the inhibitory of apoptosis protein (IAP). Anti-apoptotic members Bcl-2 and Bcl-X_L inhibit mitochondria-dependent apoptosis by preventing Bax or Bak from disrupting the integrity of the outer mitochondrial membrane. Previous studies have shown that DNA-damaging agents, serum deprivation, and endoplasmic reticulum stress agents trigger apoptosis through the mitochondria-dependent pathway. Fibroblasts from embryos of mice lacking either Bax or Bak genes, or cells that overexpress Bcl-X_L or Bcl-2, are resistant to these apoptotic agents *(48,49)*. The mechanisms by which these apoptotic stimuli converge on Bax or Bak to activate mitochondria-dependent apoptosis remain unknown.

The extrinsic pathway is initiated when a death ligand, such as FasL or TNF-α, interacts with its cell-surface receptor, Fas (CD95) or TNF receptor (TNFR1/2) *(50–52)*. This results in the formation of a death-inducing signaling complex (DISC) *(53–55)*. The formation of DISC involves adaptor proteins such as FADD (Fas-associating protein with death domain) or TRADD (TNF-α receptor associating death domain). These proteins are involved in the recruitment of pro-caspase-8 and its subsequent proteolytic activation. A variety of cell types undergoing apoptosis through this pathway show strong activation of caspase-8 and direct activation of caspase-3 *(56–58)*. In contrast, other cell types initially display a weak activation of caspase-8, which subsequently employs the mitochondria for amplification of the death signal. This process occurs by the caspase-8-dependent cleavage of Bid, a pro-apoptotic factor *(59,60)*. A truncated Bid requires either Bax or Bak to induce the loss of outer mitochondrial membrane integrity, leading to cytochrome c release and caspase-9 activation *(48)*. Thus, there is crosstalk between the extrinsic and intrinsic pathways through truncated Bid.

Several studies indicate that oxygen deprivation can induce apoptosis in a variety of cell types. This occurs in cells with oxygen levels in the range of 0–0.5%; cells with oxygen levels in the range of 1–3% do not undergo apoptosis *(60)*. As long as cells have an adequate supply of glycolytic ATP during oxygen deprivation, apoptosis can be executed *(61)*. However, if cells are deprived of both

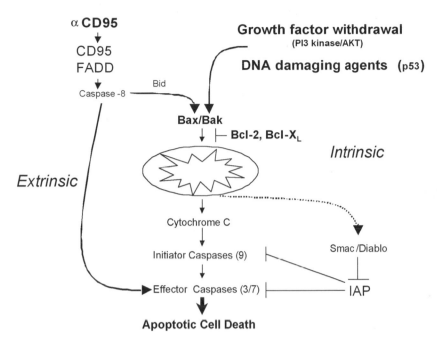

Fig. 4. Apoptotic pathways. The two best-described cell-death pathways involve the activation of caspase-3 or -7. Activation of the first pathway, the receptor-mediated pathway, occurs with engagement of a cell-surface receptor with its respective death ligand, resulting in binding of the adaptor molecule FADD (Fas-associated protein with a death domain) to the receptor. This results in the recruitment of procaspase-8, the key caspase that distinguishes the receptor-mediated apoptotic pathway. Caspase-8 can then directly activate caspase-3/7. The second pathway, the mitochondria-dependent pathway, requires the activation of pro-apoptotic Bcl-2 family members Bax or Bak, which results in outer mitochondrial membrane permeabilization and the subsequent release of pro-apoptotic proteins such as cytochrome c or apoptosis-inducing factor (AIF). Release of these proteins initiates cell death by caspase-dependent and independent mechanisms. There is communication between the receptor and mitochondrial apoptotic pathways. The receptor-mediated pathway may utilize the mitochondria as an amplification loop. Caspase-8 may cleave the pro-apoptotic protein, Bid. Truncated Bid activates Bax and/or Bak, resulting in mitochondrial permeabilization, cytochrome c release, and downstream caspase activation.

oxygen and glucose, then cells undergo necrosis. The requirement for glycolytic ATP to execute apoptosis during oxygen deprivation is attributed to energy-dependent activation of caspases. Cells overexpressing the anti-apoptotic proteins Bcl-2 or Bcl-X$_L$ have been shown to prevent oxygen deprivation–induced apoptosis by inhibiting the release of cytochrome c from the mitochondria *(61–65)*. Fibroblasts from mice lacking both Bax and Bak genes are resistant to oxygen deprivation–induced apoptosis *(61)*. Furthermore, the pro-apoptotic protein Bax translocates from the cytosol to the mitochondria during oxygen deprivation *(66)*. Cytochrome c is released and caspase-9 is activated in oxygen-deprived cells undergoing apoptosis *(61,67)*. Cytochrome c is still released in the presence of the caspase inhibitor zVAD, indicating that cytochrome c is released independent of caspase activation *(60)*. Consistent with this, Bid null fibroblasts are able to undergo apoptosis in response to oxygen deprivation, indicating that the extrinsic pathway does not contribute to oxygen deprivation-induced apoptosis (Brunelle, J. K., Chandel, N. S., unpublished data). Thus, oxygen deprivation-induced apoptosis is dependent only on the intrinsic mitochondrial pathway.

An unknown in understanding oxygen deprivation-induced apoptosis is determining the initiating mechanism by which Bax or Bak are activated to cause loss of outer mitochondrial membrane integrity. Under normal physiological conditions, the oxidation of NADH is coupled to the reduction of

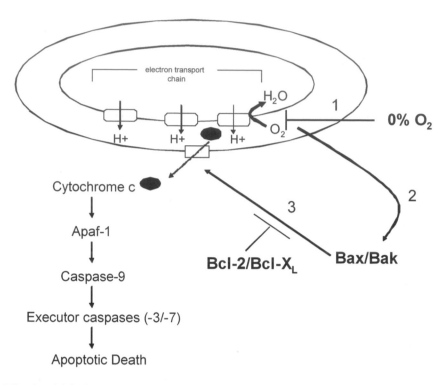

Fig. 5. Mitochondrial electron-transport chain activates Bax or Bak to initiate anoxia-induced apoptosis. Our current model proposes that oxygen deprivation inhibits the electron transport chain, which causes a fall in mitochondrial membrane potential and results in Bax or Bak activation. Activated Bax or Bak are sufficient to cause loss of outer mitochondrial membrane integrity and release of cytochrome c.

oxygen through the respiratory chain. Oxygen is reduced to water by cytochrome c oxidase. Electron transfer through the respiratory chain is coupled to the directional movement of protons across the inner mitochondrial membrane. This movement across the membrane establishes an electrochemical potential that provides the thermodynamic driving force for the F_1F_0-ATP synthase to generate ATP in the matrix. The loss of oxygen leads to an inhibition of the electron transport chain at cytochrome c oxidase, resulting in a decrease in inner mitochondrial membrane potential. This initial decrease in inner mitochondrial membrane potential due to electron transport inhibition during oxygen deprivation might be responsible for triggering Bax or Bak activation. Consistent with this hypothesis, mitochondrial membrane potential decreases in response to oxygen deprivation prior to cytochrome c release *(61)*. Cells devoid of mitochondrial DNA (ρ° cells) do not undergo cell death in response to oxygen deprivation *(60,61)*. Mitochondrial DNA encodes 13 polypeptides, including the three catalytic subunits of cytochrome c oxidase, whereas nuclear DNA encodes the pro-apoptotic protein cytochrome c. Therefore, ρ° cells do not have a functional electron transport chain and must rely only on ATP derived from anaerobic glycolysis for survival and growth. The mitochondria-dependent cell-death pathway is intact in ρ° cells, as shown by their ability to undergo death in response to a variety of apoptotic stimuli, such as doxorubicin, growth-factor withdrawal, and staurosporine treatment *(68–70)*. Based on these observations, our current model proposes that oxygen deprivation inhibits the electron transport chain, which causes a fall in mitochondrial membrane potential and results in Bax or Bak activation (*see* **Fig. 5**). Activated Bax or Bak are sufficient to cause loss of outer mitochondrial membrane integrity and release of cytochrome c.

5. CONCLUSIONS

Mammalian cells have multiple responses to low or zero oxygen concentrations. In the complete absence of oxygen, cells undergo cell death through apoptosis, and not necrosis. Apoptotic signaling during oxygen deprivation occurs through the release of cytochrome c and apaf-1-mediated caspase-9 activation. The upstream regulators of cytochrome c release are the Bcl-2 family members. Pro-apoptotic Bcl-2 family members are clearly required to initiate cytochrome c/apaf-1/caspase-9-mediated cell death during oxygen deprivation. Clearly, finding the upstream regulators of Bax or Bak is the next major step in understanding apoptotic signaling pathways in response to oxygen deprivation. A preventive strategy for cells to develop conditions resulting in absence of oxygen is to activate the HIF-1 under low oxygen concentrations. This allows cells to release factors such as VEGF to activate angiogenesis that would prevent conditions resulting in the absence of oxygen. How cells sense decreases in oxygen is not fully understood. We propose that mitochondria are the oxygen sensors. To date, our data are based on the observations that ρ° cells do not respond to low oxygen levels with respect to HIF-1 activation. The next challenge is to develop other genetic means to perturb mitochondrial function and reach conclusions similar to those that ρ° cells have provided.

ACKNOWLEDGMENTS

Supported by the Crane Asthma Center and NIH grant GM60472-05 (NSC).

REFERENCES

1. Saikumar, P., Dong, Z., Weinberg, J. M., and Venkatachalam, M. A. (1998) Mechanisms of cell death in hypoxia/reoxygenation injury. *Oncogene* **17,** 3341–3349.
2. Kang, P. M. and Izumo, S. (2000) Apoptosis and heart failure: a critical review of the literature. *Circ. Res.* **86,** 1107–1113.
3. Zipfel, G. J., Lee, J. M., and Choi, D. W. (1999) Reducing calcium overload in the ischemic brain. *N. Engl. J. Med.* **341,** 1543–1544.
4. Kantrow, S. P. and Summer, W. R. (2000) Cellular injury in sepsis. *Crit. Care Med.* **28(10),** 3569–3570.
5. Semenza, G. L. (1999) Regulation of mammalian O_2 homeostasis by hypoxia-inducible factor 1. *Annu. Rev. Cell Dev. Biol.* **15,** 551–578.
6. Iyer, N. V., Kotch, L. E., Agani, F., et al. (1998) Cellular and developmental control of O_2 homeostasis by hypoxia-inducible factor 1 alpha. *Genes* Dev. **12(2),** 149–62.
7. Yu, A. Y., Shimoda, L. A., Iyer, N. V., et al. (1999) Impaired physiological responses to chronic hypoxia in mice partially deficient for hypoxia-inducible factor 1alpha. *J. Clin. Invest.* **103(5),** 691–696.
8. Wang, G. L., Jiang, B.-H., Rue, E. A., and Semenza, G. L. (1995) Hypoxia-inducible factor 1 is a basic-helix-loop-helix-PAS heterodimer regulated by cellular O_2 tension. *Proc. Natl. Acad. Sci. USA* **92,** 5510–5514.
9. Maxwell, P. H., Wiesener, M. S., Chang, G. W., et al. (1999) The tumour suppressor protein VHL targets hypoxia inducible factors for oxygen-dependent proteolysis. *Nature* **399,** 271–275.
10. Ohh, M., Park, C. W., Ivan, M., et al. (2000) Ubiquitination of hypoxia-inducible factor requires direct binding to the beta-domain of the von Hippel-Lindau protein. *Nat. Cell Biol.* **2,** 423–427.
11. Ivan, M., Kondo, K., Yang, H., et al. (2001) HIFalpha targeted for VHL-mediated destruction by proline hydroxylation: implications for O_2 sensing. *Science* **292,** 464–468.
12. Jaakkola, P., Mole, D. R., Tian, Y. M., et al. (2001) Targeting of HIF-alpha to the von Hippel-Lindau ubiquitylation complex by O2-regulated prolyl hydroxylation. *Science* **292,** 468–472.
13. Epstein, A. C., Gleadle, J. M., McNeill, L. A., et al. (2001) *C. elegans* EGL-9 and mammalian homologs define a family of dioxygenases that regulate HIF by prolyl hydroxylation. *Cell* **107,** 43–54.
14. Goldberg, M. A., Dunning, S. P., and Bunn, H. F. (1988) Regulation of the erythropoietin gene: evidence that the oxygen sensor is a heme protein. *Science* **242(4884),** 1412–1415.
15. Srinivas, V., Zhu, X., Salceda, S., Nakamura, R., and Caro, J. (1998) Hypoxia-inducible factor 1alpha (HIF-1alpha) is a non-heme iron protein. Implications for oxygen sensing. *J. Biol. Chem.* **273(29),** 18,019–18,022.
16. Acker, H. (1994) Mechanisms and meaning of cellular oxygen sensing in the organism. *Respir. Physiol.* **95(1),** 1–10.
17. Gleadle, J. M., Ebert, B. L., and Ratcliffe, P. J. (1995) Diphenylene iodonium inhibits the induction of erythropoietin and other mammalian genes by hypoxia. Implications for the mechanism of oxygen sensing. *Eur. J. Biochem.* **234,** 92–99.
18. Chandel, N. S., Maltepe, E., Goldwasser, E., Mathieu, C. E., Simon, M. C., and Schumacker, P. T. (1998) Mitochondrial reactive oxygen species trigger hypoxia-induced transcription. *Proc. Natl. Acad. Sci. USA* **95,** 5015–5019.
19. Chandel, N. S., McClintock, D. S., Feliciano, S. E., et al. (2000) Reactive oxygen species generated at mitochondrial complex III stabilize hypoxia-inducible factor-1 during hypoxia. *J. Biol. Chem.* **275,** 25,130–25,138.

20. Agani, F. H., Pichiule, P., Chavez, J. C., and LaManna, J. C. (2000) The role of mitochondria in the regulation of hypoxia-inducible factor 1 expression during hypoxia. *J. Biol. Chem.* **275,** 35,863–35,867.
21. Williams KJ, Telfer BA, Airley RE, et al. (2002) A protective role for HIF-1 in response to redox manipulation and glucose deprivation: implications for tumorigenesis. *Oncogene* **21,** 282–290.
22. Vaux, E. C., Metzen, E., Yeates, K. M., and Ratcliffe, P. J. (2001) Regulation of hypoxia-inducible factor is preserved in the absence of a functioning mitochondrial respiratory chain. *Blood* **98,** 296–302.
23. Schroedl, C., McClintock, D. S., Scott Budinger, G. R., and Chandel, N. S. (2002) Hypoxic but not anoxic stabilization of HIF-1alpha requires mitochondrial reactive oxygen species. *Am. J. Physiol. Lung Cell Mol. Physiol.* **283(5),** L922-L931.
24. Hirota, K. and Semenza, G. L. (2001) Rac1 activity is required for the activation of hypoxia-inducible factor 1. *J. Biol. Chem.* **276,** 21,166–21,172.
25. Haddad, J. J. and Land, S. C. (2001) A non-hypoxic, ROS-sensitive pathway mediates TNF-alpha-dependent regulation of HIF-1alpha. *FEBS Lett.* **505,** 269–274.
26. Gorlach, A., Diebold, I., Schini-Kerth, V. B., et al. (2001) Thrombin activates the hypoxia-inducible factor-1 signaling pathway in vascular smooth muscle cells: role of the p22(phox)-containing NADPH oxidase. *Circ. Res.* **89,** 47–54.
27. Vaux, D. L. and Korsmeyer, S. J. (1999) Cell death in development. *Cell* **96,** 245–254.
28. Ameisen, J. C. (1996) The origin of programmed cell death. *Science* **272,** 1278–1279.
29. Evan, G. and Littlewood, T. (1998) A matter of life and cell death. *Science* **281,** 1317–1322.
30. Kerr, J. F., Wyllie, A. H., and Currie, A. R. (1972) Apoptosis: a basic biological phenomenon with wide-ranging implications in tissue kinetics. *Br. J. Cancer* **26,** 239–257.
31. Thompson, C. B. (1995) Apoptosis in the pathogenesis and treatment of disease. *Science* **267,** 1456–1462.
32. Thornberry, N. A. and Lazebnik, Y. (1998) Caspases: enemies within. *Science* **281,** 1312–1316.
33. Salvesen, G. S. and Dixit, V. M. (1997) Caspases: intracellular signaling by proteolysis. *Cell* **91,** 443–446.
34. Nicotera, P., Leist, M., and Ferrando-May, E. (1998) Intracellular ATP, a switch in the decision between apoptosis and necrosis. *Toxicol. Lett.* **102–103,** 139–142.
35. Savill, J. and Fadok, V. (2000) Corpse clearance defines the meaning of cell death. *Nature* **407,** 784–788.
36. Strasser, A., Harris, A. W., Huang, D. C., Krammer, P. H., and Cory, S. (1995) Bcl-2 and Fas/APO-1 regulate distinct pathways to lymphocyte apoptosis. *EMBO J.* **14,** 6136–6147.
37. Green, D. R. (2000) Apoptotic pathways: paper wraps stone blunts scissors. *Cell* **102,** 1–4.
38. Vander Heiden, M. G. and Thompson, C. B. (1999) Bcl-2 proteins: regulators of apoptosis or of mitochondrial homeostasis? *Nat. Cell Biol.* **1,** E209–E216.
39. Huang, D. C. and Strasser, A. (2000) BH3-Only proteins-essential initiators of apoptotic cell death. *Cell* **103,** 839–842.
40. Wang, X. (2001) The expanding role of mitochondria in apoptosis. *Genes Dev.* **15,** 2922–2933.
41. Kroemer, G. and Reed, J. C. (2000) Mitochondrial control of cell death. *Nat. Med.* **6,** 513–519.
42. Li, P., Nijhawan, D., Budihardjo, I., et al. (1997) Cytochrome c and dATP-dependent formation of Apaf-1/caspase-9 complex initiates an apoptotic protease cascade. *Cell* **91,** 479–489.
43. Zou, H., Henzel, W. J., Liu, X., Lutschg, A., and Wang, X. (1997) Apaf-1, a human protein homologous to C. elegans CED-4, participates in cytochrome c-dependent activation of caspase-3. *Cell* **90,** 405–413.
44. Du, C., Fang, M., Li, Y., Li, L., and Wang, X. (2000) Smac, a mitochondrial protein that promotes cytochrome c-dependent caspase activation by eliminating IAP inhibition. *Cell* **102,** 33–42.
45. Chai, J., Du, C., Wu, J. W., Kyin, S., Wang, X., and Shi, Y. (2000) Structural and biochemical basis of apoptotic activation by Smac/DIABLO. *Nature* **406,** 855–862.
46. Susin, S. A., Lorenzo, H. K., Zamzami, N., et al. (1999) Molecular characterization of mitochondrial apoptosis-inducing factor. *Nature* **397,** 441–446.
47. Joza, N., Susin, S. A., Daugas, E., et al. (2001) Essential role of the mitochondrial apoptosis-inducing factor in programmed cell death. *Nature* **410,** 549–554.
48. Wei, M. C., Zong, W. X., Cheng, E. H., et al. (2001) Proapoptotic BAX and BAK: a requisite gateway to mitochondrial dysfunction and death. *Science* **292,** 727–730.
49. Lindsten, T., Ross, A. J., King, A., et al. (2000) The combined functions of proapoptotic Bcl-2 family members bak and bax are essential for normal development of multiple tissues. *Mol. Cell* **6,** 1389–1399.
50. Nagata, S. and Golstein, P. (1995) The Fas death factor. *Science* **267,** 1449–1456.
51. Nagata, S. (1999) Fas ligand-induced apoptosis. *Annu. Rev. Genet.* **33,** 29–55.
52. Peter, M. E. and Krammer, P. H. (1998) Mechanisms of CD95 (APO-1/Fas)-mediated apoptosis. *Curr. Opin. Immunol.* **10,** 545–551.
53. Krammer, P. H. (2000) CD95's deadly mission in the immune system. *Nature* **407,** 789–795.
54. Hsu, H., Xiong, J., and Goeddel, D. V. (1995) The TNF receptor 1-associated protein TRADD signals cell death and NF-kappa B activation. *Cell* **81,** 495–504.
55. Chinnaiyan, A. M., O'Rourke, K., Tewari, M., and Dixit, V. M. (1995) FADD, a novel death domain-containing protein, interacts with the death domain of Fas and initiates apoptosis. *Cell* **81,** 505–512.
56. Fulda, S., Meyer, E., and Debatin, K. M. (2000) Metabolic inhibitors sensitize for CD95 (APO-1/Fas)-induced apoptosis by down-regulating Fas-associated death domain-like interleukin 1- converting enzyme inhibitory protein expression. *Cancer Res.* **60,** 3947–3956.
57. Algeciras-Schimnich, A., Shen, L., Barnhart, B. C., Murmann, A. E., Burkhardt, J. K., and Peter, M. E. (2002) Molecular ordering of the initial signaling events of CD95. *Mol. Cell. Biol.* **22,** 207–220.
58. Scaffidi, C., Fulda, S., Srinivasan, A., et al. (1998) Two CD95 (APO-1/Fas) signaling pathways. *EMBO J.* **17,** 1675–1687.

59. Li, H., Zhu, H., Xu, C. J., and Yuan, J. (1998) Cleavage of BID by caspase 8 mediates the mitochondrial damage in the Fas pathway of apoptosis. *Cell* **94,** 491–501.
60. Luo, X., Budihardjo, I., Zou, H., Slaughter, C., and Wang, X. (1998) Bid, a Bcl2 interacting protein, mediates cytochrome c release from mitochondria in response to activation of cell surface death receptors. *Cell* **94,** 481–490.
61. Santore, M. T., McClintock, D. S., Lee, V. Y., Budinger, G. R., and Chandel, N. S. (2002) Anoxia-induced apoptosis occurs through a mitochondria-dependent pathway in lung epithelial cells. *Am. J. Physiol. Lung Cell Mol. Physiol.* **282,** L727–L734.
62. McClintock, D. S., Santore, M. T., Lee, V. Y., et al. (2002) Bcl-2 family members and functional electron transport chain regulate oxygen deprivation-induced cell death. *Mol. Cell. Biol.* **22,** 94–104.
63. Parsadanian, A. S., Cheng, Y., Keller-Peck, C. R., Holtzman, D. M., and Snider, W. D. (1998) Bcl-xL is an antiapoptotic regulator for postnatal CNS neurons. *J. Neurosci.* **18,** 1009–1019.
64. Shimizu, S., Eguchi, Y., Kosaka, H., Kamiike, W., Matsuda, H., and Tsujimoto, Y. (1995) Prevention of hypoxia-induced cell death by Bcl-2 and Bcl-xL. *Nature* **374,** 811–813.
65. Graeber, T. G., Osmanian, C., Jacks, T., et al. (1996) Hypoxia-mediated selection of cells with diminished apoptotic potential in solid tumours. *Nature* **379,** 88–91.
66. Saikumar, P., Dong, Z., Patel, Y., et al. (1998) Role of hypoxia-induced Bax translocation and cytochrome c release in reoxygenation injury. *Oncogene* **17,** 3401–3415.
67. Soengas, M. S., Alarcon, R. M., Yoshida, H., et al. (1999) Apaf-1 and caspase-9 in p53-dependent apoptosis and tumor inhibition. *Science* **284,** 156–159.
68. Jacobson, M. D., Burne, J. F., King, M. P., Miyashita, T., Reed, J. C., and Raff, M. C. (1993) Bcl-2 blocks apoptosis in cells lacking mitochondrial DNA. *Nature* **361,** 365–369.
69. Wang, J., Silva, J. P., Gustafsson, C. M., Rustin, P., and Larsson, N. G. (2001) Increased in vivo apoptosis in cells lacking mitochondrial DNA gene expression. *Proc. Natl. Acad. Sci. USA* **98,** 4038–4043.
70. Marchetti, P., Susin, S. A., Decaudin, D., et al. (1996) Apoptosis-associated derangement of mitochondrial function in cells lacking mitochondrial DNA. *Cancer Res.* **56,** 2033–2038.

18

Pro-Inflammatory Signaling by Endothelial Focal Complexes in Lung

Sunita Bhattacharya

SUMMARY

Ligation of integrins or subjecting them to mechanical stress induces signaling in intracellular protein complexes known as focal complexes (FC). Such integrin-mediated responses were likely participants in our previously reported finding that the $\alpha_v\beta_3$ integrin increased lung capillary permeability. We identified underlying signaling in bovine pulmonary artery endothelial cell (BPAEC) monolayers exposed to soluble $\alpha_v\beta_3$ ligands. $\alpha_v\beta_3$ ligation induced tyrosine phosphorylation (TyrP) of FC-associated cytoskeletal proteins paxillin, cortactin, and ezrin, as well as the SH2 domain-containing proteins Shc and p125^{FAK}. During ligation, $\alpha_v\beta_3$ aggregation occurred at the apical surface of endothelial cells (EC). In parallel, $\alpha_v\beta_3$ ligation increased endothelial cytosolic Ca^{2+} concentration ($[Ca^{2+}]_i$), as determined by fura 2 ratio imaging. The $[Ca^{2+}]_i$ increase was attributable to release of Ca^{2+} from endosomal stores and Ca^{2+} influx across the plasma membrane. Underlying mechanisms were $\alpha_v\beta_3$-mediated tyrosine phosphorylation of phospholipase C-γ1 (PLC-γ1) and production of inositol (1,4,5) trisphosphate (InsP$_3$). Further studies revealed that $\alpha_v\beta_3$ ligation triggered arachidonate release, which was attributable to the simultaneous increase in $[Ca^{2+}]_i$, cPLA2 (cytosolic phospholipase A2) membrane translocation, and MAPK (mitogen-activated tyrosine kinase) TyrP. Taken together, these findings established the $\alpha_v\beta_3$ integrin in lung EC displayed inflammatory potential in vitro. To understand the relevance of these mechanisms to inflammatory signaling in lung EC *in situ*, we used a new approach. Using high tidal volume ventilation (HV) in isolated, blood-perfused rat lungs, we subjected EC to mechanical stress. After 2 h, we perfused lungs with collagenase to obtain mixed cells, which we immune sorted (4°C) to isolate fresh lung EC (FLEC). Subjection of FLEC lysates to electrophoresis and immunoblotting indicated that HV as compared to low tidal volume ventilation (LV) markedly enhanced TyrP. The tyrosine kinase blocker genistein inhibited this response. Immunofluorescent labeling of FLEC indicated HV induced FC in which aggregates of $\alpha_v\beta_3$ co-localized with FAK. Immunoprecipitation revealed HV-mediated TyrP of the FC protein paxillin, along with paxillin-associated P-selectin expression. Both responses were genistein inhibitable. However, 2-h HV did not increase lung water. These results indicate that in lung EC, the $\alpha_v\beta_3$ integrin forms FC in vitro and in vivo in association with EC TyrP. These responses are associated with $[Ca^{2+}]_i$ increase, arachidonate release, and P-selectin expression, effects capable of promoting lung leukocyte sequestration, which further enhances inflammation.

Key Words: Mechanical ventilation; cell signaling; $\alpha_v\beta_3$; FLEC; tyrosine phosphorylation; cPLA2; arachidonate; calcium.

1. INTRODUCTION

At the cell-matrix interface, proteins exist in complexes called *focal complexes* (FC). FC consist of cytoskeleton-linked molecules, such as paxillin and talin, kinases such as focal adhesion kinase

From: *Cell Signaling in Vascular Inflammation*
Edited by: J. Bhattacharya © Humana Press Inc., Totowa, NJ

(FAK), and integrins, which are transmembrane heterodimers linking extracellular matrix with focal complexes *(1,2)*. Such linkage enables matrix-integrin interactions to induce signaling in FC. Matrix glycoproteins aggregate integrins to generate second messengers in FCs *(1,2)*. Similarly, mechanical stress leading to integrin aggregation generates signal transduction in focal complexes *(3)*. Such signaling is exemplified in enhancement of TyrP, cytosolic Ca^{2+} ($[Ca^{2+}]_i$) increase, transcription-factor generation, and stress fiber formation.

Although the role of endothelial integrins in focal complexes has been discussed largely in the context of matrix-dependent functions, such as cell adhesion, angiogenesis, and wound healing *(4,5)*, their significance in the quiescent, nonproliferating lung vascular bed is undefined. Furthermore, studies of matrix-dependent responses that address functions of basal, matrix-facing integrins do not clarify the roles of apical integrins at the luminal surface. Because these luminal integrins *(6)* face the circulation, they may function as receptors for blood-borne ligands. Relevant to such a role is the $\alpha_v\beta_3$ integrin, which is abundantly distributed luminally and abluminally *(7)* in microvessels of the lung. At the luminal surface, its ability to bind pro-inflammatory molecules such as the activated complement complex SC5b-9, the thrombin–antithrombin complex, and viruses *(8–10)*, is likely to enhance capillary permeability *(11)*. The promiscuous binding property across the vast vascular surface of the lung, together with its ability to mobilize Ca^{2+} rapidly when it spreads on its ligand *(12)*, accords the luminal $\alpha_v\beta_3$ integrin a pathologic potential that warrants further study. These considerations indicate the need to investigate the underlying mechanisms of $\alpha_v\beta_3$-mediated signaling in lung inflammation and edema.

2. LUNG ENDOTHELIAL SIGNALING IN VITRO: THE ROLE OF THE $\alpha_v\beta_3$ INTEGRIN

We defined $\alpha_v\beta_3$-induced signaling responses in monolayers of bovine pulmonary artery endothelial cells (BPAEC).

2.1. $\alpha_v\beta_3$-Mediated TyrP

We first determined whether $\alpha_v\beta_3$ ligation induced EC TyrP *(8)*, since we previously observed that $\alpha_v\beta_3$-mediated increase of lung capillary permeability was TyrP dependent *(11)*. We ligated the $\alpha_v\beta_3$ integrin with the soluble glycoprotein ligands, multimeric vitronectin (Vn), or the Vn-containing complement complex SC5b-9, whose levels increase during sepsis. Alternatively, we used the anti-$\alpha_v\beta_3$ monoclonal antibody LM609, followed by crosslinking secondary antibody. Vn recognizes the $\alpha_v\beta_3$ integrin by means of its tripeptide RGD (arginine, glycine, aspartic acid) epitope *(13)*. Multimeric Vn and SC5b-9 elicited time- and concentration-dependent increases in TyrP of numerous proteins *(8)* (**Fig. 1A**). Furthermore, antibody-mediated integrin clustering induced a similar profile of protein TyrP. Antiserum against Vn, RGD peptides, and monoclonal and polyclonal anti-$\alpha_v\beta_3$ antibodies blocked the Vn- and SC5b-9-induced TyrP, while antibodies against the β_1 and $\alpha_v\beta_5$ integrins did not. These findings suggest integrin aggregation was critical for signaling. Among the proteins undergoing vitronectin-mediated TyrP were the cytoskeletal proteins paxillin, cortactin, and ezrin, as well as the SH2 domain-containing protein Shc, and p125[FAK]. The wide functional range of these responses suggested multiple signals may be activated during inflammatory conditions associated with accumulation of the $\alpha_v\beta_3$ ligand SC5b-9. Furthermore, $\alpha_v\beta_3$-mediated TyrP of FC proteins *(1,2)* suggested it played a role in the induction of FCs.

2.2. $\alpha_v\beta_3$ Aggregation

To localize the site of $\alpha_v\beta_3$ aggregation, we characterized its distribution on BPAEC monolayers at baseline and following ligation *(14)*. We exposed lightly fixed monolayers to fluorescently tagged anti-$\alpha_v\beta_3$ antibody followed by secondary crosslinking antibody. Confocal images viewed by low and high magnification revealed diffuse distribution of the $\alpha_v\beta_3$ integrin at baseline (**Fig. 1B a** and **c**). In contrast, following secondary antibody-mediated clustering, fluorescence was distributed in

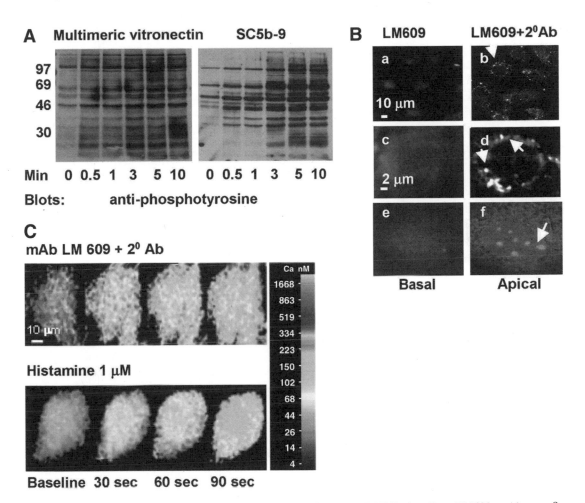

Fig. 1. $\alpha_v\beta_3$-induced bovine pulmonary artery endothelial cell (BPAEC) signaling. *LM609*, mAb to $\alpha_v\beta_3$, *2^0Ab*, secondary Ab. (**A**) Antiphosphotyrosine blots of whole-cell lysates. (**B**) Confocal microscopy of the fluorescently labeled $\alpha_v\beta_3$ integrin. Replicated three times. (**C**) Ratio imaging of time-dependent cytosolic Ca^{2+} ([Ca2+]$_i$) responses in single cells of separate, fura 2-loaded BPAEC monolayers: $\alpha_v\beta_3$ crosslinking (top panel), 1 mmol/L histamine (lower panel). Key gives [Ca^{2+}]$_i$ in nmol/L. Reproduced from refs. *8*, *14*, and *15*, with permission.

clumps, mainly at the cell periphery (**Fig. 1B b** and **d**, arrows mark aggregates). These findings indicated the potential for integrin ligation to induce integrin aggregation, which in turn leads to FC formation *(1)*. Similar aggregation followed exposure to multimeric Vn and SC5b-9. Images in the *z*-axis showed that while the apical surface displayed fluorescence in a clumped distribution (**Fig. 1B, e** and **f**), the basal surface did not *(14)*. These findings together suggested that circulating $\alpha_v\beta_3$ ligands may aggregate luminal integrins during signaling. Furthermore, distribution of $\alpha_v\beta_3$ aggregates at the lung EC periphery indicated their likely proximity to inter-endothelial junctions, where they may regulate endothelial barrier responses.

2.3. The $\alpha_v\beta_3$ Integrin in [Ca^{2+}]$_i$ Signaling

A consideration in defining mechanisms underlying $\alpha_v\beta_3$-mediated increase of capillary permeability *(11)* was the role of cytosolic Ca^{2+} concentration ([Ca^{2+}]$_i$), since [Ca^{2+}]$_i$ increase regulates cell contraction, which in turn opens interendothelial junctions *(16)*. Moreover, the rapid mobilization of endothelial Ca^{2+}, which is characteristic of inflammatory processes, suggested $[Ca^{2+}]_i$ increase may play a role in $\alpha_v\beta_3$-mediated increase of capillary permeability. To determine $[Ca^{2+}]_i$ responses to $\alpha_v\beta_3$ ligation, we used multimeric Vn, SC5b-9 and crosslinking primary anti-$\alpha_v\beta_3$, and secondary antibodies *(14)*. We quantified endothelial $[Ca^{2+}]_i$ by the fura 2 ratio imaging method of single cells in confluent BPAEC monolayers. At baseline, endothelial $[Ca^{2+}]_i$ levels remained steady at 86 nmol/L for >20 min (**Fig. 1C**). Crosslinking the $\alpha_v\beta_3$ integrin by sequential exposure of monolayers to anti-$\alpha_v\beta_3$ mAb, LM609, and secondary immunoglobulin (Ig)G resulted in a $[Ca^{2+}]_i$ increase that initiated at the cell periphery, then spread centripetally. The increase, which was 100% above baseline, commenced in <0.5 min, peaked in <2 min, and decayed to baseline in approx 5 min (**Fig. 1C**, upper panel). Similar responses occurred following the addition of vitronectin (400 µg/mL) and SC5b-9. In contrast, histamine-induced $[Ca^{2+}]_i$ increases occurred more globally and usually initiated at the cell center, then spread outward (**Fig. 1C**, lower panel).

2.4. Protein Tyrosine Phosphorylation and $[Ca^{2+}]_i$ Regulation in BPAEC

External Ca^{2+} depletion blunted the crosslinking-induced $[Ca^{2+}]_i$ increase by 60%, a response that was completely inhibited by thapsigargin pretreatment. Thus, the $[Ca^{2+}]_i$ increase was attributable partly to release of Ca^{2+} from endosomal stores, but mostly to Ca^{2+} influx across the plasma membrane. Induced aggregation of the $\alpha_v\beta_3$ integrin enhanced TyrP of phospholipase C–γ1 (PLC-γ1) and increased accumulation of inositol (1,4,5) trisphosphate (InsP$_3$). Genistein, a broad-spectrum tyrosine kinase inhibitor *(17)*, abrogated both these effects as well as the $\alpha_v\beta_3$-induced $[Ca^{2+}]_i$ increases. We concluded that aggregation of the endothelial $\alpha_v\beta_3$ integrin induced a rapid TyrP-dependent increase of $[Ca^{2+}]_i$. This response may subserve the $\alpha_v\beta_3$ integrin's inflammatory role in blood vessels.

2.5. The Role of the $\alpha_v\beta_3$ Integrin in Cytosolic Phospholipase A2 Activation

Thus far, our investigations have revealed that $\alpha_v\beta_3$ integrin aggregation induced proinflammatory processes such as EC protein TyrP and increase of $[Ca^{2+}]_i$, but an inflammatory endpoint to these signaling pathways was not clear. Since both these pathways underlie EC production of the inflammatory mediator arachidonic acid, we considered that $\alpha_v\beta_3$ ligation on lung EC may activate cytosolic phospholipase A2 (cPLA$_2$). cPLA$_2$ activation releases free arachidonic acid, which may generate prostaglandins and other oxidized compounds. Released arachidonate may cause further Ca^{2+} mobilization *(18,19)* and generate feedback effects by activating ERK *(20)*, thereby amplifying $\alpha_v\beta_3$-induced proinflammatory signaling to augment lung injury. In the family of cytoadhesive integrins, ligation of β_1 integrins has been shown to induce cPLA$_2$ activation *(21,22)*. However, these reports concern circulating or proliferating cells and do not represent responses that may be relevant to cells under stable conditions, such as those of endothelial cells of lung vessels. The role of the $\alpha_v\beta_3$ integrin, which is richly supplied in lung endothelium, was not clear in the context of cPLA$_2$ activation despite its ability to initiate the required signaling.

In confluent EC monolayers, cPLA$_2$ is located in the cytosol, but on activation, it translocates to membranes *(18)*. The translocation is attributable to an increase of EC Ca^{2+}, although activation also requires the enzyme to be phosphorylated *(18)*. Signaling pathways acting through TyrP may regulate both events, since TyrP activates the ERK (extracellular signal regulated kinase) MAPK (mitogen activated protein kinase), which phosphorylates cPLA$_2$ *(18)* and also activates phospholipase Cγ (PLCγ, leading to EC Ca^{2+} increases *(14)*. Since we showed that $\alpha_v\beta_3$ ligation induced several signaling pathways in lung EC *(8,14)*, we tested the extent to which these pathways interacted for cPLA$_2$ activation *(15)*.

2.6. Vitronectin-Induced Arachidonate Release

$\alpha_v\beta_3$ ligation with multimeric Vn caused concentration-dependent arachidonate (**Fig. 2A**) production that was inhibited by pretreating the monolayers with the anti-$\alpha_v\beta_3$ mAb LM609 *(15)*. No inhi-

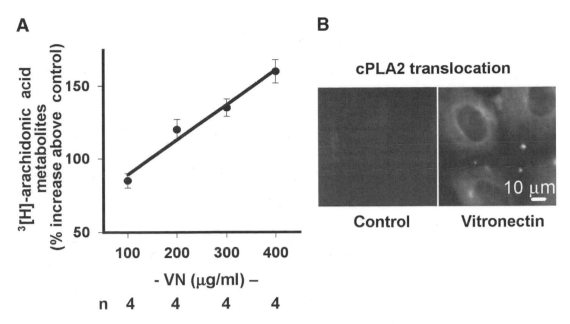

Fig. 2. $\alpha_v\beta_3$-mediated arachidonate release is associated with membrane translocation of cPLA2. *VN*, vitronectin. **(A)** Arachidonate release following the addition of different concentrations of VN was determined in [^{3}H]-arachidonate-loaded, confluent bovine pulmonary artery endothelial cell (BPAEC) monolayers. Data are mean ± SE. *n* = number of monolayers. Linear regression, *$p < 0.01$; **(B)** membrane translocation of cPLA2 in BPAEC. Monolayers were treated with buffer or vitronectin (400 mg/mL, 15 min), fixed, permeabilized, and labeled with anti-cPLA2 mAb followed by FITC antimouse immunoglobulin (Ig)G. Replicated in three experiments. Reproduced from ref. *15*, with permission.

bition occurred in the presence of the isotypic mAb PIF6 that recognizes the integrin $\alpha_v\beta_5$. The underlying mechanism of arachidonate release was activation of pathways that lead to cPLA2 activation, because membrane translocation of cPLA2 (cytosolic phospholipase A2) (**Fig. 2B**) and tyrosine phosphorylation of the MAPK (mitogen activated tyrosine kinase) ERK2 were also attributable to $\alpha_v\beta_3$ ligation. The cPLA2 inhibitor arachidonyl trifluoromethyl ketone (AACOCF$_3$), the tyrosine kinase inhibitor genistein, and the MAPK kinase inhibitor PD 98059 all blocked the induced arachidonate release. Moreover, the intracellular Ca^{2+}-chelator MAPTAM also inhibited arachidonate release. These findings indicated that ligation of apical $\alpha_v\beta_3$ in BPAEC caused ERK2 activation and an increase of intracellular Ca^{2+}, both conjointly required for cPLA2 activation and arachidonate release. This was the first instance of integrin-induced protein TyrP that initiated these dual regulatory pathways to generate a proinflammatory response.

In summary, ligating the $\alpha_v\beta_3$ integrin on BPAEC monolayers induced: (1) integrin aggregation at the apical surface, mainly at the cell periphery; (2) TyrP of multiple focal adhesion proteins; (3) tyrosine phosphorylation of PLCγ, InsP3 production, and increase of $[Ca^{2+}]_i$, chiefly attributable to entry of external Ca^{2+}; and (4) arachidonate release attributable to the confluence of $\alpha_v\beta_3$-mediated $[Ca^{2+}]_i$ increase, cPLA2 phosphorylation, and membrane translocation of cPLA2 and MAPK TyrP. Thus our in vitro findings indicated that $\alpha_v\beta_3$-mediated protein TyrP initiates proinflammatory signaling, such as increase of $[Ca^{2+}]_i$ and cPLA2-mediated arachidonate release. Because both these second messengers induce inflammatory signaling *(16,18)*, aggregating the apical $\alpha_v\beta_3$ integrin on lung EC has considerable potential for inducing lung injury. However, since these studies were conducted in vitro, the potential for $\alpha_v\beta_3$ to induce inflammatory lung endothelial signaling in vivo remains undefined, except for its ability to induce an increase of lung capillary permeability *(11)*.

Moreover, the role of lung endothelial focal complexes in lung inflammation is also not understood. In this regard, mechanical stress-induced formation of FC in vitro *(3)* indicates that similar integrin-mediated effects may occur in endothelium *in situ* when it is subjected to mechanical stress. To understand the role of integrin-mediated focal-complex formation in such stress, we studied endothelial signaling in lungs subjected to high tidal volume ventilation.

3. MECHANICAL STRESS-INDUCED LUNG ENDOTHELIAL SIGNALING *IN SITU*: RESPONSES OF THE $\alpha_V\beta_3$ INTEGRIN, FOCAL COMPLEXES, AND P-SELECTIN

Mechanical ventilation is essential for managing respiratory failure in lung injury. However, the high airway pressures and large tidal volumes that are often necessary exacerbate the injury *(23)*. Many studies indicate that lungs exposed to mechanical ventilation develop an inflammatory phenotype, characterized by increase of microvascular permeability *(24)*, secretion of cytokines *(25)*, and enhanced leukocyte sequestration *(26)*. These findings provide broad-based evidence that mechanical ventilation causes tissue stress in lungs. However, no studies have addressed the intracellular signaling mechanisms that underlie the inflammatory response to ventilation stress.

Endothelial cells (ECs) lining lung microvessels initiate inflammation by expressing the leukocyte adhesion receptor P-selectin, which induces leukocyte rolling on the EC surface *(27)*. In lung endothelium, P-selectin, a constituent of Weibel-Palade bodies (WPB), is probably restricted to extra-alveolar vessels *(28)*, although others propose a more extensive expression *(29)*. Nevertheless, a role for the receptor may be indicated in lung pathology in that P-selectin expression increases in vascular stress *(30)*.

We considered the possibility that high-volume lung ventilation (HV) may induce P-selectin expression in lung EC. Lung expansion during HV stretches the pulmonary vascular bed and is therefore likely to stretch lung ECs. In vitro studies indicate that EC monolayers subjected to stretch enhance protein TyrP and induce formation of FCs *(3)*. Although the relevance of these EC responses to lung inflammation remains unclear, there are indications from other cell types that TyrP plays a role in P-selectin responses. Thus, platelet activation is accompanied by P-selectin TyrP *(31)*, and specific tyrosine residues in the cytoplasmic tail of P-selectin determine its sorting to secretory granules in the AtT tumor cell line *(32)*. However, the extent to which TyrP induces EC expression of P-selectin is not known.

A general difficulty is that the understanding of EC signaling mechanisms has been developed through studies in vitro that may not apply to mechanisms *in situ*. Here, we used a new approach involving immunomagnetic cell recovery from ventilation-stressed lungs to determine signaling mechanisms in EC *in situ (33)*.

3.1. Ventilation Protocol and EC Isolation

We prepared isolated blood-perfused lungs as described in *(30)*. Briefly, we excised lungs from anesthetized, heparinized rats, pump-perfused them with autologous blood (37°C, 14 mL/min), and mechanically ventilated them using low (LV) or high (HV) tidal volumes of 6 or 12 mL/kg, respectively. The higher tidal volume closely corresponded to those associated with worse outcomes *(23)*. The corresponding inspiratory pressures were 11 and 22 cmH_2O. Throughout the ventilation period, ventilatory rate and end expiratory pressure were held constant at 30/min and 5 cmH_2O, respectively. After 2 h of mechanical ventilation, we chilled the lungs (4°C), prior to recovery of fresh lung EC (FLEC). To obtain FLEC, we buffer-perfused (4°C) lungs to clear them of blood, then sequentially infused collagenase, trypsin, and buffer. We filtered the mixed cell effluent (100 μm pore) and washed cells three times by repeated suspension in buffer and centrifugation. We incubated the mixed cells (4°C) with anti-factor VIIIR:Ag/vWf-labeled magnetic beads, prepared as described in *(33)*. Following incubation, EC attached to the beads were magnetically isolated. The FLEC isolate displayed 93 ± 0.6% viability with trypan blue exclusion (*n* = 4). We immunofluorescently labeled *(33)* for the

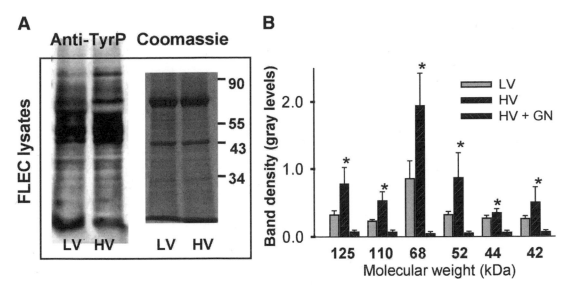

Fig. 3. Protein tyrosine phosphorylation in fresh lung endothelial cells (FLEC). *LV*, low tidal volume ventilation; *HV*, high tidal volume ventilation; *anti-TyrP*, anti-tyrosine phosphorylation; *GN*, genistein (100 mmol/L). (**A**) FLEC lysates from HV and LV were each subjected to SDS-PAGE in duplicate. Anti-tyrosine phosphorylation blots (left) and Coomassie Blue staining (right). Molecular-weight markers on right. (**B**) Quantification of band densities in A, at molecular weights indicated (*n* = 5 paired experiments). *$p < 0.05$, compared with bar on either side. Values are mean ± SE. Reproduced from ref. *33*, with permission.

EC-specific markers CD31, factor VIIIR:Ag/vWf, and acetylated low-density lipoprotein (Ac-LDL), viewing cells by both brightfield and confocal fluorescence microscopy (Zeiss, LSM 510). Fluorescence determinations on 60 cells/lung for each marker indicated positive EC phenotype in 97 ± 1% (*n* = 9 lungs).

3.2. Protein Tyrosine Phosphorylation in FLEC

Because in vitro studies indicate that mechanical challenge to cells causes the induction of protein TyrP and the formation of FCs *(3)*, we determined the extent to which these responses occurred in the present experiments. By our immunomagnetic separation protocol, we isolated $1.7 \pm 0.4 \times 10^6$ EC per rat lung. We lysed FLEC, as we reported previously for cultured EC *(8)*, then determined protein concentrations, which indicated a protein yield of 40 ± 5 µg/g lung (*n* = 14). Because approximately twice this amount was required for immunoprecipitation studies *(8)*, we combined FLEC lysates from two lungs for a single immunoprecipitation experiment. To determine TyrP in FLEC, we subjected lysates containing equal amounts of protein to gel electrophoresis in duplicate using reducing conditions. After transfer to nitrocellulose, we immunoblotted using anti-phosphotyrosine antibody as described in *(8)*. Duplicate gels were stained with Coomassie Blue. Blots were developed using enhanced chemiluminescence. In the LV group, immunoblots of FLEC lysates showed low levels of TyrP for several proteins (**Fig. 3A**). By contrast, in the HV group, TyrP was markedly enhanced for several proteins. Since this response suggested that tyrosine kinases were activated, in some experiments we infused the tyrosine kinase inhibitor genistein *(17)* in the lung's blood flow throughout the experiment. Genistein completely inhibited the enhanced TyrP (**Fig. 3B**). These findings indicated that ventilation stress enhanced protein TyrP in EC.

3.3. Focal Complexes

Because integrins constitute the link between subcellular matrix and cytoskeleton at focal adhesions, distortions at the cell-matrix interface attributable to shear and stretch induce integrin aggrega-

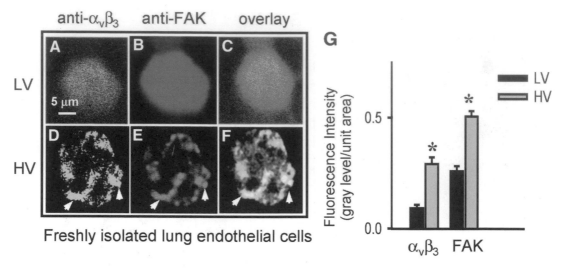

Fig. 4. Effect of high tidal volume ventilation on fresh lung endothelial cell (FLEC) expression of FAK and the $\alpha_v\beta_3$ integrin. *LV*, low tidal volume ventilation; *HV*, high tidal volume ventilation. Confocal fluorescent images of single, freshly isolated cell from LV (upper panel) and HV (lower panel) labeled for the $\alpha_v\beta_3$ integrin (**A,D**) and FAK (**B,E**), and corresponding overlay images (**C,F**). (**G**) Quantification of fluorescence intensity (digital imaging) in 50 cells/lung from three paired LV and HV experiments. *$p < 0.01$ compared with bar on left. Values are mean ± SE. Reproduced from ref. *33*, with permission.

tion and FC formation *(3)*. We used immunofluorescent labeling of the $\alpha_v\beta_3$ integrin and the focal adhesion protein FAK in FLEC to detect the extent to which these events may have occurred in the present study. To assess FC formation, we determined aggregation of FAK and of the $\alpha_v\beta_3$ integrin by confocal microscopy. We immunofluorescently labeled the $\alpha_v\beta_3$ integrin and FAK on fixed permeabilized FLEC from LV and HV. We detected immunofluorescence using confocal fluorescence microscopy (Zeiss, LSM 510). In LV, cell-surface fluorescence was weak and diffuse (**Fig. 4A,B**). By contrast, in HV (**Fig. 4D,E**), fluorescent aggregates of 2–5 μm diameter were evident over >50% of the cell surface. The merged pseudocolors in image overlays (**Fig. 4C,F**) indicated that the proteins had co-localized in the presence of ventilation stress in HV. We digitally imaged single cells to quantify fluorescence intensity (MCID-M4, Imaging Research, Brock Univ., St. Catharines, Canada). Fluorescence intensity per unit area for both proteins was greater in HV than LV (**Fig. 4G**). Since initial TyrP blots of FLEC lysates revealed a prominent band at approx 68 kD (**Fig. 3A**) that potentially indicated paxillin; in a separate group we sequentially blotted for TyrP and paxillin. Further, we immunoprecipitated paxillin from FLEC lysates. These experiments revealed that TyrP on paxillin was two times greater in HV than in LV. Both the HV-induced co-localization of the $\alpha_v\beta_3$ integrin and FAK in aggregates and the enhanced TyrP of paxillin are consistent with increased focal adhesion formation. We speculate that to promote cell anchorage, EC *in situ* developed FC to withstand mechanical stresses induced by HV.

3.4. P-Selectin Expression

To define inflammatory consequences of HV-induced EC TyrP, we determined surface expression of P-selectin, using immunofluorescence to label FLEC. We sequentially exposed FLEC to anti-P-selectin mAb and fluorescence-tagged antimouse IgG. We maintained cells at 4°C to prevent cellular uptake of the antibodies, and thereby to label surface proteins selectively. In fields of cells viewed at low power by confocal microscopy, immunofluorescence of P-selectin was weak and diffuse in LV, but extensive and present on >97% of cells in HV (**Fig. 5A**, arrows mark cells that were

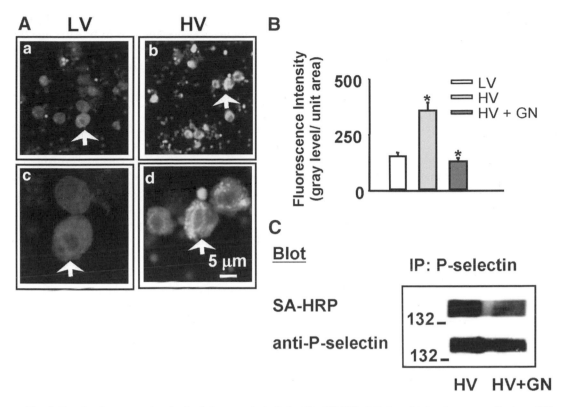

Fig. 5. P-selectin expression in fresh lung endothelial cells (FLEC). *LV*, low tidal volume ventilation; *HV*, high tidal volume ventilation; *IP*, immunoprecipitation; *SA-HRP*, streptavidin horseradish-peroxidase; *GN*, genistein (100 mmol/L). (**A**) Confocal fluorescent images of FLEC, labeled for P-selectin. (**B**) Quantification of fluorescence intensity (digital imaging of single cells), mean ± SE for 30 cells per lung ($n = 3$ paired experiments). $*p < 0.05$, compared with left bar. (**C**) SA-HRP (top) and anti-P-selectin (bottom) blots of IP of P-selectin from surface-biotinylated FLEC. Molecular-weight markers on left. $n = 3$ paired experiments. Reproduced from ref. *33*, with permission.

viewed at low [top] and high [bottom] magnifications in each group). Viewed at high magnification, most cells for HV revealed a clumped fluorescence at the cell periphery. By contrast, fluorescence was diffuse and weak for LV. Quantification by digital image analysis indicated a twofold increase of fluorescence in HV (**Fig. 5B**), reaffirming that HV increased cell-surface P-selectin expression. Inclusion of genistein in the perfusate diminished immunofluorescence of P-selectin. We also used immunoprecipitation to detect surface expression of P-selectin. We surface-biotinylated FLEC at 4°C, lysed the cells, and immunoprecipitated P-selectin. Sequential blotting of electrophoresed, transferred immunoprecipitates revealed a band at 140 kDa that was more prominent in HV than in LV on streptavidin-horseradish peroxidase blotting. Reprobing with anti-P-selectin mAb identified the band as P-selectin, indicating that surface expression of P-selectin was enhanced in HV. This blot, which also provided an assessment of the total amount of P-selectin protein in FLEC, namely that comprising the intracellular as well as the surface-expressed contents revealed bands that were consistently more pronounced in HV. This finding indicated that HV increased the overall amounts of P-selectin protein in FLEC. We reprobed the blot of immunoprecipitated P-selectin with anti-paxillin mAb. This blot also revealed a more prominent band in HV than in LV, indicating that ventilation stress increased the association of paxillin with P-selectin. Inclusion of genistein in the perfusate during HV decreased the recovery of cell-surface P-selectin by immunoprecipitation (**Fig. 5C**). These findings indicated that the HV-induced P-selectin expression was blocked by blockade of TyrP. It is proposed that TyrP of P-selectin regulates its incorporation in secretory granules *(32)*. Although the specific targets of tyrosine phosphorylation remain unclear, taken together with the reported data, our findings indicate that protein TyrP is critical in the regulation of P-selectin expression in EC.

P-selectin is stored in Weibel-Palade bodies (WPB) adjacent to the EC luminal membrane *(34)*. Activation of WPB exocytosis causes P-selectin expression and is generally attributed to increases of cytosolic Ca^{2+} *(35)*. In previous studies *(14,15)*, we showed that exposing EC to the $\alpha_v\beta_3$ ligand vitronectin causes aggregation of the $\alpha_v\beta_3$ integrin. Genistein blocks the associated induction of TyrP that leads to ER release of Ca^{2+}, but not the integrin aggregation itself. These findings suggest that $\alpha_v\beta_3$ aggregation is not determined by TyrP, although the aggregation event activates tyrosine kinases. To the extent that these mechanisms apply to the present experiments, we speculate that the present $\alpha_v\beta_3$ aggregation activated TyrP-dependent pathways to induce the Ca^{2+} increase required for WPB exocytosis.

The localization of P-selectin with paxillin points to a new mechanism underlying P-selectin expression. Paxillin, which is recruited to focal adhesions following aggregation and autophosphorylation of FAK, is increasingly regarded as an adaptor protein that forms a docking platform for signaling proteins *(1)*. Although such mechanisms remain inadequately understood in the context of inflammation, the enhanced association between paxillin and P-selectin in ventilation stress suggests that paxillin may provide a docking function for P-selectin exocytosis. Although this issue requires further investigation, the tyrosine residue on P-selectin has been previously implicated in the sorting of P-selectin to secretory vesicles *(32)*. Tyrosine kinases are implicated in some forms of exocytosis *(38)*, and tyrosine-phosphorylated adaptor proteins may act as P-selectin chaperones during WPB exocytosis.

3.5. Lung Water

To assess the extent to which pulmonary edema is associated with the HV-induced TyrP, focal adhesion formation, and P-selectin expression, we determined extravascular lung water by our standard methods *(33)*. In paired LV and HV experiments, lung water averaged 4 ± 0.1 and 4.1 ± 0.1 g/g dry (mean $\pm$ SE; $n = 4$), respectively. These values were within our established limits of normal. We point out that despite the enhanced P-selectin expression on FLEC, HV for 2 h did not increase lung water. To this extent, our findings agree with those of Frank et al. *(37)*, who showed that mechanical ventilation at tidal volume of 12 mL/kg does not cause pulmonary edema. However, the fact that proinflammatory signaling was induced in the present experiments is an indication that even in the absence of pulmonary edema, these modest levels of ventilation stress may be sufficient to initiate endothelial signaling that primes the microvascular bed for injury. Thus, Frank et al. *(37)* have shown that mechanical ventilation at 12 mL/kg exacerbates pre-existing lung injury induced by acid instillation.

In summary, freshly isolated lung EC provided novel *in situ* evidence showing high tidal volume-mediated endothelial protein TyrP, which induces P-selectin expression. Furthermore, the newly developed immunochemical and immunofluorescence assays in FLEC showed activation of several proteins in focal complexes. Among these were (a) aggregation and co-localization of the $\alpha_v\beta_3$ integrin and FAK, (b) paxillin TyrP, and (c) its association with P-selectin, whose surface expression was induced. We ruled out platelets as a source of the present P-selectin expression, because lungs were cleared of blood components with extensive buffer perfusion prior to cell isolation. Moreover, the high purity of the cell isolate and the phenotypic appearance of P-selectin expressing cells also indicated the absence of platelets. The increased P-selectin expression was blocked by inhibition of EC protein TyrP. We conclude that in ventilation stress, protein TyrP constitutes a major pathway for proinflammatory signaling in lung EC.

For the first time, these methods allow detection of signaling mechanisms in EC that are freshly isolated from experimentally treated lungs. Cell recovery at 4°C inactivated enzymatic processes and thereby preserved phosphorylation responses developed *in situ*. Immunomagnetic protocols for EC recovery have targeted CD31 or bound lectins on the cell surface *(33)*. We avoided these targets, since CD31 is nonspecific for EC and is also expressed on leukocytes *(38)*, while lectins may cause cell lysis. In EC, vWf is contained in Weibel-Palade bodies *(34)* and is secreted by WPB exocytosis *(35)*. Under nonstimulated conditions, vWf is expressed on the surface of nonpermeabilized cells *(39)* as well as of unfixed peri-alveolar capillary endothelium *(40)*. Our finding that vWf is expressed on the surface of FLEC corroborates these reports.

Microscopy of FLEC indicated that our recovery procedure yielded single as well as clumped cells. Because of clumping, these isolated cells were amenable to immunofluorescence and confocal microscopy, but not to fluorescence-activated cell sorting. Using immunofluorescent labeling for three EC-specific markers, we determined that the cells were recovered with high purity and viability. Presently, the vascular sites of origin for these cells remain undetermined. In the pulmonary circulation, extra-alveolar vessels are preferred sites of expression for both vWf and P-selectin *(39,40)*. Since our recovered EC expressed both proteins, they may be of extra-alveolar origin. This possibility is also supported by the relatively small cell recovery by our isolation methods. Thus, in both LV and HV, each lung yielded 1–2 million FLEC that constitutes a small fraction of the estimated 410×10^6 EC in rat lung *(41)*. Since the bulk of lung EC are contained in alveolar capillaries, we attribute the small FLEC yield to the possibility that capillary EC were not accessible to our isolation methods.

In conclusion, our in vitro and *in situ* lung endothelial studies suggest that the $\alpha_v\beta_3$ integrin induces FC formation that is associated with EC TyrP. Furthermore, in cultured BPAEC the $\alpha_v\beta_3$ integrin induces proinflammatory signaling such as $[Ca^{2+}]_i$ increase and arachidonate release. In lung endothelium *in situ*, mechanical stress is also proinflammatory, since HV leads to TyrP-dependent expression of the cell adhesion molecule P-selectin, as well as its association with the FC protein paxillin. Leukocyte-mediated lung injury may result from these integrin-associated FC signaling cascades.

ACKNOWLEDGMENT

This study was supported by grant HL-54157 from the National Institutes of Health, Bethesda, Maryland.

REFERENCES

1. Turner, C. E. (2000) Paxillin and focal adhesion signaling. *Nat. Cell Biol.* **2**, E231–E236.
2. Sastry, S. K. and Burridge, K. (2000) Focal adhesions: a nexus for intracellular signaling and cytoskeletal dynamics. *Exp. Cell Res.* **261**, 25–36.
3. Matthews, B. D., Overby, D. R., Alenghat, F. J., et al. (2004) Mechanical properties of individual focal adhesions probed with a magnetic microneedle. *Biochem. Biophys. Res. Commun.* **313**, 758–764.
4. Jin, Z. G., Ueba, H., Tanimoto, T., et al. (2003) Ligand-independent activation of vascular endothelial growth factor receptor 2 by fluid shear stress regulates activation of endothelial nitric oxide synthase. *Circ. Res.* **93**, 354–363.
5. Boudreau, N. J. and Varner, J. A. (2004) The homeobox transcription factor Hox D3 promotes integrin alpha5beta1 expression and function during angiogenesis. *J. Biol. Chem.* **279**, 4862–4868.
6. Cheresh, D. A. (1987) Human endothelial cells synthesize and express an Arg-Gly-Asp-directed adhesion receptor involved in attachment to fibrinogen and von Willebrand factor. *Proc. Natl. Acad. Sci. USA* **84**, 6471–6475.
7. Singh, B., Fu, C., and Bhattacharya, J. (2000) Vascular expression of the $\alpha_v\beta_3$ integrin in lung and other organs. *Am. J. Physiol.* **278**, L217–L226.
8. Bhattacharya, S., Fu, C., Bhattacharya, J., et al. (1995) Soluble ligands of the $\alpha_v\beta_3$ integrin mediate enhanced tyrosine phosphorylation of multiple proteins in adherent bovine pulmonary artery endothelial cells. *J. Biol. Chem.* **270**, 16,781–16,787.
9. Wells, M. J. and Blajchman, M. A. (1998) In vivo clearance of ternary complexes of vitronectin-thrombin-antithrombin is mediated by hepatic heparan sulfate proteoglycans. *J. Biol. Chem.* **273**, 23,440–23,447.
10. Gavrilovskaya, I. N., Shepley, M., Shaw, R., et al. (1998) β_3 integrins mediate the cellular entry of hanta viruses that cause respiratory failure. *Proc. Natl. Acad. Sci. USA* **9**, 7074–7079.

11. Tsukada, H., Ying, X., Fu, C., et al. (1995) Ligation of endothelial $\alpha_v\beta_3$ integrin increases capillary hydraulic conductivity of rat lung. *Circ. Res.* **77,** 651–659.
12. Schwartz, M. A. (1993) Spreading of human endothelial cells on fibronectin or vitronectin triggers elevation of intracellular free calcium. *J. Cell. Biol.* **120,** 1003–1010.
13. Preissner, K. T. (1991) Structure and biological role of vitronectin. *Annu. Rev. Cell. Biol.* **7,** 275–310.
14. Bhattacharya, S., Ying, X., Fu, C., et al. (2000) $\alpha_v\beta_3$ integrin induces tyrosine phosphorylation-dependent Ca2+ influx in pulmonary endothelial cells. *Circ. Res.* **86,** 456–462.
15. Bhattacharya, S., Patel, R., Sen, N., et al. (2001) Dual signaling by the $\alpha_v\beta_3$ integrin activates cPLA2 in bovine pulmonary artery endothelial cells. *Am. J. Physiol. Lung Cell. Mol. Physiol.* **280,** L1049–L1056.
16. Lum, H., Aschner, J. L., Phillips, P. G., et al. (1992) Time course of thrombin-induced increase in endothelial permeability: relationship to Ca2+ and inositol polyphosphates. *Am. J. Physiol.* **263,** L219–L225.
17. Akiyama, T. J., Ishida, S., Nakagawa, H., et al. (1987) Genistein, a specific inhibitor of tyrosine-specific protein kinases. *J. Biol. Chem.* **262,** 5592–5595.
18. Leslie, C. C. (1997) Properties and regulation of cytosolic phospholipase A2. *J. Biol. Chem.* **272,** 16,709–16,712.
19. Shuttleworth, T. J. and Mignen, O. (2003) Calcium entry and the control of calcium oscillations. *Biochem. Soc. Trans.* **Oct 31(Pt 5),** 916–919.
20. Dulin, N. O., Alexander, L. D., Harwalkar, S., et al. (1998) Phospholipase A2-mediated activation of mitogen-activated protein kinase by angiotensin II. *Proc. Natl. Acad. Sci. USA* **95,** 8098–8102.
21. Clark, E. A. and Hynes, R. O. (1996) Ras activation is necessary for integrin-mediated activation of extracellular signal-regulated kinase 2 and cytosolic phospholipase A2 but not for cytoskeletal organization. *J. Biol. Chem.* **271,** 14,814–14,818.
22. Cybulsky, A. V., Carbonetto, S., Cyr, M. D., et al. (1993) Extracellular matrix-stimulated phospholipase activation is mediated by beta 1-integrin. *Am. J. Physiol.* **64,** C323–C332.
23. Eisner, M. D., Thompson, T., Hudson, L. D., et al. (2001) Efficacy of low tidal volume ventilation in patients with different clinical risk factors for acute lung injury and the acute respiratory distress syndrome. *Am. J. Respir. Crit. Care Med.* **164,** 231–236.
24. Parker, J. C., Ivey, C. L., and Tucker, J. A. (1998) Gadolinium prevents high airway pressure-induced permeability increases in isolated rat lungs. *J. Appl. Physiol.* **84,** 1113–1118.
25. Ricard, J. D., Dreyfuss, D., and Saumon, G. (2001) Production of inflammatory cytokines in ventilator-induced lung injury: a reappraisal. *Am. J. Respir. Crit. Care Med.* **163,** 1176–1180.
26. Imanaka, H., Shimaoka, M., Matsuura, N., et al. (2001) Ventilator-induced lung injury is associated with neutrophil infiltration, macrophage activation, and TGF-beta 1 mRNA upregulation in rat lungs. *Anesth. Analg.* **92,** 428–436.
27. Gardiner, E. E., De Luca, M., McNally, T., et al. (2001) Regulation of P-selectin binding to the neutrophil P-selectin counter-receptor P-selectin glycoprotein ligand-1 by neutrophil elastase and cathepsin G. *Blood* **98,** 1440–1447.
28. McNiff, J. M. and Gil, J. (1983) Secretion of Weibel-Palade bodies observed in extra-alveolar vessels of rabbit lung. *J. Appl. Physiol.* **54,** 1284–1286.
29. Kuebler, W. M., Kuhnle, G. E., Groh, J., et al. (1997) Contribution of selectins to leucocyte sequestration in pulmonary microvessels by intravital microscopy in rabbits. *J. Physiol.* **501,** 375–86.
30. Kuebler, W. M., Ying, X., Singh, B., et al. (1999) Pressure is proinflammatory in lung venular capillaries. *J. Clin. Invest.* **104,** 495–502.
31. Crovello, C. S., Furie, B. C., and Furie, B. (1993) Rapid phosphorylation and selective dephosphorylation of P-selectin accompanies platelet activation. *J. Biol. Chem.* **268,** 14,590–14,593.
32. Modderman, P. W., Beuling, E. A., Govers, L. A., et al. (1998) Determinants in the cytoplasmic domain of P-selectin required for sorting to secretory granules. *Biochem. J.* **336,** 153–161.
33. Bhattacharya, S., Sen, N., Yiming, M. T., et al. (2003) High tidal volume ventilation induces proinflammatory signaling in rat lung endothelium. *Am. J. Resp. Cell Mol. Bio.* **28,** 218–224.
34. McEver, R. P., Beckstead, J. H., Moore, K. L., et al. (1989) GMP 140, a platelet alpha-granule membrane protein, is also also synthesized by vascular endothelial cells and is localized in Weibel-Palade bodies. *J. Clin. Invest.* **84,** 92–99.
35. Datta, Y. H., Romano, M., Jacobson, B. C., et al. (1995) Peptido-leukotrienes are potent agonists of von Willebrand factor secretion and P-selectin surface expression in human umbilical vein endothelial cells. *Circulation* **92,** 3304–3311.
36. Hartwell, D. W., Mayadas, T. N., Berger, G., et al. (1998) Role of P-selectin cytoplasmic domain in granular targeting in vivo and in early inflammatory responses. *J. Cell Biol.* **143,** 1129–1141.
37. Frank, J. A., Gutierrez, J. A., Jones, K. D., et al. (2002) Low tidal volume reduces epithelial and endothelial injury in acid-injured rat lungs. *Am. J. Respir. Crit. Care Med.* **165(2),** 242–249.
38. Ilan, N., Cheung, L., Pinter, E., et al. (2000) Platelet-endothelial cell adhesion molecule-1 (CD31), a scaffolding molecule for selected catenin family members whose binding is mediated by different tyrosine and serine/threonine phosphorylation. *J. Biol. Chem.* **275,** 21,435–21,443.
39. Wagner, D. D., Olmsted, J. B., and Marder, V. J. (1982) Immunolocalization of von Willebrand protein in Weibel-Palade bodies of human endothelial cells. *J. Cell Biol.* **95,** 355–360.
40. Jin, E., Ghazizadeh, M., Fujiwara, M., et al. (2001) Angiogenesis and phenotypic alteration of alveolar capillary endothelium in areas of neoplastic cell spread in primary lung adenocarcinoma. *Pathol. Int.* **51,** 691–700.
41. Stone, K. C., Mercer, R. R., Gehr, P., et al. (1992) Allometric relationships of cell numbers and size in the mammalian lung. *Am. J. Respir. Cell. Mol. Biol.* **6,** 235–243.

19

Hydrogen Peroxide As Intracellular Messenger

Production, Target, and Elimination

Sue Goo Rhee, Tong-Shin Chang, Yun Soo Bae, Seung-Rock Lee, and Sang Won Kang

SUMMARY

Engagement of peptide growth-factor receptors induces a transient production of low levels of H_2O_2 in various cells. The H_2O_2 response to platelet-derived growth factor requires the intrinsic tyrosine kinase activity of the receptor as well as the activation of phosphatidylinositol 3-kinase (PI 3-kinase). It appears that PtdIns(3,4,5)P3, a product of PI 3-kinase, is necessary to activate an isoform of NADPH oxidase through the small GTP-binding protein Rac. H_2O_2 thus produced propagates its signal by specifically acting on protein tyrosine phosphatases. And enhancement of protein tyrosine phosphorylation in growth factor-stimulated cells depends on the H_2O_2 production. This is probably because the activation of a receptor tyrosine kinase is not sufficient to increase the steady-state level of protein tyrosine phosphorylation in cells, and that concurrent inhibition of protein tyrosine phosphatase by H_2O_2 might be needed as well. Elimination of H_2O_2 appears to be an extensively regulated process. Peroxiredoxin I (Prx I) and Prx II, two cytosolic thioredoxin-dependent peroxidases, are inactivated at the G2-M transition through Cdc2 kinase-dependent phosphorylation.

Key Words: Hydrogen peroxide; intracellular messenger; PDGF receptor; NADPH oxidase; protein tyrosine phosphatase; peroxiredoxin; Cdc2 kinase.

1. INTRODUCTION

There is increasing evidence that hydrogen peroxide (H_2O_2) serves as an intracellular messenger mediating various cell functions, including proliferation, differentiation, apoptosis, and senescence, when produced in low amount and in a controlled fashion *(1–9)*. Ligands that elicit an H_2O_2 response include peptide growth factors such as platelet-derived growth factor (PDGF) *(10)*, epidermal growth factor (EGF) *(11)*, basic fibroblast growth factor (bFGF) *(12)*, insulin *(13)*, vascular endothelial growth factor (VEGF) *(14)*, and granulocyte-macrophage colony-stimulating factor (GMCSF) *(15)*; cytokines such as transforming growth factor-β1 *(16–18)*, interleukin (IL)-1 *(15,19,20)*, IL-3 *(15)*, IL-4 *(21)*, interferon (IFN)-γ *(20)*, and tumor necrosis factor (TNF)-α *(19,20,22)*; ligands of immune receptors such as T-cell antigen receptor ligands *(23)* and immunoglobulin (Ig)E receptor *(24)*; agonists of heterotrimeric GTP-binding protein (G protein)-coupled receptors (GPCRs), such as angiotensin IIf *(25–27)*, thrombin , thyrotropin *(20)*, parathyroid hormone *(20,28)*, lysophosphatidic acid (LPA) *(29,30)*, sphingosine 1-phosphate *(31)*, serotonin *(32,33)*, endothelin *(34)*, acetylcholine *(35)*, platelet-activating factor *(36,37)*, histamine *(38)*, and bradykinin *(39)*; and other stimulants, like leptin *(40)* and shear stress *(41)*. The addition of exogenous H_2O_2 or the intracellular production in response

From: *Cell Signaling in Vascular Inflammation*
Edited by: J. Bhattacharya © Humana Press Inc., Totowa, NJ

to receptor stimulation affect the function of various proteins, including transcription factors *(42–44)*, protein kinases *(2)*, protein tyrosine phosphatases *(45–48)*, phospholipases *(49,50)*, inositol lipid phosphatase *(51)*, ion channels *(52)*, and G proteins *(53)*. Accordingly, H_2O_2 is now recognized as a ubiquitous intracellular messenger under subtoxic conditions.

The essential role of H_2O_2 production in intracellular signaling by various receptors has been demonstrated by the observation that corresponding receptor-mediated events are abrogated by inhibiting the production of H_2O_2 with a dominant negative Rac1 (Rac1N17), an inhibitor of NADPH oxidase complex, or by blocking the accumulation of H_2O_2 with enzymes such as catalase and peroxiredoxin. Several examples are:

1. The response of rat vascular smooth-muscle cells to PDGF, which includes tyrosine phosphorylation of various cecllular proteins, activations of mitogen-activated protein kinases (MAPKs), DNA synthesis, and chemotaxis, was inhibited when the growth factor-stimulated rise in H_2O_2 concentration was blocked by incubating the cells with catalase *(10)*.
2. The elimination of H_2O_2 by catalase inhibited the EGF-induced tyrosine phosphorylation of various cellular proteins, including the EGF receptor and phospholipase C-1 in A431 cells *(11)*.
3. The angiotensin II stimulation of Akt/PKB in rat vascular smooth-muscle cells was abrogated by overexpression of catalase that blocked angiotensin II-induced intracellular H_2O_2.
4. The activation of nuclear factor (NF)κB induced by tumor necrosis factor α was blocked by overproduction of Prx II *(54)*; and the calcium oscillation induced by histamine in human aortic endothelial cells was blocked by expressing RacN17 *(38)*.

Understanding the intracellular messenger function of H_2O_2 calls for studies of how receptor occupation elicits the production of H_2O_2, what kinds of molecules are targeted by the produced H_2O_2, and how H_2O_2 is eliminated after the completion of its mission. Here, we summarize progress made in these areas of research, with emphasis on those from our own laboratory.

2. GROWTH FACTOR-INDUCED H_2O_2 PRODUCTION

H_2O_2 is generated in all aerobic organisms as a result of normal cellular metabolism. Thus, electrons that leak from the electron transport chain of mitochondria cause the univalent reduction of molecular oxygen to the superoxide anion ($O_2^{•-}$), which is then spontaneously or enzymatically dismutated to H_2O_2. Hydrogen peroxide is also generated in cells by arachidonic acid-metabolizing enzymes *(55)*, xanthine oxidase *(56)*, nitric oxide synthase *(56)*, and cytochrome P450 *(57)*, NADPH oxidase *(58)*, as well as in the cellular response to ultraviolet radiation. Some of these H_2O_2 production mechanisms have been linked to receptor activation—for example, xanthine oxidase for reactive oxygen species (ROS) produced in thrombin-activated platelets *(59)*, and 5-lipoxygenase for ROS produced in TNF-stimulated Rat-2 fibroblasts *(60)*. Even the mitochondrial production was suggested to be deliberate and responsible for ROS produced when endothelial cells were detached from a solid surface *(61)*. Among those H_2O_2-generating enzymes, however, the best studied in relation to receptor stimulation is NADPH oxidase in phagocytic cells.

Phagocytes undergo a respiratory burst in response to bacteria, resulting in robust production of ROS, which together function in bacterial killing. The multisubunit NADPH oxidase complex generates $O_2^{•-}$ via the one-electron reduction of O_2 *(62)*. The $O_2^{•-}$ is then spontaneously or enzymatically dismutated to H_2O_2. The membrane-associated catalytic moiety gp91 *phox* contains all the prosthetic groups needed to transfer electrons from NADPH to oxygen (FAD, two hemes, and a binding site for NADPH), but is catalytically inactive in the absence of regulatory proteins. Another membrane protein, p22 *phox*, complexes with gp91 *phox* to form flavocytochrome b $_{558}$ and serves as a docking site for the cytosolic regulatory proteins p47 *phox*, p67 *phox*, p40 *phox*, and the small GTPase Rac. These proteins translocate to the plasma membrane upon cell activation, and p67 *phox* activates electron flow within gp91 *phox* *(63)*.

Nonphagocytic cells generate ROS at much lower levels compared to phagocytic cells. Although it was commonly assumed that this ROS originated from mitochondria, diphenylene iodonium, an inhibitor of the respiratory burst oxidase, sometimes blocked ROS production *(17,19,27,38)*. In addition, overexpression of wild-type Rac1 or a constitutively active form of Rac1 (Rac1V12) in fibroblasts was associated with increased production of H_2O_2, suggesting the involvement of gp91 *phox*-like protein *(64,65)*.

The first homolog of gp91 *phox*, cloned from colon cDNA, is Nox1, formerly Mox1 *(66)*. Nox1 generated low levels of superoxide *(66)* and H_2O_2 when expressed in NIH 3T3 cells *(66,67)*. Additional homologs were cloned subsequently *(58,68–70)*, and the family, called Nox/Duox family, currently consists of seven human homologs. Evolutionary relationships reveal three subgroupings: The gp91 *phox* subfamily consists of Nox1, gp91 *phox*, Nox3, and Nox4. These homologs are, like gp91 *phox*, approx 65 kD. A second group, the Duox enzymes, are 180 kD, in which two domains are present in addition to the C-terminal gp91 *phox* homology domain: an N-terminal peroxidase homology domain, and a central domain containing two EF-hand calcium-binding motifs. Thus, for Duox, both the catalytic moiety that generates the hydrogen peroxide and the one that uses the hydrogen peroxide as substrate are incorporated into the same polypeptide. The Nox5 group exists in two splice variants: The short form is similar in size to gp91 *phox*, and the long forms, like Duox, also contain a calcium-binding domain.

In addition to the well-established host defense function, ROS produced by the members of Nox/Duox family were shown to play the roles of intracellular messenger and oxygen sensor *(58)*. In support of the messenger role, Nox1 was induced in vascular smooth muscle by platelet-derived growth factor, angiotensin II, and phorbol esters *(66,71)*, and Nox1 overexpression produced a cancer phenotype of NIH 3T3 and epithelial cells *(66,72)*. The ROS production induced by angiotensin II and PDGF in vascular smooth muscle, which normally expresses Nox1, was blocked by antisense-Nox1, and the Nox1-antisense cells exhibited a slower growth phenotype *(71)*.

We studied the mechanism of PDGF-mediated generation of H_2O_2. The binding of PDGF to its receptors results in receptor autophosphorylation on specific tyrosine residues. These phosphotyrosine residues initiate cellular signaling by acting as high-affinity binding sites for the Src homology 2 (SH2) domains of various effector proteins. In the PDGF β receptor (PDGFβR), seven autophosphorylation sites have been identified as specific binding sites for Src family tyrosine kinases (Tyr^{579} and Tyr^{581}), phosphatidylinositol 3-kinase (PI3K) (Tyr^{740} and Tyr^{751}), the GTPase-activating protein of Ras (GAP) (Tyr^{771}), SH2 domain-containing protein tyrosine phosphatase-2 (SHP-2) (Tyr^{1009}), and phospholipase C-γ1 (PLC-γ1) (Tyr^{1021}). A series of PDGFβR mutants was previously constructed that includes a kinase-deficient mutant and receptors in which the binding sites for PI3K, GAP, SHP-2, and PLC γ1 were changed individually or in various combinations to phenylalanine *(73)*. To characterize the mechanism of H_2O_2 production in nonphagocytic cells, we measured PDGF-dependent H_2O_2 generation in human hepatoma HepG2 cells expressing these various PDGFβR mutants. PDGF failed to increase H_2O_2 production in cells expressing either the kinase-deficient mutant or a receptor in which the two Tyr residues required for the binding of PI3K were replaced by Phe. In contrast, PDGF-induced H_2O_2 production in cells expressing a receptor in which the binding sites for GAP, SHP-2, and PLC-γ1 were all mutated was slightly greater than that in cells expressing the wild-type receptor. Only the PI3K binding site was alone sufficient for PDGF-induced H_2O_2 production. The effect of PDGF on H_2O_2 generation was blocked by the PI3K inhibitors LY294002 and wortmannin or by overexpression of Rac1N17. Furthermore, expression of the membrane-targeted p110 subunit (p110-CAAX) of PI3K was sufficient to induce H_2O_2 production. These results suggest that a product of PI3K is required for PDGF-induced production of H_2O_2 in nonphagocytic cells, and that Rac1 mediates signaling between the PI3K product and the putative NADPH oxidase.

Our observation that Rac1N17 blocked the Y740/751 receptor-induced generation of H_2O_2 indicates that Rac1 acts downstream of PI3K in the signaling pathway that leads to activation of NADPH oxidase. Moreover, signaling by this pathway appears independent of activation of GAP, SHP-2, and PLC-γ1. Additional evidence suggests that Rac functions downstream of PI3K *(74)*. Thus, the ex-

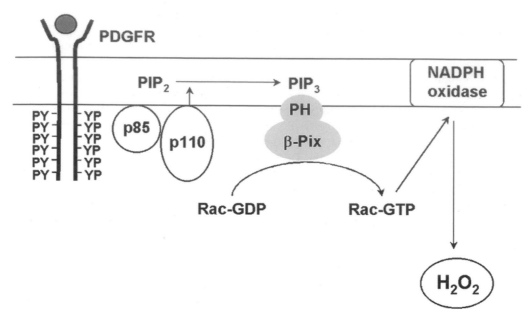

Fig. 1. The mechanism of platelet-derived growth factor-induced H_2O_2 production.

change of Rac-bound GDP for GTP catalyzed by guanine nucleotide exchange factors (GEFs) is stimulated by phosphatidylinositol 3,4,5-trisphosphate (PI[3,4,5]P$_3$), a product of the action of PI3K. A family of GEF proteins that mediate the activation of Rac-related proteins has been identified. All members of this family, including Vav, Sos, and βPix, contain a pleckstrin homology (PH) domain that binds inositol-containing phospholipids such as PI(4,5)P$_2$ and PI(3,4,5)P$_3$ *(74,75)*. PI(4,5)P$_2$, when bound to the PH domain of Vav, inhibited activation of Vav GEF activity by the protein tyrosine kinase Lck, whereas PI(3,4,5)P$_3$ enhanced phosphorylation and activation of Vav by Lck *(76)*. Thus, the activation of PI3K might serve to convert a Vav inhibitor to an activator, resulting in a rapid transformation of inactive, GDP-bound Rac to its active, GTP-bound form. Our unpublished results indicate that βPix might be the Rac GEF responsible for the activation of Nox1. Thus, βPix physically associated with Nox1 protein, and PDGF-induced H_2O_2 production was significantly reduced when βPix expression was reduced by RNA interference in several different cell lines.

Figure 1 depicts the mechanism of PDGF-induced H_2O_2 production. The essential role of PI3K is likely to provide PI(3,4,5)P$_3$ that recruits and activates βPix by interacting with its PH domain. The PI(3,4,5)P$_3$-bound βPix then converts GDP-bound Rac to GTP-bound form, which induces NADPH oxidase activity in both phagocytes and nonphagocytic cells.

3. REVERSIBLE INACTIVATION OF PROTEIN TYROSINE PHOSPHATASES IN CELLS STIMULATED WITH GROWTH FACTORS

H_2O_2 itself is a mild oxidant and is relatively inert to most biomolecules. However, H_2O_2 is able to oxidize cysteine (Cys-SH) residues in proteins to Cys sulfenic acid or disulfide, both of which are readily reduced back to Cys-SH by various cellular reductants. The cysteine thiolate anion (Cys-S$^-$) is more readily oxidized by H_2O_2 than is the Cys sulfhydryl group (Cys-SH). Because the pK_a values of most protein Cys-SH residues are approx 8.5 *(77)*, few proteins would be expected to possess a Cys-SH residue that is readily susceptible to oxidation by H_2O_2 in cells. Protein Cys residues exist as thiolate anions at neutral pH, often because the negatively charged thiolate is stabilized by salt bridges to positively charged amino acid residues.

Proteins with low-pK_a cysteine residues include protein tyrosine phosphatases (PTPs). All PTPs contain an essential cysteine residue (pK_a = 4.7 to 5.4) in the signature active site motif His-Cys-X-X-Gly-X-X-Arg-Ser/Thr (where X is any amino acid), which exists as a thiolate anion at neutral pH *(78)*. This thiolate anion contributes to formation of a thiol-phosphate intermediate in the catalytic mechanism of PTPs. The active-site cysteine is the target of specific oxidation by various oxidants, including H_2O_2, and this modification can be reversed by incubation with thiol compounds such as dithiothreitol (DTT) and reduced glutathione. These observations suggested that PTPs might undergo H_2O_2-dependent inactivation in cells. However, such evidence was not available until we demonstrated the ability of intracellularly produced H_2O_2 to oxidize PTP1B in EGF-stimulated A431 cells *(45)*.

We followed the oxidation of PTP1B in EGF-stimulated cells by taking advantage of the fact that H_2O_2 and [^{14}C]iodoacetic acid (IAA) selectively and competitively react with cysteine residues that exhibit a low pK_a. A431 cells were stimulated with EGF (200 ng/mL) and then lysed in a buffer containing 2 mM [^{14}C]IAA. PTP1B was precipitated from the cell lysates with a specific mAb, and the decrease in [^{14}C] radioactivity associated with the immunoprecipitated PTP1B was taken as the measure of its oxidation. The amount of oxidatively inactivated PTP1B was maximal (approx 40%) 10 min after exposure of cells to EGF and returned to baseline values by 40 min, suggesting that the oxidation of this phosphatase by H_2O_2 is reversible in cells. With the use of the recombinant 37-kDa form of PTP1B, we also showed that the site of oxidation by H_2O_2 was the essential residue Cys^{215}.

The oxidized products of cysteine include sulfenic acid (Cys-SOH), disulfide (Cys-S-S-Cys), sulfinic acid (Cys-SO_2H), and sulfonic acid (Cys-SO_3H). The oxidative product of PTP1B was proposed to be sulfenic acid. The disulfide intermediate was excluded as the H_2O_2-modified form of PTP1B on the basis of the observation that only one out of six DTNB (5,5'-dithiobis-2-nitorbenzoic acid)-sensitive residues was lost after H_2O_2 oxidation, and the sulfinic and sulfonic acid intermediates on the basis of the observation that the oxidized PTP1B could be reduced back to its original state by DTT. Cysteine sulfenic acid is highly unstable and readily undergoes condensation with a thiol. However, the sulfenic-acid intermediate of PTP1B is likely stabilized by the fact that, according to the X-ray structure of the 37-kDa form of PTP1B *(79)*, no cysteine residues are located near Cys^{215}. Furthermore, the sulfenate anion (Cys-SO$^-$) is also likely stabilized by a salt bridge to Arg^{221}, which was shown to stabilize the thiolate anion of Cys^{215} and consequently to reduce its pK_a. Alternatively, Cys^{215}-SOH might react with glutathione, as Chock's laboratory detected glutathionylated PTP-1B in A431 cells treated with EGF *(46)*. Deglutathionylation of PTP1B is most likely catalyzed by glutaredoxin (thioltranferase).

Experiments with purified PTP1B suggest that the sufenic acid-containing PTP1B is reactivated more effectively by thioredoxin (Trx) than by glutaredoxin or glutathione at the physiological concentrations of these reductants. Thus, Trx might be a physiological electron donor for PTP1B, as well as other protein tyrosine phosphatases, when the oxidized enzymes are not glutathionylated.

Insulin stimulation also induces the production of intracellular H_2O_2 *(13)*. Goldstein's laboratory demonstrated the reversible oxidation of PTP1B and possibly other PTPs in insulin-stimulated cells by directly measuring the catalytic activity of PTPase activity in cell homogenates under strictly anaerobic conditions *(47)*. About 62% of total cellular PTPase activity was found to be reversibly inactivated in 3T3-L1 adipocytes and hepatoma cells stimulated with insulin. PTP1B, selectively immunoprecipitated from cell homogenates, was inhibited up to 88% following insulin stimulation. These results suggested that H_2O_2 produced in response to insulin contributes to the insulin-stimulated cascade of protein tyrosine phosphorylation by oxidatively inactivating PTP1B and other PTPs.

Tonks's laboratory developed another method to reveal reversible oxidation of PTPs in cells *(48)*. This method is based on the fact that those PTPs with the oxidized Cys-SOH at their active site are resistant to alkylation by IAA and can be reactivated by treatment with DTT, whereas any PTPs that had not been oxidized by H_2O_2 in the cell became irreversibly inactivated by alkylation with IAA. To visualize active PTPs, an aliquot of cell lysate that had been prepared under anaerobic conditions was subjected to sodium dodecyl sulfate (SDS)-polyacrylamide gel electrophoresis (PAGE) containing a radioactively labeled substrate, and proteins in the gel were renatured in the presence of DTT. Under these conditions, the activity of the PTPs in which the active-site Cys had been subjected to H_2O_2 oxidation to sulfenic acid was recovered, whereas those that were not oxidized in response to the initial stimulus and were irreversibly alkylated in the lysis step remained inactive. The bands corresponding to activated PTPs were then detected by dephosphorylation of a [^{32}P]phosphate-labeled poly Glu-Tyr. Using this in-gel assay, Tonks's laboratory showed that the SH2 domain containing PTP, SHP-2, was reversibly oxidized in Rat-1 cells treated with PDGF. As in the case of PTP1B, the oxidation of SHP-2 was reversible.

SHP-2 is a ubiquitously expressed cytosolic PTP that contains two SH2 domains and a PTP catalytic domain. The crystal structure revealed that SHP-2 exists in an inactive conformation in which the active site is occluded by the N-terminal SH2 domain *(80)*. Binding of autophosphorylated PDGF receptor promotes adoption of an open, active conformation in which the catalytic site of SHP-2 is free to interact with substrates *(80)*. Thus, one would anticipate that following binding of SHP-2 to autophosphorylated receptor, tyrosine phosphorylation of the PDGF receptor would be decreased. However, the peak of PDGF receptor autophosphorylation occurred during the time in which SHP-2 was associated with the receptor. These seemingly contradictory observations can be explained if the PDGF receptor–bound SHP-2 is temporarily inhibited. It is likely that the temporary inhibition is achieved through H_2O_2 produced in response to PDGF stimulation, and SHP-2 becomes reactivated after the intracellular concentration of H_2O_2 declines.

The results summarized above clearly indicate that H_2O_2 produced in response to growth-factor stimulation is capable of causing a reversible oxidation of PTPs in cells. These results, together with the observation that increased levels of PDGF-, EGF-, or insulin-induced protein tyrosine phosphorylation requires H_2O_2 production *(10,11,47,48)*, indicate that the activation of receptor protein tyrosine kinase (RTK) per se by binding of the corresponding growth factor may not be sufficient to increase the steady-state level of protein tyrosine phosphorylation in cells. Rather, the concurrent inhibition of PTPs by H_2O_2 may also be required. This suggests that the extent of autophosphorylation of RTKs and their substrates would return to basal values after degradation of H_2O_2 and the subsequent reactivation of PTPs by electron donors. The proposed role of H_2O_2 in growth factor–induced protein tyrosine phosphorylation is depicted in **Fig. 2**.

4. CONTROLLED ELIMINATION OF INTRACELLULAR H_2O_2 VIA PEROXIREDOXIN

As exemplified by cyclic nucleotides and inisitol 1,4,5-trisphosphate, timely elimination of second messengers after completion of their functions is critical for cellular signaling. Thus, in general, elimination as well as production of intracellular messengers is a highly controlled process. This would seem especially true for H_2O_2, which is readily converted to deleterious hydroxyl radicals. Enzymes that are capable of eliminating H_2O_2 include catalase and glutathione peroxidase, as well as peroxiredoxin (Prx). There is no evidence that the activities of the two conventional enzymes catalase and glutathione peroxidase are regulated.

Prx is a novel family of peroxidases that are present in organisms from all kingdoms *(81)*. All Prx enzymes contain a conserved cysteine residue at the amino-terminal region, which is the primary site of oxidation by H_2O_2. Mammalian Prx exists as at least six isoforms, which can be divided into three subgroups—namely, 2-Cys, atypical 2-Cys, and 1-Cys subgroups *(54,82,83)*. The 2-Cys members, which include Prx I, II, II, and IV, contain an additional conserved cysteine at the carboxy-terminal region, whereas Prx V and Prx VI, the members of the atypical 2-Cys and 1-Cys subgroups, respectively, do not contain this second conserved cysteine. The amino acid sequence identity among the three subgroup members is low (<20%), whereas that among the 2-Cys subgroup members is 60–80%. Prx isoforms are differently distributed in organelles: Prx I and II are in the cytosol; Prx III is

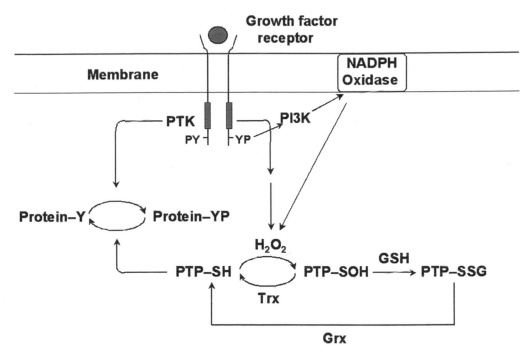

Fig. 2. Oxidative inhibition of PTP by H_2O_2 in growth factor-stimulated cells and reactivation by thioredoxin (Trx) or glutaredoxin (Grx)

expressed with the mitochondrial targeting sequence and exclusively localized in the mitochondria; Prx IV contains the amino-terminal signal sequence for secretion and is found in the endoplasmic reticulum as well as in the extracellular space; Prx V is expressed in the long and short forms that are found in the mitochondria and peroxisomes, respectively *(83)*; and Prx VI is found in the cytosol *(84,85)*. When overexpressed in various cells, Prx enzymes efficiently reduced the intracellular level of H_2O_2 produced in the cells stimulated with platelet-derived growth factor or TNF-α, inhibited NFκB activation induced by TNF-α, and blocked the apoptosis induced by ceramide *(84,86)*, indicating that Prx enzymes serve as a component of signaling cascades by removing H_2O_2.

Prx 1 contains a consensus site (Thr^{90}-Pro-Lys-Lys^{93}) for phosphorylation by cyclin-dependent kinases (Cdks). We recently showed that Prx I and Prx II can be phosphorylated specifically at Thr^{90} by several Cdks, including Cdc2 kinase *(87)*. Prx I phsphorylation at Thr^{90} caused a decrease in peroxidase activity by more than 80%. To monitor Prx I phosphorylation in cells, we prepared antibodies specific to Prx I phosphorylated at Thr90. Experiments with HeLa cells arrested at various stages of the cell cycle show that Prx I phosphoryaltion at Thr^{90} occurs in parallel to the activation of Cdc2 kinase. Prx I phosphoryaltion was observed in cells in mitotic phase but not in interphase, despite the fact that Prx I can be phosphorylated by other Cdk isoforms in vitro. This is probably because Prx I, a cytosolic protein, can encounter activated Cdks only after the nuclear envelope breaks down during mitosis, and because Cdc2 kinase is the Cdk that is activated in mitotic phase. Both the in vitro and in vivo phosphorylation of Prx I at Thr^{90} was inhibited by roscovitine, an inhibitor of Cdks. Prx II also can be phosphorylated, albeit more weakly than is Prx I, by Cdc2 kinase in vitro. Prx II is also a cytosolic protein. Therefore, Cdc2 kinase-dependent phosphorylation and inactivation of Prx II are likely to occur in mitosis.

Inactivation of Prx I and Prx II is expected to result in an increase in the intracellular concentration of H_2O_2. The significance of the temporary increase of H_2O_2 concentration during mitosis is not

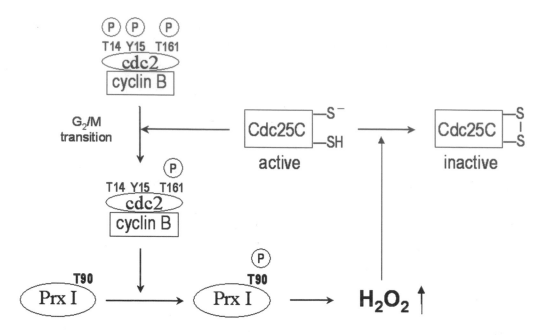

Fig. 3. Regulation of Prx I peroxidase activity through Cdc2 kinase-dependent phosphorylation and inactivation of Cdc25C by H_2O_2.

clear. One of the potential target molecules on which H_2O_2 acts to propagate its signal is Cdc25C dual phosphatase, an important regulator of Cdc2 kinase. At the onset of mitosis, the Cdc25C phosphatase activates Cdc2 kinase by dephosphorylating Thr14 and Tyr15 (88,89). The Cdc25C phosphatase is weakly active during interphase and fully activated during mitosis. Control of Cdc25C itself is also a highly regulated process, which involves phosphorylation and dephosphorylation: Cdc25C is phosphorylated and activated by several kinases, including Cdc2 kinase, and inactivated by OA-sensitive phosphatases (90). Therefore, the small amount of active Cdc2 kinase produced by Cdc25C is expected to stimulate further Cdc2 kinase activation, creating a positive feedback effect. Like other protein tyrosine phosphatases, Cdc25 phosphatases contain an essential cysteine residue in the His-Cys-X-X-X-X-X-Arg motif (91). Cdc25C was shown to be sensitive to oxidation and requires the presence of reducing agents for its activity (92,93). Exposure of Cdc25 to H_2O_2 promotes an intramolecular disulfide bond between the active site Cys^{330} and another invariant Cys^{377}. This disulfide bond formation altered the binding of Cdc25 with 14-3-3 and hence the subcellular localization of the protein (93).

Taken together, we speculate that as mitosis progresses to prometaphase, the nuclear envelope breaks down, and Prx I, likely Prx II also, becomes phosphorylated by Cdc2 kinase that had been activated at the stage of G_2 to M transition. As the result of phosphorylation, the two cytosolic Prx enzymes become inactive, allowing accumulation of H_2O_2 in cells. The resulting H_2O_2 causes inactivation of Cdc25C, which in turn serves as a mechanism to halt the positive feedback loop of Cdc25 phosphatase and Cdc2 kinase. Thus, H_2O_2 might serve as an inhibitor of Cdc25C phosphatase throughout later stages of mitosis and cooperate with cyclin B degradation to promote the exit from mitosis.

Irrespective of whether or not CDC25C is a target of H_2O_2 during the cell cycle, our results clearly demonstrate that peroxidase activity of Prx I is regulated through phosphorylation (**Fig. 3**). This is the first example that any of the H_2O_2 eliminating enzymes—catalase, glutathione peroxidase, and peroxiredoxin—is regulated through posttranslational modification. The Prx phosphorylation is consistent with the thesis that intracellular concentration of H_2O_2 is strictly regulated through the fine control of processes involved in the production as well as elimination.

5. CONCLUDING REMARKS

Increasing evidence now qualifies H_2O_2 to join the ranks of cAMP, Ca^{2+}, inositol 1,4,5-trisphosphate, and NO in its role as an intracellular messenger. However, unlike the other second messengers, very little is known about the pathway by which H_2O_2 is generated in response to receptor stimulation and what molecules are direct targets of the H_2O_2 messenger function. We have described how H_2O_2 production by PDGF involves signaling molecules like PI3K, Rac1, a Rac GEF called βPix, and Nox1, an isoform of NADPH oxidase. Evidence suggests that lipoxygenases and cyclooxygenases are also involved in receptor-mediated H_2O_2 generation. Considering that stimulation of numerous (cytokine, growth factor, G protein-coupled) receptors induces H_2O_2 production, as with other second messengers, various protein kinases and phosphatases, heterotrimeric and small G proteins, adaptor proteins, and scaffolding proteins are likely to be involved in the production of H_2O_2. Additionally, these components are expected to be subject to control by other second messenger-generating cascades.

We have proposed that H_2O_2 can propagate its signal by oxidizing active-site cysteines of PTPs that are sensitive to oxidation by H_2O_2 because their pK_as are lower than those of other cysteines. In addition, many protein kinases, transcriptional factors, and ion channels have been proposed to be controlled by H_2O_2 through oxidation of their H_2O_2-sensitive cysteine residues.

A lot less is known about the termination of H_2O_2 messenger function. H_2O_2 has long been considered an undesirable byproduct of respiration and thought to be removed by the passive action of enzymes like catalase and glutathione peroxidase. With our result that Prx I and Prx II can be regulated through Cdc2 kinase-dependent phosphorylation, we are finding evidence for the active participation of H_2O_2-eliminating enzymes in intracellular signaling.

REFERENCES

1. Rhee, S. G. (1999) Redox signaling: hydrogen peroxide as intracellular messenger. *Exp. Mol. Med.* **31**, 53–59.
2. Rhee, S. G., Bae, Y. S., Lee, S. R., and Kwon, J. (2000) Hydrogen peroxide: A key messenger that modulates protein phosphorylation through cysteine oxidation. *Science's stke* pe1.
3. Finkel, T. (1998) Oxygen radicals and signaling. *Curr. Opin. Cell. Biol.* **10**, 248–253.
4. Adler, V., Yin, Z., Tew, K. D., and Ronai, Z. (1999) Role of redox potential and reactive oxygen species in stress signaling. *Oncogene* **18**, 6104–6111.
5. Suzuki, Y. J. and Ford, G. D. (1999) Redox regulation of signal transduction in cardiac and smooth muscle. *J. Mol. Cell. Cardiol.* **31**, 345–353.
6. Griendling, K. K. and Ushio-Fukai, M. (2000) Reactive oxygen species as mediators of angiotensin II signaling. *Regul. Pept.* **91**, 21–27.
7. Patel, R. P., Moellering, D., Murphy-Ullrich, J., Jo, H., Beckman, J. S., and Darley-Usmar, V. M. (2000) Cell signaling by reactive nitrogen and oxygen species in atherosclerosis. *Free Radic. Biol. Med.* **28**, 1780–1794.
8. Forman, H. J. and Torres, M. (2001) Signaling by the respiratory burst in macrophages. *IUBMB Life* **51**, 365–371.
9. Thannickal, V. J. and Fanburg, B. L. (2000) Reactive oxygen species in cell signaling. *Am. J. Physiol. Lung Cell. Mol. Physiol.* **279**, L1005–L1028.
10. Sundaresan, M., Yu, Z. X., Ferrans, V. J., Irani, K., and Finkel, T. (1995) Requirement for generation of H_2O_2 for platelet-derived growth factor signal transduction. *Science* **270**, 296–299.
11. Bae, Y. S., Kang, S. W., Seo, M. S., et al. (1997) Epidermal growth factor (EGF)-induced generation of hydrogen peroxide. Role in EGF receptor-mediated tyrosine phosphorylation. *J. Biol. Chem.* **272**, 217–221.
12. Lo, Y. Y. and Cruz, T. F. (1995) Involvement of reactive oxygen species in cytokine and growth factor induction of c-fos expression in chondrocytes. *J. Biol. Chem.* **270**, 11,727–11,730.
13. May, J. M. and de Haen, C. (1979) Insulin-stimulated intracellular hydrogen peroxide production in rat epididymal fat cells. *J. Biol. Chem.* **254**, 2214–2220.
14. Abid, M. R., Tsai, J. C., Spokes, K. C., Deshpande, S. S., Irani, K., and Aird, W. C. (2001) Vascular endothelial growth factor induces manganese-superoxide dismutase expression in endothelial cells by a Rac1-regulated NADPH oxidase-dependent mechanism. *FASEB J.* **15**, 2548–2550.
15. Sattler, M., Winkler, T., Verma, S., et al. (1993) Hematopoietic growth factors signal through the formation of reactive oxygen species. *Blood* **93**, 2928–2935.

16. Ohba, M., Shibanuma, M., Kuroki, T., and Nose, K. (1994) Production of hydrogen peroxide by transforming growth factor-beta 1 and its involvement in induction of egr-1 in mouse osteoblastic cells. *J. Cell. Biol.* **126,** 1079–1088.

17. Thannickal, V. J. and Fanburg, B. L. (1995) Activation of an H_2O_2-generating NADH oxidase in human lung fibroblasts by transforming growth factor beta 1. *J. Biol. Chem.* **270,** 30,334–30,338.

18. Thannickal, V. J., Aldweib, K. D., and Fanburg, B. L. (1998) Tyrosine phosphorylation regulates H_2O_2 production in lung fibroblasts stimulated by transforming growth factor beta1. *J. Biol. Chem.* **273,** 23,611–23,615.

19. Meier, B., Radeke, H. H., Selle, S., et al. (1989) Human fibroblasts release reactive oxygen species in response to interleukin-1 or tumour necrosis factor-alpha. *Biochem. J.* **263,** 539–545.

20. Krieger-Brauer, H. I. and Kather, H. (1995) The stimulus-sensitive H_2O_2-generating system present in human fat-cell plasma membranes is multireceptor-linked and under antagonistic control by hormones and cytokines. *Biochem. J.* **307,** 543–548.

21. Lee, Y. W., Kuhn, H., Hennig, B., Neish, A. S., and Toborek, M. (2001) IL-4-induced oxidative stress upregulates VCAM-1 gene expression in human endothelial cells. *J. Mol. Cell Cardiol.* **33,** 83–94.

22. Deshpande, S. S., Angkeow, P., Huang, J., Ozaki, M., and Irani, K. (2000) Rac1 inhibits TNF-alpha-induced endothelial cell apoptosis: dual regulation by reactive oxygen species. *FASEB J.* **14,** 1705–1714.

23. Tatla, S., Woodhead, V., Foreman, J. C., and Chain, B. M. (1999) The role of reactive oxygen species in triggering proliferation and IL- 2 secretion in T cells. *Free Radic. Biol. Med.* **26,** 14–24.

24. Kitai, S. T., Shepard, P. D., Callaway, J. C., and Scroggs, R. (1999) Afferent modulation of dopamine neuron firing patterns. *Curr. Opin. Neurobiol.* **9,** 690–697.

25. Zafari, A. M., Ushio-Fukai, M., Akers, M., et al. (1998) Role of NADH/NADPH oxidase-derived H_2O_2 in angiotensin II-induced vascular hypertrophy. *Hypertension* **32,** 488–495.

26. Du, J., Peng, T., Scheidegger, K. J., and Delafontaine, P. (1999) Angiotensin II activation of insulin-like growth factor 1 receptor transcription is mediated by a tyrosine kinase-dependent redox- sensitive mechanism. *Arterioscler. Thromb. Vasc. Biol.* **19,** 2119–2126.

27. Ushio-Fukai, M., Alexander, R. W., Akers, M., et al. (1999) Reactive oxygen species mediate the activation of Akt/ protein kinase B by angiotensin II in vascular smooth muscle cells. *J. Biol. Chem.* **274,** 22,699–22,704.

28. Kimura, T., Okajima, F., Sho, K., Kobayashi, I., and Kondo, Y. (1995) Thyrotropin-induced hydrogen peroxide production in FRTL-5 thyroid cells is mediated not by adenosine 3',5'-monophosphate, but by Ca2+ signaling followed by phospholipase-A2 activation and potentiated by an adenosine derivative. *Endocrinology* **136,** 116–123.

29. Chen, Q., Olashaw, N., and Wu, J. (1995) Participation of reactive oxygen species in the lysophosphatidic acid- stimulated mitogen-activated protein kinase activation pathway. *J. Biol. Chem.* **270,** 28,499–28,502.

30. Sekharam, M., Cunnick, J. M., and Wu, J. (2000) Involvement of lipoxygenase in lysophosphatidic acid-stimulated hydrogen peroxide release in human HaCaT keratinocytes. *Biochem. J.* **346 Pt 3,** 751–758.

31. Okajima, F., Tomura, H., Sho, K., et al. (1997) Sphingosine 1-phosphate stimulates hydrogen peroxide generation through activation of phospholipase C-Ca2+ system in FRTL-5 thyroid cells: possible involvement of guanosine triphosphate-binding proteins in the lipid signaling. *Endocrinology* **138,** 220–229.

32. Mukhin, Y. V., Garnovskaya, M. N., Collinsworth, G., et al. (2000) 5-Hydroxytryptamine1A receptor/Gibetagamma stimulates mitogen-activated protein kinase via NAD(P)H oxidase and reactive oxygen species upstream of src in chinese hamster ovary fibroblasts. *Biochem. J.* **347 Pt 1,** 61–67.

33. Greene, E. L., Houghton, O., Collinsworth, G., et al. (2000) 5-HT(2A) receptors stimulate mitogen-activated protein kinase via H(2)O(2) generation in rat renal mesangial cells. *Am. J. Physiol. Renal Physiol.* **278,** F650–F658.

34. Galle, J., Lehmann-Bodem, C., Hubner, U., Heinloth, A., and Wanner, C. (2000) CyA and OxLDL cause endothelial dysfunction in isolated arteries through endothelin-mediated stimulation of O(2)(-) formation. *Nephrol. Dial. Transplant.* **15,** 339–346.

35. Naarala, J., Tervo, P., Loikkanen, J., and Savolainen, K. (1997) Cholinergic-induced production of reactive oxygen species in human neuroblastoma cells. *Life Sci.* **60,** 1905–1914.

36. Gardner, C. R., Laskin, J. D., and Laskin, D. L. (1993) Platelet-activating factor-induced calcium mobilization and oxidative metabolism in hepatic macrophages and endothelial cells. *J. Leukoc. Biol.* **53,** 190–196.

37. Goldman, R., Moshonov, S., and Zor, U. (1999) Calcium-dependent PAF-stimulated generation of reactive oxygen species in a human keratinocyte cell line. *Biochim. Biophys. Acta* **1438,** 349–358.

38. Hu, Q., Yu, Z., Ferrans, V., Takeda, K., Irani, K., and Ziegelstein, R. C. (2002) Critical role of NADPH oxidase-derived reactive oxygen species in generating calcium oscillation in human aortic endothelial cells stimulated by histamine. *J. Biol. Chem.* **277,** 32,546–32,551.

39. Greene, E. L., Velarde, V., and Jaffa, A. A. (2000) Role of reactive oxygen species in bradykinin-induced mitogen-activated protein kinase and c-fos induction in vascular cells. *Hypertension* **35,** 942–947.

40. Yamagishi, S. I., Edelstein, D., Du, X. L., Kaneda, Y., Guzman, M., and Brownlee, M. (2001) Leptin induces mitochondrial superoxide production and monocyte chemoattractant protein-1 expression in aortic endothelial cells by increasing fatty acid oxidation via protein kinase A. *J. Biol. Chem.* **276,** 25,096–25,100.

41. Yeh, L. H., Park, Y. J., Hansalia, R. J., et al. (1999) Shear-induced tyrosine phosphorylation in endothelial cells requires Rac1-dependent production of ROS. *Am. J. Physiol.* **276,** C838–C847.

42. Janssen-Heininger, Y. M., Poynter, M. E., and Baeuerle, P. A. (2000) Recent advances towards understanding redox mechanisms in the activation of nuclear factor kappaB. *Free Radic. Biol. Med.* **28,** 1317–1327.

43. Hsu, T. C., Young, M. R., Cmarik, J., and Colburn, N. H. (2000) Activator protein 1 (AP-1)- and nuclear factor kappaB (NF-kappaB)- dependent transcriptional events in carcinogenesis. *Free Radic. Biol. Med.* **28,** 1338–1348.

44. Arrigo, A. P. (1999) Gene expression and the thiol redox state. *Free Radic. Biol. Med.* **27,** 936–944.

45. Lee, S. R., Kwon, K. S., Kim, S. R., and Rhee, S. G. (1998) Reversible inactivation of protein-tyrosine phosphatase 1B in A431 cells stimulated with epidermal growth factor. *J. Biol. Chem.* **273**, 15,366–15,372.
46. Barrett, W. C., DeGnore, J. P., Keng, Y. F., Zhang, Z. Y., Yim, M. B., and Chock, P. B. (1999) Roles of superoxide radical anion in signal transduction mediated by reversible regulation of protein-tyrosine phosphatase 1B. *J. Biol. Chem.* **274**, 34543–34546.
47. Mahadev, K., Zilbering, A., Zhu, L., and Goldstein, B. J. (2001) Insulin-stimulated hydrogen peroxide reversibly inhibits protein- tyrosine phosphatase 1b in vivo and enhances the early insulin action cascade. *J. Biol. Chem.* **276**, 21,938–21,942.
48. Meng, T. C., Fukada, T., and Tonks, N. K. (2002) Reversible oxidation and inactivation of protein tyrosine phosphatases in vivo. *Mol. Cell* **9**, 387–399.
49. Wang, X. T., McCullough, K. D., Wang, X. J., Carpenter, G., Holbrook, N. J. (2001) Oxidative stress-induced phospholipase C-gamma 1 activation enhances cell survival. *J. Biol. Chem.* **276**, 28,364–28,371.
50. Min, D. S., Kim, E. G., and Exton, J. H. (1998) Involvement of tyrosine phosphorylation and protein kinase C in the activation of phospholipase D by H_2O_2 in Swiss 3T3 fibroblasts. *J. Biol. Chem.* **273**, 29,986–29,994.
51. Lee, S. R., Yang, K. S., Kwon, J., Lee, C., Jeong, W., and Rhee, S. G. (2002) Regulation of PTEN by superoxide and H_2O_2 through the reversible formation of a disulfide between Cys124 and Cys71. *J. Biol. Chem.* **277**, 20,336–20,342.
52. Kourie, J. I. (1998) Interaction of reactive oxygen species with ion transport mechanisms. *Am. J. Physiol.* **275**, C1–C24.
53. Nishida, M., Schey, K. L., Takagahara, S., et al. (2002) Activation mechanism of Gi and Go by reactive oxygen species. *J. Biol. Chem.* **277**, 9036–9042.
54. Kang, S. W., Chae, H. Z., Seo, M. S., Kim, K., Baines, I. C., and Rhee, S. G. (1998) Mammalian peroxiredoxin isoforms can reduce hydrogen peroxide generated in response to growth factors and tumor necrosis factor-alpha. *J. Biol. Chem.* **273**, 6297–6302.
55. Funk, C. D. (2001) Prostaglandins and leukotrienes: advances in eicosanoid biology. *Science* **294**, 1871–1875.
56. Saugstad, O. D. (1996) Role of xanthine oxidase and its inhibitor in hypoxia: reoxygenation injury. *Pediatrics* **98**, 103–107.
57. Bernhardt, R. (1996) Cytochrome P450: structure, function, and generation of reactive oxygen species. *Rev. Physiol. Biochem. Pharmacol.* **127**, 137–221.
58. Lambeth, J. D. (2002) Nox/Duox family of nicotinamide adenine dinucleotide (phosphate) oxidases. *Curr. Opin. Hematol.* **9**, 11–17.
59. Wachowicz, B., Olas, B., Zbikowska, H. M., and Buczynski, A. (2002) Generation of reactive oxygen species in blood platelets. *Platelets* **13**, 175–182.
60. Woo, C. H., Eom, Y. W., Yoo, M. H., et al. (2000) Tumor necrosis factor-alpha generates reactive oxygen species via a cytosolic phospholipase A2-linked cascade. *J. Biol. Chem.* **275**, 32,357–32,362.
61. Li, A. E., Ito, H., Rovira, I. I., et al. (1999) A role for reactive oxygen species in endothelial cell anoikis. *Circ. Res.* **85**, 304–310.
62. Babior, B. M. (1999) NADPH oxidase: an update. *Blood* **93**, 1464–1476.
63. Nisimoto, Y., Motalebi, S., Han, C. H., and Lambeth, J. D. (1999) The p67(phox) activation domain regulates electron flow from NADPH to flavin in flavocytochrome b(558). *J. Biol. Chem.* **274**, 22,999–23,005.
64. Sundaresan, M., Yu, Z. X., Ferrans, V. J., et al. (1996) Regulation of reactive-oxygen-species generation in fibroblasts by Rac1. *Biochem. J.* **318**, 379–382.
65. Joneson, T. and Bar-Sagi, D. (1998) A Rac1 effector site controlling mitogenesis through superoxide production. *J. Biol. Chem.* **273**, 17,991–17,994.
66. Suh, Y. A., Arnold, R. S., Lassegue, B., et al. (1999) Cell transformation by the superoxide-generating oxidase Mox1. *Nature* **401**, 79–82.
67. Arnold, R. S., Shi, J., Murad, E., et al. (2001) Hydrogen peroxide mediates the cell growth and transformation caused by the mitogenic oxidase Nox1. *Proc. Natl. Acad. Sci. USA* **98**, 5550–5555.
68. De Deken, X., Wang, D., Many, M. C., et al. (2000) Cloning of two human thyroid cDNAs encoding new members of the NADPH oxidase family. *J. Biol. Chem.* **275**, 23,227–23,233.
69. Geiszt, M., Kopp, J. B., Varnai, P., and Leto, T. L. (2000) Identification of renox, an NAD(P)H oxidase in kidney. *Proc. Natl. Acad. Sci. USA* **97**, 8010–8014.
70. Yang, S., Madyastha, P., Bingel, S., Ries, W., and Key, L. (2001) A new superoxide-generating oxidase in murine osteoclasts. *J. Biol. Chem.* **276**, 5452–5458.
71. Lassegue, B., Sorescu, D., Szocs, K., et al. (2001) Novel gp91(phox) homologues in vascular smooth muscle cells : nox1 mediates angiotensin II-induced superoxide formation and redox- sensitive signaling pathways. *Circ. Res.* **88**, 888–894.
72. Arbiser, J. L., Petros, J., Klafter, R., et al. (2002) Reactive oxygen generated by Nox1 triggers the angiogenic switch. *Proc. Natl. Acad. Sci. USA* **99**, 715–720.
73. Valius, M. and Kazlauskas, A. (1993) Phospholipase C-gamma 1 and phosphatidylinositol 3 kinase are the downstream mediators of the PDGF receptor's mitogenic signal. *Cell* **73**, 321–334.
74. Rameh, L. E. and Cantley, L. C. (1999) The role of phosphoinositide 3-kinase lipid products in cell function. *J. Biol. Chem.* **274**, 8347–8350.
75. Leevers, S. J., Vanhaesebroeck, B., and Waterfield, M. D. (1999) Signalling through phosphoinositide 3-kinases: the lipids take centre stage. *Curr. Opin. Cell. Biol.* **11**, 219–225.
76. Han, J., Luby-Phelps, K., Das, B., et al. (1998) Role of substrates and products of PI 3-kinase in regulating activation of Rac-related guanosine triphosphatases by Vav. *Science* **279**, 558–560.

77. Besse, D., Siedler, F., Diercks, T., Kessler, H., and Moroder, L. (1997) The redox potential of Selenocysteine in unconstrained cyclic peptides. *Angew. Chem. Int. Ed. Engl.* **36,** 883–885.
78. Lohse, D. L., Denu, J. M., Santoro, N., and Dixon, J. E. (1997) Roles of aspartic acid-181 and serine-222 in intermediate formation and hydrolysis of the mammalian protein-tyrosine-phosphatase PTP1. *Biochemistry* **36,** 4568–4575.
79. Barford, D., Flint, A. J., and Tonks, N. K. (1994) Crystal structure of human protein tyrosine phosphatase 1B. *Science* **263,** 1397–1404.
80. Hof, P., Pluskey, S., Dhe-Paganon, S., Eck, M. J., and Shoelson, S. E. (1998) Crystal structure of the tyrosine phosphatase SHP-2. *Cell* **92,** 441–450.
81. Chae, H. Z., Robison, K., Poole, L. B., Church, G., Storz, G., and Rhee, S. G. (1994) Cloning and sequencing of thiol-specific antioxidant from mammalian brain: alkyl hydroperoxide reductase and thiol-specific antioxidant define a large family of antioxidant enzymes. *Proc. Natl. Acad. Sci. USA* **91,** 7017–7021.
82. Rhee, S. G., Kang, S. W., Chang, T. S., Jeong, W., and Kim, K. (2001) Peroxiredoxin, a novel family of peroxidases. *IUBMB Life* **52,** 35–41.
83. Seo, M. S., Kang, S. W., Kim, K., Baines, I. C., Lee, T. H., and Rhee, S. G. (2000) Identification of a new type of mammalian peroxiredoxin that forms an intramolecular disulfide as a reaction intermediate. *J. Biol. Chem.* **275,** 20,346–20,354.
84. Kang, S. W., Baines, I. C., and Rhee, S. G. (1998) Characterization of a mammalian peroxiredoxin that contains one conserved cysteine. *J. Biol. Chem.* **273,** 6303–6311.
85. Matsumoto, A., Okado, A., Fujii, T., et al. (1999) Cloning of the peroxiredoxin gene family in rats and characterization of the fourth member. *FEBS Lett.* **443,** 246–250.
86. Zhang, P., Liu, B., Kang, S. W., Seo, M. S., Rhee, S. G., and Obeid, L. M. (1997) Thioredoxin peroxidase is a novel inhibitor of apoptosis with a mechanism distinct from that of Bcl-2. *J. Biol. Chem.* **272,** 30,615–30,618.
87. Chang, T. S., Jeong, W., Choi, S. Y., Yu, S., and Rhee, S. G. (2002) Regulation of peroxiredoxin I activity by Cdc2-mediated phosphorylation. *J. Biol. Chem.* **277,** 25,370–25,376.
88. Norbury, C. and Nurse, P. (1992) Animal cell cycles and their control. *Annu. Rev. Biochem.* **61,** 441–470.
89. Morgan, D. O. (1995) Principles of CDK regulation. *Nature* **374,** 131–134.
90. Hoffmann, I., Clarke, P. R., Marcote, M. J., Karsenti, E., and Draetta, G. (1993) Phosphorylation and activation of human cdc25-C by cdc2–cyclin B and its involvement in the self-amplification of MPF at mitosis. *EMBO J.* **12,** 53–63.
91. Fauman, E. B., Cogswell, J. P., Lovejoy, B., et al. (1998) Crystal structure of the catalytic domain of the human cell cycle control phosphatase, Cdc25A. *Cell* **93,** 617–625.
92. Dunphy, W. G. and Kumagai, A. (1991) The cdc25 protein contains an intrinsic phosphatase activity. *Cell* **67,** 189–196.
93. Savitsky, P. A. and Finkel, T. (2002) Redox regulation of Cdc25C. *J. Biol. Chem.* **277,** 20,535–20,540.

20

Calcium-Inhibited Adenylyl Cyclase (AC$_6$) Controls Endothelial Cell Barrier Function

Troy Stevens

SUMMARY

For many years, investigators have recognized that inflammatory mediators increase cytosolic calcium in endothelial cells, which triggers intercellular gap formation and increased permeability. However, this calcium-mediated increase in permeability occurs only when cAMP levels are not also increased. Indeed, a rise in cAMP prevents inflammatory mediators from increasing permeability, and it even reverses tissue edema that has already been initiated. Studies examining the crosstalk between cytosolic calcium and cAMP reveal an inverse relationship, where increased cytosolic calcium decreases cAMP. Endothelial cell expression of a type 6 (calcium-inhibited) adenylyl cyclase is responsible for this action, so that calcium entry across the cell membrane decreases cAMP synthesis. Eliminating calcium inhibition of cAMP prevents inflammatory mediators from increasing endothelial cell permeability, indicating that crosstalk between these intracellular messengers is necessary for the endothelium to change its shape.

Key Words: cAMP; cytosolic calcium; signal transduction; permeability; lung.

1. INTRODUCTION

Under normal conditions, endothelium represents a semipermeable barrier to water, solutes, molecules, and circulating cells. This barrier is maintained by cell–cell and cell–matrix adhesions, and opposed by a constitutive inward tension. In response to various inflammatory stimuli, transient intercellular gaps form, allowing delivery of plasma-rich constituents to underlying tissue. Such a breach in barrier function involves both an increase in centripetally directed tension and a decrease in cell–cell and cell–matrix tethering (reviewed in refs. *1–7*). Understanding the molecular events that underlie endothelial cell gap formation and resolution are of significant interest, because prolonged disruption of the endothelial cell barrier results in tissue edema that compromises organ function.

Studies from the 1950 to the 1990s clearly implicated two signaling pathways in control of endothelial cell barrier function (reviewed in ref. *8*). Physiological transitions in cytosolic calcium ($[Ca^{2+}]_i$) induce interendothelial cell gaps. Majno and Palade *(9)* were among the first investigators to lay such groundwork, utilizing electron microscopy to describe histamine- and serotonin-induced intercellular gaps selectively arising in postcapillary venules. Many subsequent studies confirmed these findings, and further demonstrated that gap formation is accompanied by an increase in protein and fluid flux across the barrier. It is now a well-accepted idea that physiological transitions in $[Ca^{2+}]_i$ are sufficient to disrupt the endothelial cell barrier and increase permeability.

Studies from other investigator groups resolved that an increase in adenosine 3'5'-cyclic monophosphate (cAMP) strengthens endothelial cell barrier function (reviewed in ref. *8*). Since its original description *(10)*, several physiological roles have been described for cAMP, though none are more

From: *Cell Signaling in Vascular Inflammation*
Edited by: J. Bhattacharya © Humana Press Inc., Totowa, NJ

convincing than its dominant control of endothelial cell barrier function *(8)*. cAMP directly activates several signaling molecules, including cyclic nucleotide-gated cation channels *(11)* and EPAC *(12)*, but its best-accepted mode of action is through activation of the cAMP-dependent protein kinase (PKA) *(13)*. PKA phosphorylates the endothelial cell myosin light chain kinase to reduce centripetally directed tension *(14)*, and is also resolved within sites of cell–cell adhesion. At this time, PKA substrates within sites of cell-cell and cell-matrix tethering are poorly described, but recent findings suggest that cAMP elevations intensely increase endothelial cell adhesion *(15)*. Indeed, we have come to find that physiological transitions in $[Ca^{2+}]_i$ increase permeability only if cAMP concentrations do not rise *(8)*, leading to the idea that cAMP plays a dominant role in the control of endothelial cell barrier function.

If $[Ca^{2+}]_i$ transitions increase endothelial cell permeability only in the absence of a rise in cAMP, then it stands to reason that crosstalk between these signaling pathways must contribute critically to the cell's response to inflammatory agonists. Our group addressed this idea in the mid-1990s, and we have resolved that Ca^{2+} influx across the endothelial cell membrane directly inhibits type 6 adenylyl cyclase (AC_6) *(16)*. Inhibition of AC_6 reduces cAMP, absolutely necessary for endothelial cell barrier disruption. This review details studies leading up to the current-day thinking regarding such physiological crosstalk between $[Ca^{2+}]_i$ and cAMP signaling pathways in control of endothelial cell barrier function.

2. PULMONARY ARTERY ENDOTHELIUM

Some of the earliest work in postcapillary venules revealed that inflammatory agonists that increase $[Ca^{2+}]_i$ promote intercellular gap formation. While this observation was initially made using histamine as a model, later work resolved similar endothelial gaps formed in response to thrombin, brakykinin, ATP, ADP, substance P, and other inflammagens *(8)*. These agonists share in common the ability to couple through their receptors to activation of G_q proteins and, in turn, phospholipase C. Phospholipase C hydrolyzes phosphatidyl inositol 4,5-bisphosphate into two products: inositol 1,4,5-trisphosphate ($InsP_3$) and diacylglycerol. $InsP_3$ diffuses to the nearby endoplasmic reticulum, where it promotes Ca^{2+} release that transiently depletes Ca^{2+} in the store. Such Ca^{2+} depletion from endoplasmic reticulum activates a Ca^{2+} entry pathway generally referred to as store-operated Ca^{2+} entry *(17–25)*. The signaling complexity associated with G_q activation of store-operated channel (SOC) entry can be simplified using thapsigargin, a plant alkaloid that inhibits the sarcoplasmic/endoplasmic reticulum Ca^{2+} ATPase (SERCA) *(26)*. Direct inhibition of SERCA prevents Ca^{2+} reuptake into the endoplasmic reticulum, and depletes Ca^{2+} stores. Although $InsP_3$-induced Ca^{2+} store depletion is transient (because released Ca^{2+} is rapidly re-sequestered by SERCA) whereas thapsigargin-induced Ca^{2+} store depletion is prolonged (because Ca^{2+} reuptake is inhibited), both of these agonists activate SOC entry. In nonexcitable cells like endothelia, SOC entry is thought to represent the principal mode of Ca^{2+} entry across the cell membrane *(8,18,20,27)*.

Recent studies utilized thapsigargin, or other agents that directly inhibit SERCA activity, to assess the contribution of SOC entry to endothelial cell barrier function. Using mostly conduit-derived endothelial cells like pulmonary artery endothelial cells (PAECs), several studies reported thapsigargin dose-dependently increases $[Ca^{2+}]_i$ and macromolecular permeability *(16,28–33)* over an identical concentration range. Moreover, increased permeability required the presence of physiological extracellular Ca^{2+} concentrations; decreasing extracellular Ca^{2+} to 100 nM prevented thapsigargin from increasing permeability (**Fig. 1**) *(16,28,31,33)*. To confirm this idea, recalcification experiments were performed, where thapsigargin was applied in low extracellular Ca^{2+} *(30–32)*. Under such conditions, thapsigargin induces Ca^{2+} release from the endoplasmic reticulum and opens SOC entry channels. However, since extracellular Ca^{2+} is not present to permeate the plasma membrane, Ca^{2+} does not enter through SOC channels. Replenishing extracellular Ca^{2+} promotes immediate Ca^{2+} entry through already open channels, resulting in a sustained rise in $[Ca^{2+}]_i$ (**Fig. 2A**). Interestingly,

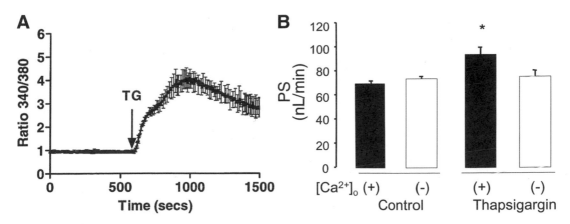

Fig. 1. Activation of store-operated Ca^{2+} entry increases pulmonary artery endothelial cells (PAECs) permeability. **(A)** Activation of store-operated Ca^{2+} entry using thapsigargin (TG; 1 μM) increases $[Ca^{2+}]_i$, reflected as an increase in the 340/380 ratio in fura-2-loaded cells. Adapted from ref. *33*. **(B)** Thapsigargin increased PAEC macromolecular permeability, as indicated by the diffusive capacity (PS) values for 23-Å dextran macromolecules. This effect of thapsigargin requires normal extracellular Ca^{2+} ($[Ca^{2+}]_o$). Adapted from ref. *32*.

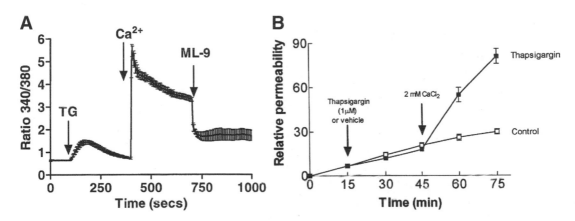

Fig. 2. Ca^{2+} entry across the cell membrane is required for thapsigargin to increase endothelial cell permeability. **(A)** Thapsigargin (TG; 1 μM) was applied to fura-loaded pulmonary artery endothelial cells (PAECs) incubated in 100 nM extracellular Ca^{2+}. Under these conditions, thapsigargin induced a small, transient rise in $[Ca^{2+}]_i$ (reflected by an increase in the 340/380 ratio) as a result of passive Ca^{2+} release from the endoplasmic reticulum. Subsequently adding 2 mM extracellular Ca^{2+} resulted in a large, sustained rise in $[Ca^{2+}]_i$ owing to entry across the plasmalemma through open channels. In this study, Ca^{2+} entry was inhibited using a myosin light chain kinase inhibitor, ML-9. Adapted from *(33)*. **(B)** Using a similar re-calcification protocol, thapsigargin-induced Ca^{2+} release did not alter endothelial cell permeability. However, re-addition of extracellular Ca^{2+} induced an abrupt, large increase in PAEC permeability. Adapted from ref. *30*.

thapsigargin does not increase endothelial cell permeability until extracellular Ca^{2+} is replenished to allow for entry through SOC entry channels (**Fig. 2B**). These findings are compatible with the idea that Ca^{2+} entry through SOC entry channels is sufficient to increase endothelial cell permeability.

Because rises in $[Ca^{2+}]_i$ increase endothelial cell permeability only if intracellular cAMP does not also increase, we examined the impact of thapsigargin on cAMP concentrations. Thapsigargin acutely decreased cAMP in intact PAECs *(16)*. Similar Ca^{2+} inhibition of cAMP was observed when the

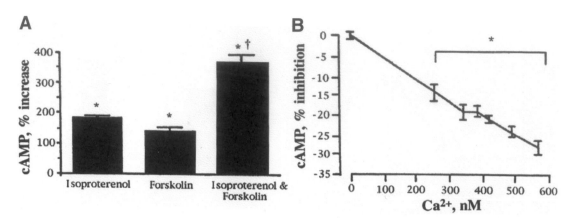

Fig. 3. Submicromolar Ca^{2+} concentrations inhibit adenylyl cyclase activity in pulmonary artery endothelial cells (PAECs). **(A)** PAEC membranes were enriched using a 30–40% sucrose gradient. Application of isoproterenol and forskolin each increased cAMP, indicating the presence of adenylyl cyclase activity. Isoproterenol and forskolin stimulation together produced an additive rise in cAMP. Adapted from ref. *16*. **(B)** Exposure of isoproterenol- and forskolin-stimulated PAEC membranes to increasing Ca^{2+} concentrations revealed adenylyl cyclase activity was inhibited within submicromolar concentration ranges. These findings are consistent with the presence of a Ca^{2+}-inhibited adenylyl cyclase, AC_6, in PAECs. Adapted from ref. *16*.

PAEC membrane was permeabilized to allow access of extracellular Ca^{2+} to the intracellular compartment. Inhibition of constitutive Ca^{2+} leak into the cells increased cAMP, and prevented thapsigargin from decreasing cAMP. Collectively, these early observations suggested that Ca^{2+} entry across the cell membrane regulated either cAMP synthesis or degradation.

Two enzyme systems control cAMP pools in living cells, including adenylyl cyclases that synthesize cAMP and phosphodiesterases that degrade cAMP. Each enzyme family has a large number of members that exhibit unique regulatory properties, although appreciation for such diversity was not fully realized until the mid-1990s. Cooper and coworkers discovered an adenylyl cyclase that was inhibited by submicromolar Ca^{2+} concentrations, e.g., AC_6 *(34)*. We screened PAECs for the presence of this enzyme and found AC_6 was expressed in lung endothelium, both in vitro and in vivo *(16,28)*. AC_6 was found to be enriched in lipid rafts and caveolae that are isolated in a 30–40% sucrose gradient. PAEC membranes isolated from the 30–40% sucrose gradient exhibited adenylyl cyclase activity that could be stimulated by isoproterenol and forskolin, and potentiated by phosphodiesterase inhibition *(16,35)*. Moreover, cAMP synthesized in isolated membranes was inhibited by submicromolar Ca^{2+} concentrations, consistent with the presence of a high-affinity Ca^{2+} binding site that reduced enzyme catalytic activity (**Fig. 3**) *(34,36)*. Thus, PAECs express an AC_6 that is inhibited specifically by SOC entry pathways, providing a plausible mechanism by which inflammatory Ca^{2+} agonists reduce cAMP necessary for inter-endothelial cell gap formation and increased endothelial cell permeability.

Type 1 phosphodiesterase is activated by rises in $[Ca^{2+}]_i$. Thompson and colleagues *(37)* have examined the expression and activity of PAEC phosphodiesterases and found expression of types 3,4, and 5. The dominant cAMP hydrolyzing enzyme is type 4 phosphodiesterase, which is inhibited by rolipram. Thus, at the present time neither expression nor activity of type 1 phosphodiesterase has been observed in endothelia, suggesting that the principal mechanism by which SOC entry reduces cAMP is by inhibition of AC_6.

To begin to address the physiological significance of AC_6 in control of endothelial cell barrier function, forskolin (direct adenylyl cyclase activator), rolipram (type 4 phosphodiesterase inhibitor), or their combination were applied to PAEC monolayers before thapsigargin *(16,28)*. As in earlier

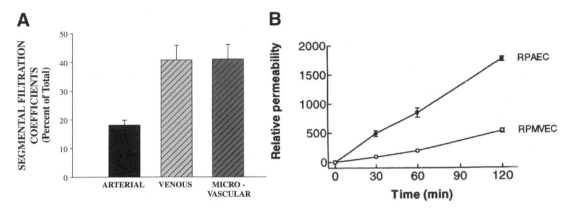

Fig. 4. Lung microvascular endothelial cells possess a more restrictive barrier than do pulmonary artery and vein endothelial cells. (**A**) Segmental permeability measurements in an isolated perfused rat lung reveals that venous and microvascular endothelial cell segments contribute equally to the basal filtration across the lung circulation, whereas arterial segments contribute less significantly. Standardization of these measurements to total surface area indicates that microvascular endothelial cells possess a substantially enhanced barrier function. Adapted from ref. *42*. (**B**) Macromolecular (12,000 mol wt FITC-dextran) permeability is greater across cultured pulmonary artery endothelial cells (PAECs) than across cultured PMVECs, indicating further that microvascular endothelial cells possess enhanced barrier function when compared with their macrovascular counterparts. Adapted from ref. *30*.

reports, cAMP elevating agents were profoundly barrier protective. However, these studies were significantly limited by an inability to precisely control physiological cAMP concentrations. Indeed, forskolin and rolipram induce substantial increases in cAMP and do not therefore answer the real question of whether a *decrease* in cAMP is necessary for barrier disruption to proceed.

3. PULMONARY MICROVASCULAR ENDOTHELIUM

While most permeability studies are conducted using conduit endothelium, control of microvascular endothelial cell barrier function is of the greatest physiological interest, as it directly pertains to efficiency of gas exchange across the alveolar-capillary unit. This issue has become exceedingly important as we now realize that pulmonary artery and microvascular endothelium likely arise from distinct precursor cell types in the course of development, where macrovascular endothelium arises from angiogenesis of the pulmonary truncus and microvascular endothelium arises from vasculogenesis of the lung bud *(38,39)*. These epigenetically distinct cells give rise to large and small vessels, respectively, that do not fuse to form a continuous circulation until mid-gestation in the late pseudoglandular phase of lung development. It appears such divergent origins—e.g., epigenetic origins—confer long-lasting attributes that functionally distinguish macrovascular and microvascular endothelium *(40,41)*.

One functional difference between PAECs and pulmonary microvascular endothelial cells (PMVECs) is their barrier function. PMVECs form a tighter, more restrictive barrier than do their macrovascular counterparts, both in vitro and in vivo (**Fig. 4**) *(29,30,42)*. Under basal conditions, fluid and macromolecular flux is greatly attenuated in PMVECs. Such enhanced PMVEC barrier function is likely required to protect the lung's gas exchange area from fluid and protein accumulation, to optimize gas exchange.

We examined the ability of thapsigargin to increase PMVEC permeability first using an isolated perfused rat lung model, in which hydraulic conductivity was measured as an index for permeability *(28,29)*. Thapsigargin induced a dose-dependent increase in permeability with an EC_{50} approx 30 nM (**Fig. 5**), identical to the EC_{50} for thapsigargin to inhibit SERCA and identical to its ability to increase

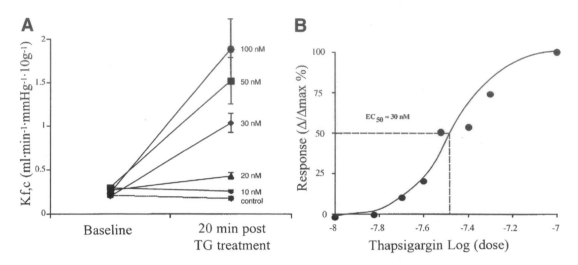

Fig. 5. Thapsigargin increases lung permeability. **(A)** Re-circulation of thapsigargin (TG) in an isolated perfused rat lung preparation dose-dependently increases permeability, estimated by the filtration coefficient. Adapted from ref. *29*. **(B)** Dose response reveals an EC_{50} = 30 n*M*, similar to the IC_{50} of thapsigargin for the sarcoplasmic/endoplasmic reticulum Ca^{2+} ATPase (SERCA). Adapted from ref. *29*.

endothelial cell $[Ca^{2+}]_i$. Thus, thapsigargin increases lung permeability by activating SOC entry. Moreover, either reducing extracellular Ca^{2+} to 10 μ*M* or increasing endothelial cell cAMP prevented thapsigargin from increasing permeability, compatible with the idea that activation of SOC entry reduces cAMP necessary for barrier disruption—just as in the PAEC models described above.

In isolated perfused lung studies, the measurement endpoint is Kfc, or capillary filtration coefficient. Partly because of the lung's large surface area, filtration across the capillaries is thought to dominate this index. However, light microscopy revealed that the thapsigargin-induced increase in permeability was accompanied by substantial perivascular cuffing with only limited degrees of alveolar-capillary engorgement, with no sign of alveolar fluid accumulation or atelectasis (**Fig. 6A**) *(29)*. Ultra-structural studies further supported this finding, demonstrating prominent intercellular gaps in arteries and veins larger than 100 μ*M* (**Fig. 6B**). In these larger vessels, interstitial spaces were hydrated, consistent with the presence of fluid throughout the interstitium and in perivascular compartments. In stark contrast, gaps between capillary and microvascular endothelial cells were not observed.

We therefore sought to determine whether the apparent insensitivity to thapsigargin in PMVECs was a result of the cell type *per se* or, rather, a function of the microvascular environment in vivo. Thapsigargin was applied to PMVECs in culture and macromolecular flux examined *(30)*. Just as in studies in the isolated perfused lung, activation of SOC entry did not increase macromolecular permeability and did not induce inter-PMVEC gap formation (**Fig. 7**). It appears, therefore, that a principal difference between PAEC and PMVECs—even under identical environmental conditions—is coupling between activation of SOC entry and formation of intercellular gaps.

One explanation for such a discrepancy is that PMVECs just possess a lower $[Ca^{2+}]_i$ response to thapsigargin. We examined this possibility and, indeed, found that while each cell type exhibited a similar sensitivity to thapsigargin, the magnitude of the increase in $[Ca^{2+}]_i$ was substantially lower in PMVECs than in PAECs *(30,43)*. Recalcification experiments revealed that maximal activation of SOC entry in PMVECs induced an extremely high rise in $[Ca^{2+}]_i$—albeit still slightly lower than the maximal $[Ca^{2+}]_i$ response in PAECs (**Fig. 8A**). Under these conditions, maximal activation of SOC entry still did not increase PMVEC permeability (**Fig. 8B**), suggesting either an uncoupling of $[Ca^{2+}]_i$

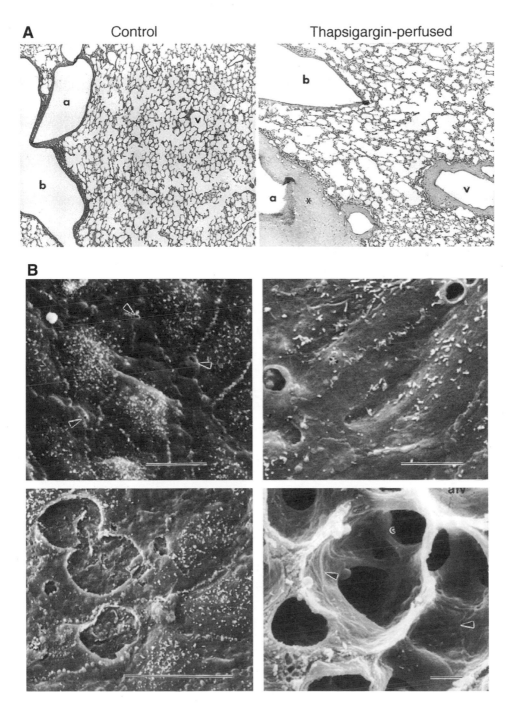

Fig. 6. Thapsigargin increased lung macrovascular and not microvascular permeability. **(A)** Histological analysis of thapsigargin-perfused lung vessels revealed prominent perivascular cuffing and limited interstitial hydration along capillary segments, consistent with increased permeability of macrovascular segments. a denotes arteriole; b denotes bronchiole; v denotes vein. Adapted from ref. *29.* **(B)** Ultrastructural analysis of lung segments demonstrated clearly delimited endothelial cell-cell borders in control-perfused vessels (upper left panel). However, in thapsigargin-perfused lungs, intercellular gaps were observed in pulmonary vein (upper right panel) and artery (lower left panel) segments. Similar gaps were not observed in microvascular lung segments (lower right panel), again consistent with the idea that thapsigargin increased permeability across larger vascular segments. Arrowheads denote cell–cell borders. Adapted from ref. *29.*

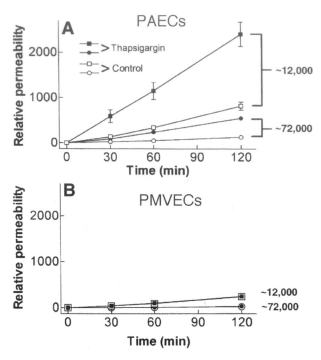

Fig. 7. Thapsigargin increases permeability across pulmonary artery endothelial cell (PAEC) and not pulmonary microvascular endothelial cell (PMVEC) monolayers. (**A**) Macromolecular (dextran) permeability across confluent cell monolayers demonstrates that thapsigargin increases PAEC and not PMVEC permeability. Adapted from ref. *30*.

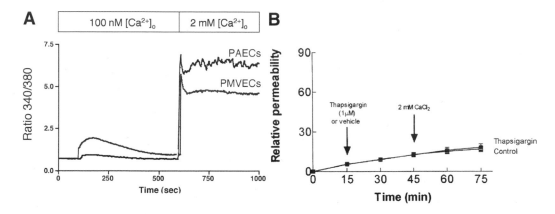

Fig. 8. Large increases in $[Ca^{2+}]_i$ are not sufficient to increase pulmonary microvascular endothelial cell (PMVEC) permeability. (**A**) Re-calcification experiment demonstrates that re-addition of extracellular Ca^{2+} induces a large rise in $[Ca^{2+}]_i$ in PMVECs. However, this large rise in $[Ca^{2+}]_i$ is still lower than that observed in pulmonary artery endothelial cells. (**B**) The large $[Ca^{2+}]_i$ rise observed using the re-calcification protocol was not sufficient to increase PMVEC macromolecular (dextran) permeability. Adapted from ref. *30*.

from cytoskeletal elements that mediate barrier disruption or the relative absence of a critical channel that uniquely couples SOC entry to barrier disruption.

Thapsigargin activates multiple ion channels, which collectively result in a global rise in $[Ca^{2+}]_i$. These channels are both Ca^{2+} selective and nonselective, and can be distinguished electrophysiologically *(44–46)*. We utilized a fura-based approach developed by Zweifach *(47)* to examine ion selectivity of SOC entry channels in PAECs and PMVECs. These findings revealed that thapsigargin activated common nonselective cation entry pathways in PAECs and PMVECs. However, it appeared that Ca^{2+} permeation was higher in PAECs than in PMVECs, suggesting that PMVECs may not possess the Ca^{2+} selective pathway activated by thapsigargin (Stevens, unpublished). Indeed, electrophysiological recordings indicated that while thapsigargin activates a Ca^{2+}-selective current (I_{SOC}) in PAECs, this current is normally absent in PMVECs (Stevens, unpublished). Thus, while contributing a relatively minor portion of the global $[Ca^{2+}]_i$ response to thapsigargin, activation of I_{SOC} appears to be a critical stimulus that disrupts endothelial cell barrier function.

Because of the implied role of AC_6 in translating physiological $[Ca^{2+}]_i$ transitions into barrier disruption, we investigated whether activation of I_{SOC} decreased cAMP. PMVECs possess an approx 10-fold greater cAMP turnover rate than do PAECs, largely the result of active type 4 phosphodiesterase activity *(43)*. Currently, the mechanism for such enhanced phosphodiesterase hydrolytic activity is unknown, but has been implicated in establishing cAMP gradients within the cell, where the plasma membrane possesses an approx 12-fold greater cAMP concentration than the bulk cytosolic compartments *(48,49)*. Acute thapsigargin application did not reduce global cAMP concentrations in PMVECs, as we observed in PAECs *(35)*. However, isolated PMVEC membranes possessed high-affinity Ca^{2+} inhibition of AC_6 activity, and these studies indicated that AC_6 represents the dominant adenylyl cyclase isoform in microvascular cells *(35)*. Inhibition of type 4 phosphodiesterase activity amplified the global cAMP response, and revealed inhibition of cAMP by thapsigargin. Interestingly, rolipram also translocated endoplasmic reticulum to the abluminal cell membrane, and unmasked activation of I_{SOC} (Stevens, unpublished). Presently, the mechanism(s) responsible for this rolipram-induced translocation of endoplasmic reticulum is (are) unknown. We have not resolved whether rolipram reveals Ca^{2+} inhibition of AC_6 because it allows thapsigargin to activate I_{SOC}, or because it amplifies the membrane-associated cAMP pool so that currently available assessment methods can resolve an inhibition. Nonetheless, rolipram—which translocates endoplasmic reticulum to the cell's abluminal surface, allows I_{SOC} activation, and reveals AC_6 inhibition—also unmasks intercellular gap formation in response to thapsigargin (Stevens, unpublished). These findings therefore support the idea that endoplasmic reticulum coupling to the plasma membrane is critical for I_{SOC} channels to become activated following Ca^{2+} store depletion. Close coupling between the endoplasmic reticulum and basolateral membrane unmasks thapsigargin-induced I_{SOC} activation, which serves as a prerequisite for AC_6 inhibition and intercellular gap formation.

To specifically test this role of AC_6 in mediating PMVEC gap formation, it is necessary to prevent Ca^{2+} from inhibiting enzyme function. At this time, the high-affinity Ca^{2+} binding site on AC_6 is unknown, although inhibition does not require calmodulin or other Ca^{2+}-binding proteins *(36,50)*. Until the high-affinity Ca^{2+} binding site on AC_6 is resolved, site-directed mutagenesis to eliminate AC_6 Ca^{2+} sensitivity is not possible. We therefore adapted an approach developed by Cooper and colleagues *(51)* to express a Ca^{2+}-stimulated adenylyl cyclase, and convert Ca^{2+} inhibition of cAMP into Ca^{2+} stimulation of cAMP. The type 8 adenylyl cyclase (AC_8) was heterologously expressed using an adenoviral approach *(15)*. Virtually 100% of PMVECs expressed AC_8, limited specifically to a punctate staining pattern on the apical and basolateral membrane surfaces with enrichment at cell-cell borders (**Fig. 9A,B**). Enzyme expression did not change basal cAMP levels (data not shown). Whereas thrombin normally reduced cAMP, in PMVECs heterologously expressing AC_8 thrombin slightly increased cAMP. Moreover, whereas thrombin application rapidly induced very large intercellular gaps (**Fig. 9C**), in PMVECs heterologously expressing AC_8 thrombin did not induce significant gap formation (**Fig. 9D**). The magnitude of this effect was striking, and indicated convincingly that membrane-associated cAMP possesses profound barrier enhancing capacity—even only small cAMP rises. Time-lapse movies further demonstrated that thrombin induces inward cell tension in cells expressing AC_8, suggesting cAMP's barrier-enhancing effect is likely due to its ability to

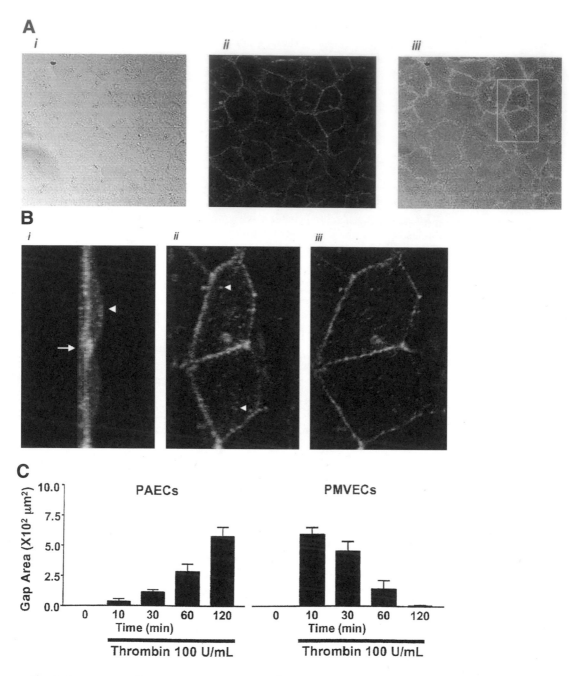

Fig. 9. Converting Ca^{2+} inhibition of cAMP to Ca^{2+} stimulation of cAMP prevents thrombin from inducing gap formation in pulmonary microvascular endothelial cells (PMVECs). (A) Adenoviral expression of a Ca^{2+}-stimulated isoform of adenylyl cyclase AC$_8$ as a YFP fusion revealed nearly 100% infection efficiency. Phase contrast (i) and fluorescent (ii) images of infected cells demonstrate enrichment of YFP-AC$_8$ at cell-cell borders. Overlay (iii) reveals the high level of expression efficiency. Adapted from ref. *15*. (B) Three-dimensional reconstruction of cells in white box from A demonstrate YFP-AC$_8$ is enriched at cell–cell borders, with punctate staining apparent on both apical and basolateral cells aspects. (i) Sideview (arrow denotes AC$_8$ expression at cell–cell borders and arrowhead denotes cell's lumical aspect); (ii) tilted view (arrowheads denote punctate staining; and (iii) top view. Adapted from *(15)*. (C) Application of thrombin to confluent pulmonary artery endothelial cell (PAEC) and PMVEC monolayers revealed distinct responses. In PAECs, gaps were slowly

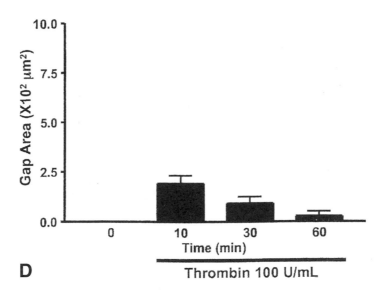

D

Fig. 9. (*continued*) developing and progressive. In PMVECs, gaps appeared and resolved quickly. This graph standardizes gap size between cell types to illustrate the different thrombin responses. Overall, however, thrombin induced larger gaps in PMVECs than in PAECs. Adapted from ref. *15*. (**D**) Heterologous expression of AC_8 prevented thrombin from inducing gaps in PMVECs. Only infrequent, small gaps appeared. These gaps re-sealed very quickly, demonstrating pronounced barrier-protective effects of membrane-associated cAMP concentrations. Adapted from ref. *15*.

strengthen cell-cell adhesions. These findings provided the first direct evidence implicating Ca^{2+} inhibition of cAMP—e.g., Ca^{2+} inhibition of AC_6—in development of interendothelial cell gaps.

4. CONCLUSION

For many years now, endothelial cell biologists have recognized the mutually opposing actions of physiological transitions in $[Ca^{2+}]_i$ and cAMP in control of endothelial cell barrier function. A rise in $[Ca^{2+}]_i$ disrupts the endothelial cell barrier, whereas a rise in cAMP strengthens the endothelial cell barrier. Only recently have we developed an understanding for crosstalk mechanisms between $[Ca^{2+}]_i$ and cAMP in endothelium, which represent a normal physiological signaling response to inflammatory mediators. Indeed, G_q agonists that increase $[Ca^{2+}]_i$ inhibit AC_6 activity and reduce membrane-associated cAMP. Such inhibition of cAMP is essential for intercellular gap formation, placing AC_6 as a key upstream signaling molecule that intensely controls endothelial cell barrier function.

REFERENCES

1. Lum, H. and Malik, A. B. (1996) Mechanisms of increased endothelial permeability. *Can. J. Physiol. Pharmacol.* **74**, 787–800.
2. Lum, H. and Malik, A. B. (1994) Regulation of vascular endothelial barrier function. *Am. J. Physiol.* **267**, L223–L241.
3. Curry, F. E and Adamson, R. H. (1999) Transendothelial pathways in venular microvessels exposed to agents which increase permeability: the gaps in our knowledge. *Microcirculation* **6**, 3–5.
4. Curry, F. E. (1992) Modulation of venular microvessel permeability by calcium influx into endothelial cells. *FASEB J.* **6**, 2456–2466.
5. Bogatcheva, N. V., Garcia, J. G., and Verin, A. D. (2002) Molecular mechanisms of thrombin-induced endothelial cell permeability. *Biochemistry (Mosc.)* **67**, 75–84.
6. Garcia, J. G., Verin, A. D., and Schaphorst, K. L. (1996) Regulation of thrombin-mediated endothelial cell contraction and permeability. *Semin. Thromb. Hemost.* **22**, 309–315
7. Garcia, J. G., Pavalko, F. M., and Patterson, C. E. (1995) Vascular endothelial cell activation and permeability responses to thrombin. *Blood Coagul. Fibrinolysis.* **6**, 609–626.

8. Moore, T. M., Chetham, P. M., Kelly, J. J., and Stevens, T. (1998) Signal transduction and regulation of lung endothelial cell permeability. Interaction between calcium and cAMP. *Am. J. Physiol.* **275,** L203–L222.
9. Majno, G. and Palade, G. E. (1961) Studies on inflammation. I. The effect of histamine and serotonin on vascular permeability: an electron microscopic study. *J. Biophys. Biochem. Cytol.* **11,** 571–605
10. Robison, G. A., Butcher, R. W., and Sutherland, E. W. (1968) Cyclic AMP. *Annu. Rev. Biochem.* **37,** 149–174
11. Kaupp, U. B. and Seifert, R. (2002) Cyclic nucleotide-gated ion channels. *Physiol. Rev.* **82,** 769–824.
12. Quilliam, L. A., Rebhun, J. F., and Castro, A. F. (2002) A growing family of guanine nucleotide exchange factors is responsible for activation of Ras-family GTPases. *Prog. Nucleic Acid Res. Mol. Biol.* **71,** 391–444
13. Robinson-White, A. and Stratakis, C. A. (2002) Protein kinase A signaling: "cross-talk" with other pathways in endocrine cells. *Ann. NY Acad. Sci.* **968,** 256–270.
14. Garcia, J. G., Lazar, V., Gilbert-McClain, L. I., Gallagher, P. J., and Verin, A. D. (1997) Myosin light chain kinase in endothelium: molecular cloning and regulation. *Am. J. Respir. Cell. Mol. Biol.* **16,** 489–494.
15. Cioffi, D. L., Moore, T. M., Schaack, J., Creighton, J. R., Cooper, D. M., and Stevens, T. (2002) Dominant regulation of interendothelial cell gap formation by calcium- inhibited type 6 adenylyl cyclase. *J. Cell. Biol.* **157,** 1267–1278.
16. Stevens, T., Nakahashi, Y., Cornfield, D. N., McMurtry, I. F., Cooper, D. M., and Rodman, D. M. (1995) Ca(2+)-inhibitable adenylyl cyclase modulates pulmonary artery endothelial cell cAMP content and barrier function. *Proc. Natl. Acad. Sci. USA* **92,** 2696–2700.
17. Venkatachalam, K., van Rossum, D. B., Patterson, R. L., Ma, H. T., and Gill, D. L. (2002) The cellular and molecular basis of store-operated calcium entry. *Nat. Cell. Biol.* **4,** E263–E272.
18. Bauer, N. N. and Stevens, T. (2002) Putative role for a myosin motor in store-operated calcium entry. *Cell. Biochem. Biophys.* **37,** 53–70
19. Zitt, C., Halaszovich, C. R., and Luckhoff, A. (2002) The TRP family of cation channels: probing and advancing the concepts on receptor-activated calcium entry. *Prog. Neurobiol.* **66,** 243–264.
20. Nilius, B. and Droogmans, G. (2001) Ion channels and their functional role in vascular endothelium. *Physiol. Rev.* **81,** 1415–1459.
21. Sanders, K. M. (2001) Invited review: mechanisms of calcium handling in smooth muscles. *J. Appl. Physiol.* **91,** 1438–1449.
22. Putney, J. W., Jr., Broad, L. M., Braun, F. J., Lievremont, J. P., and Bird, G. S. (2001) Mechanisms of capacitative calcium entry. *J. Cell. Sci.* **114,** 2223–2229.
23. Dutta, D. (2000) Mechanism of store-operated calcium entry. *J. Biosci.* **25,** 397–404.
24. Petersen, O. H., Burdakov, D., and Tepikin, A. V. (1999) Regulation of store-operated calcium entry: lessons from a polarized cell. *Eur. J. Cell. Biol.* **78,** 221–223.
25. Parekh, A. B. and Penner, R. (1997) Store depletion and calcium influx. *Physiol Rev.* **77,** 901–930.
26. Thastrup, O., Cullen, P. J., Drobak, B. K., Hanley, M. R., and Dawson, A. P. (1990) Thapsigargin, a tumor promoter, discharges intracellular Ca^{2+} stores by specific inhibition of the endoplasmic reticulum Ca2(+)-ATPase. *Proc. Natl. Acad. Sci. USA* **87,** 2466–2470.
27. Tran, Q. K., Ohashi, K., and Watanabe, H. (2000) Calcium signalling in endothelial cells. *Cardiovasc. Res.* **48,** 13–22.
28. Chetham, P. M., Guldemeester, H. A., Mons, N., et al. (1997) Ca(2+)-inhibitable adenylyl cyclase and pulmonary microvascular permeability. *Am. J. Physiol.* **273,** L22–L30.
29. Chetham, P. M., Babal, P., Bridges, J. P., Moore, T. M., and Stevens, T. (1999) Segmental regulation of pulmonary vascular permeability by store- operated Ca^{2+} entry. *Am. J. Physiol.* **276,** L41–L50.
30. Kelly, J. J., Moore, T. M., Babal, P., Diwan, A. H., Stevens, T., and Thompson, W. J. (1998) Pulmonary microvascular and macrovascular endothelial cells: differential regulation of Ca^{2+} and permeability. *Am. J. Physiol.* **274,** L810–L819.
31. Moore, T. M., Brough, G. H., Babal, P., Kelly, J. J., Li, M., and Stevens, T. (1998) Store-operated calcium entry promotes shape change in pulmonary endothelial cells expressing Trp1. *Am. J. Physiol.* **275,** L574–L582.
32. Moore, T. M., Norwood, N. R., Creighton, J. R., et al. (2000) Receptor-dependent activation of store-operated calcium entry increases endothelial cell permeability. *Am. J. Physiol. Lung Cell Mol. Physiol.* **279,** L691–L698.
33. Norwood, N., Moore, T. M., Dean, D. A., Bhattacharjee, R., Li, M., and Stevens, T. (2000) Store-operated calcium entry and increased endothelial cell permeability. *Am. J. Physiol. Lung Cell Mol. Physiol.* **279,** L815–824.
34. Yoshimura, M. and Cooper, D. M. (1992) Cloning and expression of a Ca(2+)-inhibitable adenylyl cyclase from NCB-20 cells. *Proc. Natl. Acad. Sci. USA* **89,** 6716–6720.
35. Creighton, J., Masada, N., Cooper, D. M. F., and Stevens, T. (2003) Coordinate regulation of membrane cAMP by calcium inhibited adenylyl cyclase and phosphodiesterase activities. *Am. J. Physiol.* **284,** L100–L107
36. Guillou, J. L., Nakata, H., and Cooper, D. M. (1999) Inhibition by calcium of mammalian adenylyl cyclases. *J. Biol. Chem.* **274,** 35,539–35,545.
37. Thompson, W. J., Ashikaga, T., Kelly, J. J., et al. (2002) Regulation of cyclic AMP in rat pulmonary microvascular endothelial cells by rolipram-sensitive cyclic AMP phosphodiesterase (PDE4). *Biochem. Pharmacol.* **63,** 797–807.
38. deMello, D. E. and Reid, L. M. (2000) Embryonic and early fetal development of human lung vasculature and its functional implications. *Pediatr. Dev. Pathol.* **3,** 439–449.
39. deMello, D. E., Sawyer, D., Galvin, N., and Reid, L. M. (1997) Early fetal development of lung vasculature. *Am. J. Respir. Cell Mol. Biol.* **16,** 568–581.
40. King, J., Hamil, T., Creighton, J., et al. (2003) Structural and functional characteristics of lung macro- and microvascular endothelial cell phenotypes. *Microvasc. Res.* **67,** 139–151.
41. Stevens, T., Rosenberg, R., Aird, W., et al. (2001) NHLBI workshop report: endothelial cell phenotypes in heart, lung, and blood diseases. *Am. J. Physiol. Cell Physiol.* **281,** C1422–C1433.

42. Parker, J. C. and Yoshikawa, S. (2002) Vascular segmental permeabilities at high peak inflation pressure in isolated rat lungs. *Am. J. Physiol. Lung Cell Mol. Physiol.* **283,** L1203–L1209.
43. Stevens, T., Creighton, J., and Thompson, W. J. (1999) Control of cAMP in lung endothelial cell phenotypes. Implications for control of barrier function. *Am. J. Physiol.* **277,** L119–L126.
44. Brough, G. H., Wu, S., Cioffi, D., et al. (2001) Contribution of endogenously expressed Trp1 to a Ca2+-selective, store-operated Ca^{2+} entry pathway. *FASEB J.* **15,** 1727–1738.
45. Wu, S., Moore, T. M., Brough, G. H., et al. (2000) Cyclic nucleotide-gated channels mediate membrane depolarization following activation of store-operated calcium entry in endothelial cells. *J. Biol. Chem.* **275,** 18,887–18,896.
46. Wu, S., Sangerman, J., Li, M., Brough, G. H., Goodman, S. R., and Stevens, T. (2001) Essential control of an endothelial cell ISOC by the spectrin membrane skeleton. *J. Cell. Biol.* **154,** 1225–1233.
47. Zweifach, A. (2000) Target-cell contact activates a highly selective capacitative calcium entry pathway in cytotoxic T lymphocytes. *J. Cell. Biol.* **148,** 603–614.
48. Rich, T. C., Fagan, K. A., Nakata, H., Schaack, J., Cooper, D. M., and Karpen, J. W. (2000) Cyclic nucleotide-gated channels colocalize with adenylyl cyclase in regions of restricted cAMP diffusion. *J. Gen. Physiol.* **116,** 147–161.
49. Rich, T. C., Fagan, K. A., Tse, T. E., Schaack, J., Cooper, D. M., and Karpen, J. W. (2001) A uniform extracellular stimulus triggers distinct cAMP signals in different compartments of a simple cell. *Proc. Natl. Acad. Sci. USA* **98,** 13,049–13,054.
50. Gu, C. and Cooper, D. M. (2000) Ca(2+), Sr(2+), and Ba(2+) identify distinct regulatory sites on adenylyl cyclase (AC) types VI and VIII and consolidate the apposition of capacitative cation entry channels and Ca(2+)-sensitive ACs. *J. Biol. Chem.* **275,** 6980–6986.
51. Fagan, K. A., Graf, R. A., Tolman, S., Schaack, J., and Cooper, D. M. (2000) Regulation of a Ca^{2+}-sensitive adenylyl cyclase in an excitable cell. Role of voltage-gated versus capacitative Ca2+ entry. *J. Biol. Chem.* **275,** 40,187–40,194.

Index